Ceramics in Orthopaedics

HARTMUT ZIPPEL
MARTIN DIETRICH
Editors

Bioceramics in Joint Arthroplasty

8th BIOLOX® Symposium

Berlin, March 28-29, 2003

Proceedings

with 120 Figures
and 25 Tables

STEINKOPFF DARMSTADT

ISBN-13: 978-3-7985-1417-1 **e-ISBN-13: 978-3-642-85763-8**
DOI: 10.1007/978-3-642-85763-8

Cataloging-in-Publication Data applied for
A catalog record for this book is available from the Library of Congress.
Bibliographic information published by Die Deutsche Bibliothek
Die Deutsche Bibliothek lists this publication in the Deutsche Nationalbibliografie, detailed bibliographic data is available in the Internet at <http://dnb.ddb.de>.

Steinkopff Verlag Darmstadt
a member of BertelsmannSpringer Science+Business Media GmbH

http://www.steinkopff.springer.de

Cover Design: TOP DESIGN, Thomas Schuster, Waiblingen

Production and Typesetting: druckerei justus kuch GmbH, Nürnberg

SPIN 10927311 105/7231-543210 - Printed on acid-free paper.

Preface

Dear Colleague and Participant of Bioceramics in Joint Arthroplasty
8th Biolox® Symposium

It is a pleasure for us to be able to present you with the proceedings of this Symposium. This is something that we are very proud of, as it is the first time that we have been able to achieve our objective of distributing this collection of all presentations made at this Symposium in a printed form at this time. The achievement of this goal was reached in great part as a result of the excellent cooperation of all of the speakers as well as the commitment of the publishing house to assist us in every way possible to meet the strict deadlines imposed. Additionally, a special thanks must also be given to some very special people who diligently worked to make sure our objective was met. They are: Gertrud Volkert, M.D. and Petra Elster of the Steinkopff Verlag Publishing company and our own Symposium Administrator, Hedi Kissinger.

We believe that you will find this book to be a valuable and useful addition to your reference library. We hope that within its covers, you will find the most up to date scientific and clinical information regarding the use of ceramic solutions to address wear related problems in Orthopedic Surgery.

This Symposium also marks a very special and long awaited event for many of the speakers, participants and the CeramTec Medical Product Division, the approval for sale of the Biolox Wear couple by the Food and Drug Administration. This approval was made possible by the overwhelming proof of Safety and Effectiveness compiled by the clinical investigators and the American Orthopedic Implant companies over the last 7 years. We are convinced that this will be a significant step forward towards the increasing acceptance of ceramic solutions in the USA.

The Symposium also pays tribute to the fact that this is the first time that we have held this scientific venue outside of Stuttgart. We think that the excellence of the presentations, the fruitful discussions, the quality of the organization, the depth of knowledge of the participants and even the City of Berlin will have all worked together to make this a very special event in the pursuit of increased recognition of the benefits of Biolox ceramic technology by the Orthopedic Surgical community.

Hartmut Zippel
Symposium President
Chairman of the Orthopedic Clinic
Charité Berlin

Martin Dietrich
Managing Director
CeramTec Medical Products

CeramTec wishes to express its deepest appreciation to Prof. Dr. med. Zippel and all of the many people that have contributed to the success of this 8th Biolox® Symposium.

Ceramics in Orthopaedics

8th BIOLOX® Symposium
Proceedings

Edited by
HARTMUT ZIPPEL
MARTIN DIETRICH

List of contents

SESSION 1

Basics of Ceramic Components in Hip Arthroplasty

SESSION 2

Adverse Reactions in Total Joint Replacement: Infections, Allergic Reactions and others

SESSION 3

Future Ceramic Materials in Joint Arthroplasty

SESSION 4

Computer Assisted Knee Surgery: Development and Evaluation

SESSION 5

Clinical Results in Hip Arthroplasty

SESSION 6

Complications in THR using Ceramics

SESSION 7

Quality and Regulatory Issues

List of contributors

RAINER BADER, Dr. med. Dipl.-Ing.
Technische Universität München
Klinik für Orthopädie und Sportorthopädie
Connollystraße 32
80809 München, Germany

B. SONNY BAL, MD, MBA
University of Missouri-Columbia
One Hospital Drive, MC-213
65212 Columbia, MO, USA

ANTONIO BERIZZI, MD
U.O.A., Ortopedia e Traumatologia
Citadella, Italy

BENJAMIN BIERBAUM, MD
New England Bone and Joint Institute
125 Parker Hill Avenue
02120 Boston, MA, USA

M. BOEHLER, MD
Herz Jesu Hospital
Wien, Austria

GOTTFRIED H. BUCHHORN, Dipl.-Ing.
Georg-August-University of Göttingen
Dept. of Orthopaedics
Robert-Koch-Straße 40
37075 Göttingen, Germany

WOLFGANG BURGER, Dr.
CeramTec AG
Fabrikstraße 23-29
73207 Plochingen, Germany

GIOVANNI CASTIELLO, MD
U.O.A., Ortopedia e Traumatologia
Citadella, Italy

IAN C. CLARKE, PhD
Loma Linda University Medical Center
Peterson Tribology Lab.,
Dept. Orthopaedics
12340 Anderson St.
92350 Loma Linda, CA, USA

LUIGI COLOGNESE, MD
U.O.A., Ortopedia e Traumatologia
Citadella, Italy

VINCENZO DE SANTIS, MD
Catholic University of Rome
Largo F. Vito 1
00168 Rom, Italy

MARTIN DIETRICH, Dr.
CeramTec AG
Fabrikstraße 23-29
73207 Plochingen, Germany

HOWARD S. DOBBS, Dr.
HSD Consulting
36 Alexandra Road
RG1 5PF Reading, United Kingdom

JOHN H. DUMBLETON, PhD, DSc
Consultancy in Medical Devices
512 E. Saddle River Road
07450 Ridgewood, NJ, USA

ROBERT W. EBERLE, MD
Clinical Information Consultants, Inc.
Apex, NC, USA

TOM H. EICKMANN, MD
Loma Linda University Medical Center
12340 Anderson St.
92350 Loma Linda, CA, USA

AFSHIN FAYYAZI, PD Dr. med.
Georg-August-University of Göttingen
Dept. of Pathology
Robert-Koch-Straße 40
37075 Göttingen, Germany

JONATHAN P. GARINO, MD
University of Pennsylvania
Dept. of Orthopedic Surgery
3400 Spruce Street, Silverstein Two
19104-4283 Philadelphia, PA, USA

KERSTIN GESCHWILL, Dr.
University of Aachen
Dept. of Orthopaedic Surgery
Pauwelsstraße 30
52074 Aachen, Germany

ROBERTO GIACOMETTI CERONI, Prof.
1st Ortop. Galeazzi
Via R. Galeazzi 4
85112 Milano, Italy

SASCHA GOEBEL, MD
Würzburg University
Dept. of Orthopaedics
Brettreichstraße 11
97074 Würzburg, Germany

GÖTZ GRIESMAYR
CeramTec AG
Fabrikstraße 23-29
73207 Plochingen, Germany

G. ALLEN GUSTAFSON, MD
Ascend Orthopaedic Office
92354 Loma Linda, CA, USA

CHRISTIAN HENDRICH, MD
Würzburg University
Dept. of Orthopaedics
Brettreichstraße 11
97074 Würzburg, Germany

MONIKA HUBER, Dr.
Otto Wagner-Spital
Pathologisch-Bakteriologisches Institut
Baumgatner Höhe 1
1145 Wien, Austria

JOSHUA J. JACOBS, MD
Rush Medical College
Dept. of Orthopedic Surgery
1653 W. Congress Parkway
60612 Chicago, Illinois, USA

KURT P. JUDMANN, Prof. Dipl.-Ing. Dr.
Vienna University of Technology
Dept. of Computer Technology
Gußhausstraße 27-29
1040 Wien, Austria

JÜRGEN KASPROWITSCH
CeramTec AG
Fabrikstraße 23-29
73207 Plochingen, Germany

LUC KERBOULL, Dr.
Clinique Moventis
Directeur
36, bd Saint Marcel
75005 Paris, France

STEFAN KIRSCHNER, MD
Würzburg University
Dept. of Orthopaedics
Brettreichstraße 11
97074 Würzburg, Germany

DIETMAR PIERRE KÖNIG, PD Dr. med.
Klinik und Poliklinik für Orthopädie
des Klinikums der Universität zu Köln
Joseph-Stelzmann-Straße 9
50924 Köln, Germany

KARSTEN LABS, MD, PhD
University Hospital Berlin,
Charité Dept. of Orthopaedics
Schumannstraße 20/21
10117 Berlin, Germany

JEAN-YVES LAZENNEC, Prof. Dr.
Hopital de la Pitié Salpetrière
47-83, bd. De l'Hopital
75651 Paris Cedex 13, France

STEFAN LEYEN, Dipl.-Ing.
CeramTec AG
Fabrikstraße 23-29
73207 Plochingen, Germany

GERNOT LIEBENTRITT, MSc
Centerpulse Orthopedics Ltd.
PO Box 65
8404 Winterthur, Switzerland

FELIX LINTNER, Prim. Univ. Prof. Dr.
Otto Wagner-Spital
Pathologisch-Bakteriologisches Institut
Baumgatner Höhe 1
1145 Wien, Austria

GIULIO MACCAURO, MD
Catholic University of Rome
Largo F. Vito 1
00168 Rom, Italy

M. MANAKA, MD
Loma Linda University Medical Center
Peterson Tribology Lab.,
Dept. Orthopaedics
12340 Anderson St.
92350 Loma Linda, CA, USA

MICHAEL T. MANLEY, PhD
Stryker Howmedica Osteonics
Chief Scientific Advisor
300 Commerce Ct.
07430 Mahwah, NJ, USA

JOHN M. MARTELL, MD
The University of Chicago
Medical Center
Dept. of Surgery
5841 S. Maryland Avenue, Room E309
60637 Chicago, Illinois, USA

GEORG MATZIOLIS, MD
University Hospital Berlin, Charité
Dept. of Orthopaedics
Schumannstraße 20/21
10117 Berlin, Germany

PATRICIE MERKERT, Dr.
CeramTec AG,
Fabrikstraße 23-29
73207 Plochingen, Germany

J. WESLEY MESKO, MD
2901 Stabler Street Lower Level
48910 Lansing, Michigan, USA

JÖRN MICHAEL, Dr. med.
Klinik und Poliklinik für Orthopädie
des Klinikums der Universität zu Köln
Joseph-Stelzmann-Straße 9
50924 Köln, Germany

WOLFRAM MITTELMEIER, PD Dr. med.
Technische Universität München
Klinik für Orthopädie und
Sportorthopädie
Connollystraße 32
80809 München, Germany

GREGOR MÖCKEL, Dr. med.
Charité University Hospital
Dept. of Orthopedics
Schumannstraße 20/21
10117 Berlin, Germany

FRANCESCO MURATORI, MD
Catholic University of Rome
Largo F. Vito 1
00168 Rom, Italy

STEPHEN B. MURPHY, MD
Boston Orthopedic Group Inc.
1269 Beacon Street
02446 Brookline, MA, USA

CHRISTOPHER NIEDHART, Dr.
University of Aachen
Dept. of Orthopaedic Surgery
Pauwelsstraße 30
52074 Aachen, Germany

FRITZ UWE NIETHARD, Prof. Dr.
University of Aachen
Dept. of Orthopaedic Surgery
Pauwelsstraße 30
52074 Aachen, Germany

H. OONISHI, MD
Tominaga Hospital
H. Oonishi Memorial Joint Center
Osaka, Japan

ANDREAS PAUSCHITZ, Dipl.-Ing. Dr.
University of Technology
Dept. of Micro-Technique
and Precision Engineering
Floragasse 7
1040 Wien, Austria

CARSTEN PERKA, MD, PhD
University Hospital Berlin, Charité
Dept. of Orthopaedic
Schumannstraße 20/21
10117 Berlin, Germany

CORRADO PICONI, Dr.
Catholic University of Rome
Largo F. Vito 1
00168 Rom, Italy

GEORG REINISCH, Dipl.-Ing.
Biomechanische Forschungs-GmbH
Institut zur Prüfung und Entwicklung
biomechanischer Produkte
Rechte Wienzeile 5/2
1040 Wien, Austria

CLAUDE RIEKER, PhD
Centerpulse Orthopedics Ltd.
Vice President Tribology
PO Box 65
8404 Winterthur, Switzerland

CHRISTIAN ROLLER, MD
Würzburg University
Dept. of Orthopaedics
Brettreichstraße 11
97074 Würzburg, Germany

HENNING RÜDEN, Prof. Dr. med.
University Hospital Benjamin Franklin
Institute of Hygiene
Hindenburgdamm 27
12203 Berlin, Germany

MICHAEL SAX, Dipl.-Ing.
University of Aachen
Dept. of Ceramic Engineering
Mauerstraße 5
52064 Aachen, Germany

GERHARD SCHELLER, PD Dr.
Orthopädische Universitätsklinik Mannheim
Theodor-Kutzer-Ufer 1-3
68167 Mannheim, Germany

HANS SCHMOTZER, Dr.
PI Precision Implants AG
Schachenallee 29
5001 Aarau, Switzerland

ROGER SCHOLZ, Dr. med.
Universität Leipzig
Klinik und Poliklinik für Orthopädie
Semmelweis-Straße 10
04103 Leipzig, Germany

ROLF SCHÖN, MSc
Centerpulse Orthopedics Ltd.
PO Box 65
8404 Winterthur, Switzerland

UTE SCHREINER, Dr. med.
Städtisches Klinikum
Theodor-Kutzer-Ufer 1-3
68167 Mannheim, Germany

PAUL SEREKIAN
Stryker Howmedica Osteonics
Vice President - Advanced Technology
300 Commerce Ct.
07430 Mahwah, NJ, USA

JOHN H. SHAW, Dr.
Biosciences and Implants Unit
Medical Devices Agency
Hannibal House / Elephant and Castle
SE1 6TQ London, United Kingdom

T. SHISHIDO, MD
Tokyo Medical University
Department of Orthopaedics
Tokyo, Japan

MARTIN SIMNACHER, Dr.
PI Precision Implants AG
Schachenallee 29
5001Aarau, Switzerland

ERWIN STEINHAUSER, Dr.-Ing.
Technische Universität München
Klinik für Orthopädie
und Sportorthopädie
Connollystraße 32
80809 München, Germany

BURKHARD SUMMER, Dipl.-Biol.
Klinik und Poliklinik für Dermatologie
und Allergologie der
Ludwig-Maximilians Universität München
Frauenlobstraße 9-11
80337 München, Germany

RAINER TELLE, Prof. Dr.
University of Aachen
Dept. of Ceramic Engineering
Mauerstraße 5
52064 Aachen, Germany

PETER THOMAS, PD Dr. med.
Klinik und Poliklinik für Dermatologie
und Allergologie der
Ludwig-Maximilians-Universität München
Frauenlobstraße 9-11
80337 München, Germany

ROBERT M. URBAN
Rush-Presbyterian-St. Luke's Medical Center
Dept. of Orthopedic Surgery
1653 W. Congress Parkway
60612 Chicago, Illinois, USA

AIGUO WANG, PhD
Stryker Howmedica Osteonics
Director of Bearing Technology
300 Commerce Ct.
07430 Mahwah, NJ, USA

KLAUS WEIST, MD
University Hospital Benjamin Franklin
Hospital Epidemiologist
Hindenburgdamm 27
12203 Belin, Germany

HANS-G. WILLERT, Prof. Dr.
Orthopädische Universitätsklinik
Direktor
Robert-Koch-Straße 40
37075 Göttingen, Germany

GERD WILLMANN, Prof. Dr. rer.nat.
CeramTec AG
Fabrikstraße 23-29
73207 Plochingen, Germany

LUIGI ZAGRA, Dr.
Divisione Istituto Ortopedico Galeazzi
Via R. Galeazzi 4
85112 Milano, Italy

SUSANNE ZIMMERMANN, cand. med.
Technische Universität München
Klinik für Orthopädie und Sportorthopädie
Connollystraße 32
80809 München, Germany

MARCEL ZUBERBÜHLER, Dipl.-Ing.
PI Precision Implants AG
Schachenallee 29
5001Aarau, Switzerland

KARL ZWEYMÜLLER, Prim. Univ. Prof. Dr.
Orthopädisches Krankenhaus Gersthof
Wielemansgasse 28
1180 Wien, Austria

SESSION 1

Basics of Ceramic Components in Hip Arthroplasty

1.1 Tribological and Material Properties for all-Alumina THR -Convergence with Clinical Retrieval Data

I.C. Clarke, M. Manaka, T. Shishido, H. Oonishi, G.A. Gustafson and M. Boehler

Introduction

Pierre Boutin MD in France was the first to describe the very low wear-rates with all-ceramic (COC) total hip replacements (THR). By April 1970 his first alumina ball and cup concept had been developed and implanted in concert with Daniel Blanquaert of Ceraver Inc [1]. Subsequent collaborations at the University of Paris between Drs. Boutin, Witvoet and Sedel furthered the development and analyses of their all-alumina THR. Beginning in 1977, they incorporated the taper-lock ball design and the hemispherical alumina cups of the cemented and press-fit THR types (Fig. 1).

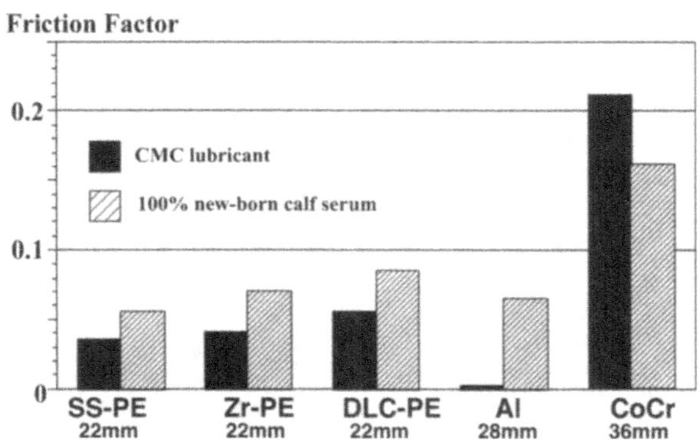

Figure 1: A 30-year road map for ceramic THR history, starting with the introduction by Boutin MD in France (1970) of the monoblock ceramic cup to this year's FDA approval (Jan. 31st, 2003) for the first metal-backed, modular ceramic cups (Strycher and Wright Medical Technology).

While Sedel's group in Paris have now provided an impressive series of publications over a 25 year period detailing results in both young and old patients [2-6], their original fixation concepts with monoblock alumina cups were not successful. However one satisfaction was that due to the ultra-low wear-rates with COC, they rarely experienced the wear debris effects that produced osteolytic phenomena [6]. Therefore their cup revision cases were uncomplicated by major bone loss.

In Germany, Peter Griss and Heinz Mittelmeier [7, 8] introduced concepts of a taper-locked, alumina balls combined with varied designs of non-cemented, monoblock alumina cups. In Austria Salzer and colleagues [9] developed a 3-peg monoblock cup design similar to Boutin's press-fit concept [1]. In Germany the 'Mittelmeier' THR concepts developed by Erhard Doerre (originally Feldmuhle Inc, now CeramTec Inc) represented the only ceramic THR to gain FDA approval in the early 1980's (AutophorTM; XenophorTM). However popularity waned rapidly in USA and by 1985 or so the unacceptably high revision rates had been well documented (Table 1). Regardless of this fact, this unique ceramic experience for the USA paved the way for a down-classification by the FDA in 1989 for the ceramic-UHMWPE concept (Fig. 1).

Date Publication	1st Author	Clinical (N)	Retrieval (N)	Linear Wear	Revisions (%)
1981	Plitz	120	15	0-0.9mm	
1984	Griss			0-2mm	
1988	Frankel	60			10%
1990	Kummer		6	10um-3mm	
1990	Mahoney	42	2	10um	35%
1992	Mittelmeier	3000		2-5um	1% - 22%
1994	Ivory	38			16%
1996a	Huo	112			44%
1996b	Huo	28			3%
1996	Hyder	26			20%
1997	Refior		54	30um - 3.7mm	
2001	Nevelos		11:11	1un - 0.5mm	

Table 1:
Summary of ceramic wear reports in Europe and the USA featuring both 'micro' and 'macro' wear of alumina balls.

Thus, THR designs from the pioneering groups of Boutin, Salzer and Mittelmeier formed the foundation for what we know today regarding clinical and wear performance of COC implants. From a frictional performance standpoint it also appeared that COC were the optimal rigid-rigid bearings (Fig. 2). In one of the rare detailed studies of THR frictional torque, it was noted that the frictional factors for ceramic-on-ceramic were equivalent to the Charnley THR and 2.5 times less than metal-on-metal bearings when run with either serum or synovial fluid as the lubricant [10].

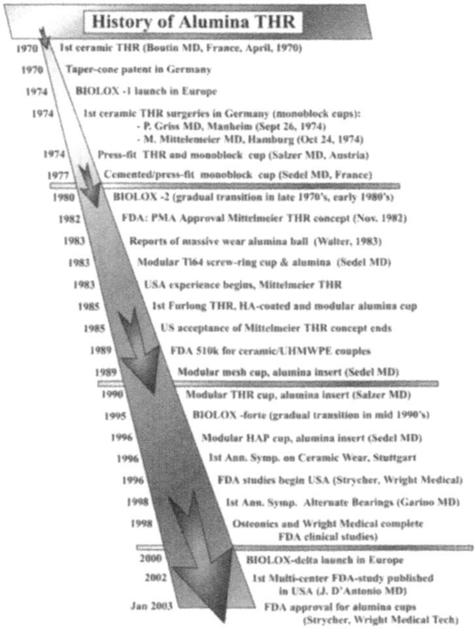

Figure 2:
Comparison of THR friction factors for 22mm UHMWPE cups, 28mm Al/Al THR and 36mm CoCr/CoCr in varied lubricants such as carboxymethyl cellulose (CMC) and 100% calf serum [10]. The 28mm COC implants were in the same range as the Charnley THR with UHMWPE cups.

In 1997, two American orthopaedic companies began the 1st FDA approved, multi-center clinical studies of ceramic-ceramic THR in the USA. By the middle of 1998, Osteonics Inc and Wright Medical Inc had enrolled more than 500 and 300 patients, respectively [11]. These clinical results with metal-backed ceramic liners have been published [12]. As of Friday January 31st, 2003, there was a historic announcement by the FDA regarding their approval for these two companies to market the first modular ceramic cups in the USA. Along with these milestones (Fig. 1) in clinical developments of ceramic THR, considerable progress has also been made in laboratory wear analyses of COC combinations. Therefore the objective of this report was to bring together the known laboratory, material and clinical wear performance for alumina-alumina THR combinations.

Clinical COC Wear Experiences

From the beginning alumina balls bearing on alumina cups have had an enviable reputation for ultra-low wear [1]. However from the world literature we can see several interesting features (Table 1). The first is that the bulk of clinical and retrieval literature reflected the basically sub-optimal performance of the Mittelmeier THR first in Europe and then in the USA. In implants retrieved for other than subluxation/tilting problems and migration, the average wear was of the order to 2 to 5 um/year [13, 14]. In some cases the original machined marks could still be seen after more than a decade of use. Since the average grain size of this historical alumina could be in the 3-4 um range, these data implied that only the surface row of 4um size grains was worn off with each year of use in the patient (Fig. 3a). For scale of comparison, a red blood cell is about 7 um in diameter (Fig. 3b).

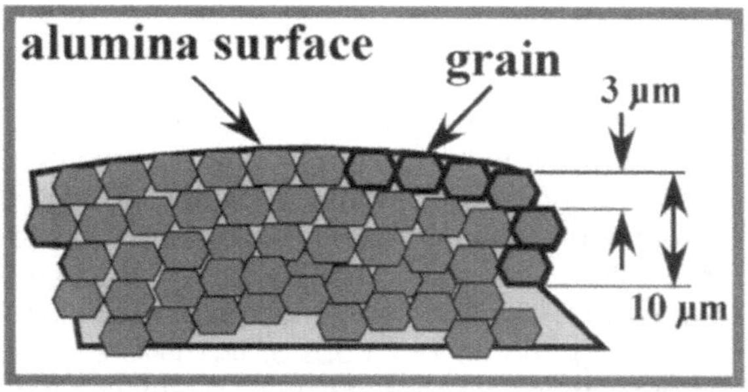

Figure 3a) Diagrammatic sketch of 5 layers of alumina grains forming the articular surface, each about 3-4 um average size. A 5 to 10 um depth of alumina wear [13, 14] would correspond to about 2-3 layers of alumina grains, and for a size comparison

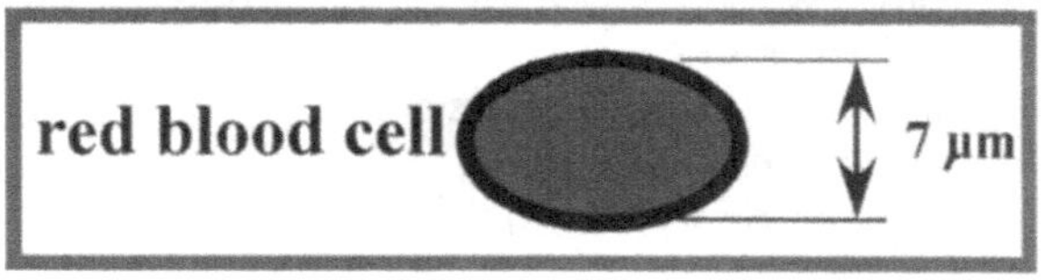

Figure 3b) the dimensions of a red blood cell are of the same magnitude as this depth of wear zone.

The second feature was that the ceramic wear scars most visible occurred as narrow "stripes" on the femoral ball and narrow zone of rim-wear in the acetabular cups [13, 16]. A third inescapable fact was that wear of some alumina implants (4 retrieval studies) was recorded much higher than the values listed above. Two of the retrievals with tilted Ceraver cups showed wear in the range 5 to 36 um/year on the balls [13]. However, comparisons of the pioneering range 5 to 36 um/year on the balls [13]. However, comparisons of the pioneering Austrian monoblock cup and a later design of modular cup provided wear rates of 39 um/year and 27 um/year, respectively [15]. Such cup wear was in the range reported by the French experience for their problem-tilted cups [13]. This implied that 6 to 10 layers of alumina grains were worn off each year (Fig. 4a). However, wear in 4 retrieval studies was recorded as high as 0.9 mm to 3.7 mm (Table 1). Photographs from a few of the pioneering studies have shown on occasion a few very misshapen alumina balls [16]. The extent of alumina grain excavation in such cases would have been really quite extraordinary (Fig. 4b).

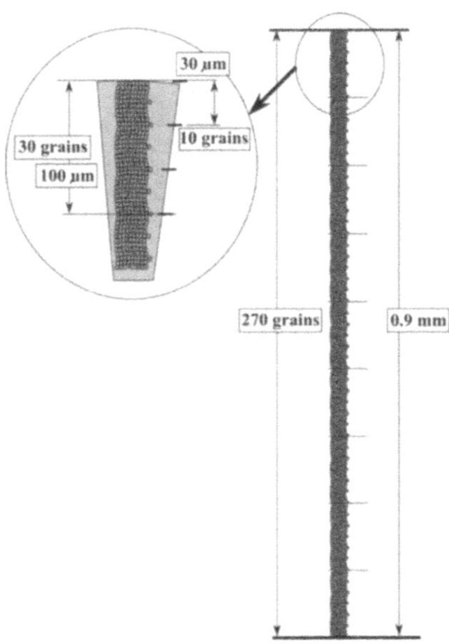

Figure 4:
Clinical COC wear rates reported as:

a) an alumina wear depth of 30 to 40 µm/year [15], corresponding to erosion of the equivalent of 10-15 layers of alumina grains

b) an alumina wear depth of 0.9 mm/year [35], corresponding to erosion of the equivalent of 270-300 layers of alumina grains. Note that maximum recorded wear of 3.7 mm on alumina ball [Table 1] would have corresponded to about 1,200 layers of alumina grains being eroded.

Unfortunately the early clinical history does not give a clear record of what was actually the problem in these patients. Sedel's extensive experience indicated that some ceramic cups which had tilted (while the patient continued to function on them) could contribute to massive wear of the alumina ball over time [17]. Thus it is to be hoped that such severe wear problems reflected early design and fixation problems (cup migration and tilting) unique to these pioneering, monoblock cups of the 1970 era. Thus the advantage of ultra-low ceramic wear [1] was offset in pioneering series by problems that were a combination of

a) bulky alumina cup design,
b) poor fixation to bone,
c) generally poor range of motion.

The most recent clinical wear study came from a series of over 1,500 cases [18]. This comprised an analysis of 16 retrieved COC implants from 3rd generation THR (Howmedica-Osteonics Inc). These were short-term cases with 0.2 to 2.5 years follow-up. A remarkable contribution from this study was their first detailed reporting of volumetric wear on retrieved ceramic implants. Eleven heads and 8 liners (BIOLOX-forte™, Ceramtec Inc) were identified at surgery by macroscopic evidence of wear (stripe wear) during various revision operations. It was noted that the wear stripes were posteriorly inclined (Fig. 5a) with average tilt 20° and latitudinal location averaging 47° above the equator (in implants defined as stable). The explanation offered was that the wear scars were formed during repetitively loaded, flexion activities (Fig. 5b). Ranking of the stripe data showed that mild wear on balls ranged from 0.1 to 0.5 mm^3/year [19]. The higher-wear cases ranged from 0.7 to 1.9 mm^3/year (average 1.1 mm^3/year year). These initial volumetric wear data for COC patients in the Australian study with up to 2 years follow-up are of great interest to the scientists developing the simulator wear studies.

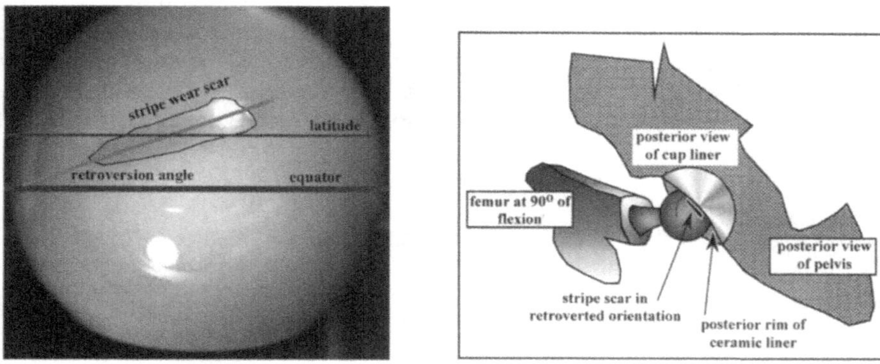

Figure 5:
Peripheral wear scar (stripe) as observed on retrieved alumina ball (with up to 2 years use) from clinical retrieval study in Sydney [18]:
a) latitude, angle and dimensions of wear scars were documented.
b) With the hip flexed to approximately 90o, such as in stair-climbing or chair-sitting activities, the stripe zone of ball-cup rim contact was angled retroverted and was sited higher on the ball dome in stable cases.

Laboratory Wear Experiences – Standard Test Modes (STD)

With the increasing interest in ceramic implants (FDA approved two ceramic cup designs, January 31st, 2003) it is imperative that a scientific foundation be laid for evaluation of the ceramic THR as well as alternate materials. A beginning has been made with the current ISO standard for hip simulation but this does not nearly address the many experimental variables in the contemporary simulator research [19].

It is readily apparent that laboratory wear machines reflect much simplicity of the human hip environment. The meaningful test parameters are seldom discerned in advance of actual patient experience and may not always be capable of duplication even when so identified. The limitations of the simple wear tester are numerous since it cannot emulate the geometrical and lubrication characteristics characteristic of the human hip joint. Even with hip simulators that can test the actual hip implants under reasonable kinematics and loading characteristics unique to the human hip joint [20-24], the features and repeatability of these computer-controlled machine may not mimic all essential features of the patient's hip performance. In addition, the test protocols, lubricants and wear-measurement methods used around the world have been quite variable. The orthopaedic surgeon can be forgiven if he becomes frustratedwith the confusion and controversy in laboratory wear simulations and the apparent lack of continuity with what he perceives as his clinical reality. However it also a mistake to be overly critical of the historical efforts to simulate all possible design features and all possible patient activities.

Until comparatively recently, THR wear studies did not include any simulation of the micro-separation ball-cup test mode. These historical studies shall be referred to as using the standard (STD) kinematics simulator mode. The Leeds Tribology group pioneered the use of micro-separation test modes and this shall be referred to as the new MSX mode. There is also a challenge in modeling the ultra-low wear magnitudes evident in COC bearings. The initial onset of wear in the first half million cycles (i.e. 0.5 million cycles, perhaps 6 months use by the patient) will be the highest and subsequent wear will be much reduced (Fig. 6). Thus the run-in phase should be easier to quantify since it will have a much larger wear magnitude than the steady-state phase. It was also noted that some studies only measured cup wear where as some provided wear for both ball and cup (total THR wear).

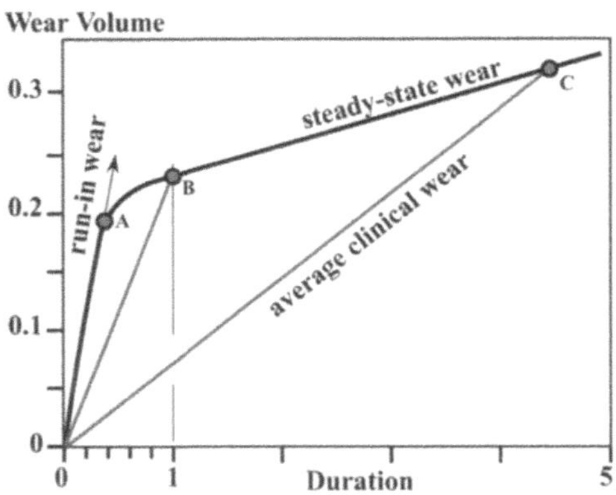

Figure 6:
Schematic illustration of biphasic wear for COC bearings. Laboratory studies can provide a detailed wear sequence from the transition of run-in to the steady-state phase. Retrieval studies can only estimate the "average" wear-rate over the lifetime of the implant. Thus the "average" clinical wear will always appear lower than the "run-in" simulator value but higher than "steady-state" value. Also the predicted "run-in" wear will vary in simulator studies depending on the datum where it was assessed, i.e. at 0.5, 0.75, 1, or 1.5 Mc durations, etc [31].

Boutin in France [1] was the first to study the low wear rates in all-ceramic (COC) total hip replacements (THR) and described the run-in and much lower steady-state response, i.e. biphasic wear of COC implants. For example in a hip simulator study (using water lubrication) of alumina ball and cup implants, the initial (run-in) phase averaged linear wear as low as 0.01 mm (< 10 um) during the first million cycles (1 Mc). Thereafter the ball wear appeared undetectable to 7.5 million cycles duration in the simulator. Later investigators using water or saline as the lubricant of choice confirmed this ultra-low, linear wear [20-24].

The STD simulator studies of alumina THR have typically provided ultra-low wear-rates. In Japan the wear-rate was 0.02 mm^3/Mc for BIOCERAM™ cups run in saline lubrication [22]. Thus the THR (total) wear may have approximated 0.04 mm^3/Mc. The wear-rates determined by Endolab using BIOLOX-forte and delta™ run with calf serum were in the same range [25]. However, these studies did not show much of a transition between run-in and any steady-state phase. In contrast, Kaddich and Pfaff [26] had reported a sharp transition into steady-state phase with their ZTA ceramic study. Their THR run-in wear-rate averaged 0.29 mm^3/Mc. In the Leeds STD study [27], THR run-in wear-rates averaged 0.14 mm^3/Mc(BIOLOX ™). A subsequent USA study described higher run-in wear of the order 0.51 mm^3/Mc for BIOLOX-forte™ cups [28]. The THR wear would have approximated perhaps 1 mm^3/Mc. The LLUMC study made a special point of detailing the transition from run-in to steady-state wear modes [29]. The COC run-in wear-rates averaged 0.5 mm^3/Mc to 0.8 Mc duration and then decreased sharply. Thus in recent STD simulator studies with standard kinematics, run-in wear-rates appeared to have varied by two orders of magnitude, from a low of 0.02 to a high of 1 mm^3/Mc with perhaps 0.5 mm^3/Mc being fairly representative.

Steady-state wear rates for ceramic THR are much more difficult to quantify being in the ultra low range. Thus most simulator studies simply reported alumina steady-state wear as "undetectable" [1, 23, 24, 28, 30]. However recent STD simulator studies have been successful in quantifying steady-state wear. The Endolab study with ZTA bearings produced 0.026 mm^3/Mc, representing an 11-fold reduction from their run-in value [26]. The Leeds Group measured a steady-state THR wear-rate of 0.05 mm^3/Mc for BIOLOX with alumina cups inclined at both 45° and 60° angles [27]. This was 3-fold less than with the run-in wear of 0.14 mm^3/Mc and no difference was detected with either cup orientation. In the LLUMC studies run out to 6 Mc and 14 Mc durations the steady-state BIOCERAM™ THR wear averaged 0.02 mm^3/Mc, a 25-fold reduction from run-in wear [29]. Thus with standard kinematics, steady-state COC wear-rates appeared to be as low as 0.02 to 0.05 mm^3/Mc. From a historical point of view, the long-term wear rates for UHMWPE cups (gamma-air) have averaged around 75 to 80 mm^3 per year. With such a comparison, the steady-state wear rate with alumina cups (STD simulator test mode) represented a potential for 1,600 to 4,000-fold reduction.

Laboratory Wear Experiences – Non-Standard Test Modes

The focus of recent simulator work has included the main topics of:

a) Standard hip kinematics with varied lubricants
b) Elevated loading (ELV) during swing phase of gait
c) Micro-separation kinematics (MSX)

The Leeds Group studied COC lubrication effects using a 25% gelatin based. low-protein solution (Gelfusive™), a 100% calf serum, water alone and also examined the 'dry' state [31]. It was noted that wear rates were reduced approximately 50% with Gelfusive and a still further 50% reduction appeared in water. Only the 'dry' wear condition produced accelerated ceramic damage (catastrophic). Thus bovine serum appeared the choice for adequate wear of alumina. However this conclusion may depend on the precise test conditions and choice of ceramic implants. Studies of THR frictional torque showed the lowest frictional effect with Al/Al in water (Fig. 2) compared to the 32-fold increase in frictional effort with 100% calf serum [10]. At LLUMC, the water-lubricated mode appeared more severe for both all-metal and all-ceramic THR compared to the test-modes with much diluted serum solutions [32-34]. Clearly more work is needed in this area to understand the importance of protein concentrations for friction and wear phenomena relative to both the human joint and the wear simulator.

In STD test mode, the Leeds Group had routinely used 0.05 kN load during the swing-phase of gait. As an elevated test mode (ELV), they added a 20-fold increase in loading during the swing-phase duration (1 kN load). The average wear trend for BIOLOX-forte was 0.11 mm^3/mc in STD mode and rose to 0.15

mm^3/Mc in ELV mode, i.e. an apparent increase of 30% [35]. However due to experimental factors these results were not statistically significant.

The Leeds Group was also the first to introduce micro-separation into the simulator kinematics during swing-phase and this created much higher COC wear-rates [36]. This also created the peripheral wears scars (stripes) seen on some retrieved implants [7, 13, 16, 37]. In their "severe" MSX mode, the COC run-in wear increased to 4 mm^3/Mc and the steady state to 1.3 mm^3/Mc (Table 2). Compared to their prior STD data, this "severe" MSX mode had increased steady

Test Mode	Run-in (mm^3/Mc)	Steady-state (mm^3/Mc)
STD (no distraction)	0.11	0.05
MSX "mild" distraction	0.55	0.10
MSX "severe" distraction	4.00	1.30

Table 2:
Summary of MSX simulator data from Leeds Group [20]. Their COC run-in wear increased to 0.6 mm^3/Mc for "mild" and 4 mm^3/Mc for "severe" test modes respectively (7-fold increase from mild to severe mode; run-in). Their steady-state data increased to 0.1 mm^3/Mc in "mild" MSX mode and 1.3 mm^3/Mc in the "severe" MSX mode, respectively (13-fold increase from mild to severe mode; steady-state). Compared to their prior STD data, the "severe" MSX mode had increased steady state wear 26-fold.

state wear some 26-fold (wear included main wear-zone and stripe wear-zones). A subsequent study with "severe" MSX mode for Al/Al provided wear-rates of over 2 mm^3/Mc in tests to 5 Mc duration, and for ZTA/Al combinations wear varied from 1 to 1.7 mm^3/Mc [38]. These were of similar magnitude to their earlier studies (Table 3).

Test Mode	Wear Vol (mm^3/Mc)	Run-in	Steady-state	Average
STD	ball + cup	0.38	0.011	0.078
MSX	ball + cup	1.74	0.39	0.66
	Ratio MSX/STD	4.6	35.5	8.5

Table 3:
Summary of MSX simulator data from LLUMC Group [19, 40] showing over 4-fold increase in run-in phase and 35-foldl increase in steady-state phase.

Thus with micro-separation kinematics (MSX), steady-state COC wear-rates trends averaged 1 to 2 mm^3/Mc. Compared to the 75 to 80 mm^3 per year wear-rates for UHMWPE cups, these COC wear-rates under "severe" simulator mode (MSX) represented a 40 to 80-fold reduction and were also comparable to the high-wear THR cases from the most recent retrieval study [18].

LLUMC Wear Experiences – MSX Test Mode

In our COC implant retrievals at LLUMC, the wear scars were mapped by light microscopy and SEM. Three examples with 16 to 22 years follow-up showed a central superior wear scar and varied shapes of peripheral wear scars (Fig. 7). For comparison between clinical and simulator wear maps, the alumina wear progression was ranked into 5 grades (Fig. 8) by SEM observations of surface burnishing and pitting [39]. The main wear zone was generally grade # 4 and the peripheral wear zones showed more damage at grade# 5. The gray surface discoloration turned out to contain Co and Cr, i.e. wear debris contaminants from fretting by the tip of the femoral stem against endosteal bone.

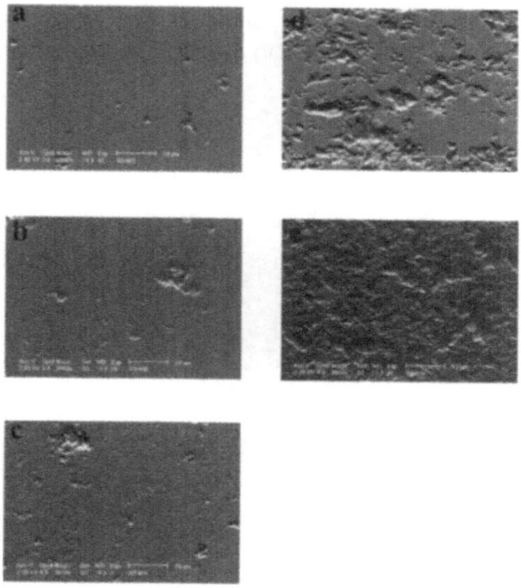

Figure 7:
Retrieved alumina ball heads with 16 to 22 years follow-up in 1st generation COC implants [38]. The bearing surfaces still retained some of their original shine with some discoloration due to smeared Co and Cr layers. The main wear zone and varied peripheral wear zones were mapped by SEM study. Narrow gray=stripes across the surfaces may have been made during the revision procedures.

Progression of surface roughness (wear) in STD simulator test [38] ranked as 5 types:
Grade# 1. Original machine tracks from the manufacturer with occasional small pits evident **(a)**
Grade# 2. Burnishing of machine tracks with more small pits appearing and some grain pull-out obvious by the larger pitting. Some grain etching becomes apparent. **(b)**
Grade# 3: Most of the machine tracks polished burnished off, appearance of numerous etched grains with some more pitting but surface gives appearance of mainly intact. **(c)**
Grade# 4: Surface now very smooth but broken up into small islands as evidence of considerable grain pull-out. **(d)**
Grade#5: Polished surface islands now gone and worn surface has a roughened granular appearance. **(e)**

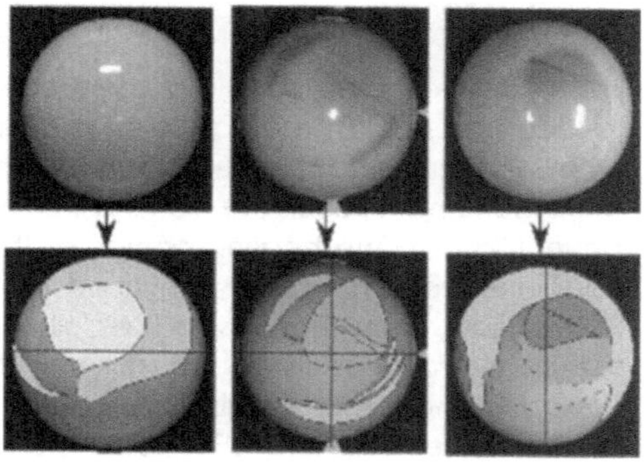

Figure 8:
Retrieved alumina ball heads with 16 to 22 years follow-up in 1st generation COC implants [38]. The bearing surfaces still retained some of their original shine with some discoloration due to smeared Co and Cr layers. The main wear zone and varied peripheral wear zones were mapped by SEM study. Narrow gray=stripes across the surfaces may have been made during the revision procedures.

At LLUMC we followed the Leeds Group's example and modified our simulators to run micro-separation wear studies [40]. The BIOLOX-forte implants (diameters 28mm, 32mm and 36mm) were studied in a 12-station, SWM hip simulator using 50% alpha-calf serum as the lubricant. The metal-backed ceramic liners (Trident, Howmedica-Osteonics) were inclined at a 50o degree inclination in the anatomical test fixtures. The MSX test mode was triggered during the swing phase of each load cycle when the joint loading reversed. A coiled-spring mechanism provided a transverse distraction of 0.5 mm with the concomitant vertical distraction constrained to 1 mm. At onset of heel strike the cup rim impinged on the ball and re-located during stance phase actions (Fig. 9a).

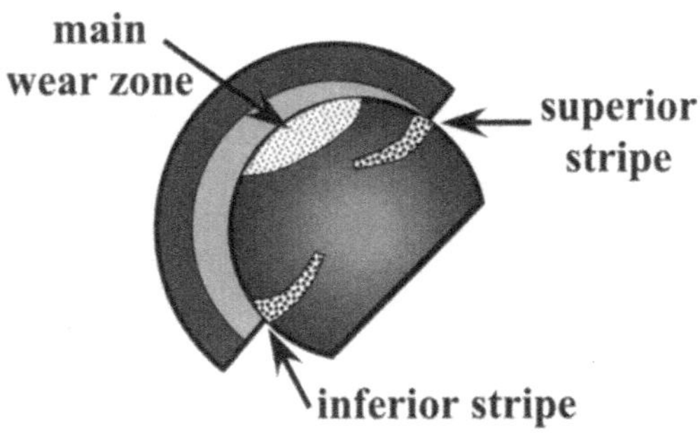

Figure 9:
Schematic of wear scars from MSX simulator study [39]:

a) Balls have standard central wear scar (main wear zone) and twp stripe scars. These correspond to inferior cup-rim contact on ball during micro-separation and superior cup-rim contact on ball reduction during heel-strike phase.

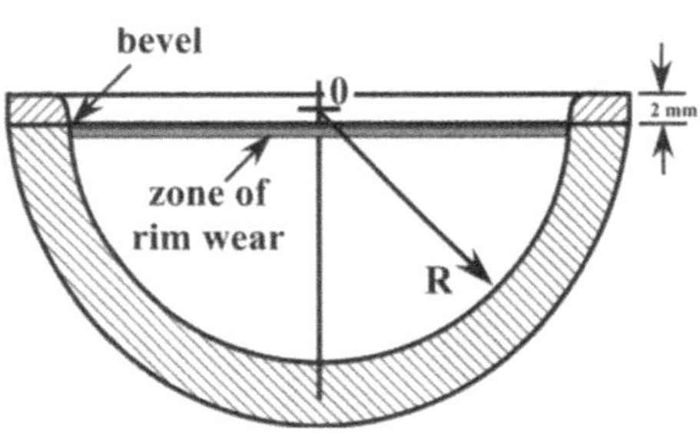

b) Schematic of ceramic insert showing region of rim wear (shaded) at junction of bearing surface and cup bevel where bearing surface is 1mm less than a hemisphere.

Two peripheral wear scars were visible on the balls within the first half million cycles and corresponded to a) the inferior cup rim impinging on ball surface during distraction phase and b) the superior cup rim impinging on ball during the re-location phase. These started off as scars about 9 mm long and approximately 1mm wide and had doubled in size by the end of the study (5 Mc duration). The corresponding wear on the alumina liner was a narrow strip bordering on the cup bevel (Fig. 10). The bearing portion of the cup ended about 1mm less than a hemisphere and the bevel continued 1 mm beyond the hemisphere.

The micro-wear features on the balls were studied by SEM (Fig. 10a) and then the wear study was continued at 1 Mc intervals to 5 Mc duration. At the end of the study, the femoral balls were characterized for surface roughness and the cups were sectioned for SEM study. The peripheral wear scars (Fig. 10b) always showed a more severe grade of wear than the main wear zone (Fig. 10a). In this study the final wear rankings were grade #3 for the main wear zone (Fig. 10c) and #4 for the stripe scar after 5 Mc duration. In the 20-year retrievals the corresponding grades were #4 and #5 [39]. Clearly the micro-separation simulator mode made a significant contribution to ceramic wear rates and created peripheral wear zones somewhat indicative of the retrievals. In our MSX study the "average" COC wear rates were 0.66 mm3/Mc for comparison with clinical data [18].

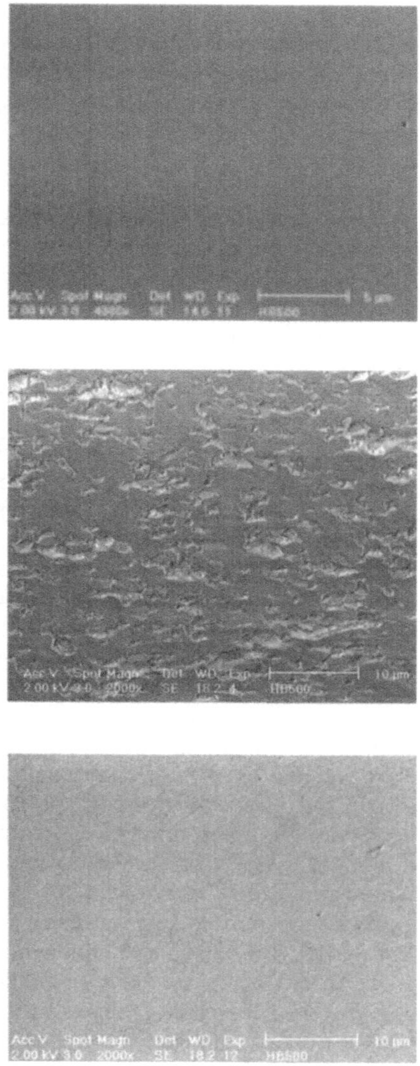

Figure 10:
SEM studies of wear progression on central and peripheral wear zones of Biolox-forte balls run under MSX mode in 50% calf serum to 5 Mc duration:

a) slightly burnished surfaces typical of main wear zone by 600,000 cycles (run-in phase)

b) partially-eroded surface typical of peripheral wear zone formed by 600,000 cycles

c) slightly burnished surfaces typical of main wear zone after 5,000,000 cycles in steady-state phase.

Discussion and Conclusions

The historical record of wear measured on retrieved 1st generation types of COC implants has varied from reports of a few microns of linear wear per year to some cases involving several millimeters of catastrophic wear. Recent Australian retrieval data with just 6 to 34 months follow-up of 3rd generation designs provided 5 THR cases with stripe wear total < 0.6 mm^3/year and 3 cases with stripe wear in the range 1.2 to 3.5 mm^3/year It was not clear what made the difference in these cases.

Looking over the history of STD simulator studies, there was also a large variation in COC wear trends. Typically there was a steep run-in phase over the first half million cycles and then a rapid transition into the steady-state phase that featured a considerably lower wear rate. The turning point for the biphasic wear trend was generally between 0.5 and 0.8 million cycles. However this biphasic wear trend did not appear in all studies and it was not clear why there was this dichotomy. The run-in wear-rates have varied by an orders of magnitude, from under 0.1 mm^3/Mc to 1 mm^3/Mc. A typical conservative value for run-in wear could be considered as 0.5 mm^3/Mc. In the steady-state mode, the STD simulator wear rates were an order of magnitude lower in the range 0.02 mm^3/Mc to 0.05 mm^3/Mc. In terms of predicting the relative wear with alumina cups compared to UHMWPE cups, the COC steady state wear rate represented a potential for a 1,600 to 4,000-fold reduction in wear debris.

With the new micro-separation (MSX) simulator kinematics, the COC wear rates have risen by an order of magnitude. In both the Leeds and the LLUMC studies, the run-in wear increased 4-fold but steady-state wear showed an approximately 30-fold increase. Run-in wear rates varied from 0.5 to 4 mm^3/Mc and steady-state wear-rates trends averaged 0.7 to 2 mm^3/Mc. The peripheral wear zones were long and narrow at 5 million cycle duration and appeared similar to those wear stripes identified in the recent Australian retrieval study with 6 to 34 months follow-up. The peripheral wear scars mapped in retrievals at 16 to 22 years were longer, broader and connected, indicative of the gait variations over 2 decades of use. The simulator MSX mode of wear scars were well formed at 600,000 cycles duration (run-in) and did not appear remarkably different by 5 million cycles duration. However the stripe wear was always a wear-grade greater than the main wear zone.

In overview, a well performing alumina ball and cup should be able to maintain steady-state THR wear rates less than 0.05 mm^3/Mc. This would represent over 1,000-fold wear reduction compared to historical UHMWPE wear-rates. In patients with peripheral wear scars forming from cup rim-contact on the femoral head, the wear rates could be an order of magnitude higher. In some cases it could be as high as 3 to 4 mm^3/Mc as measured in both simulator studies and clinical retrievals. This would still represent a 20-fold wear reduction compared to historical UHMWPE wear-rates. What is not clear is whether this wear trend will continue or whether it will become self-limiting once the alumina-alumina bearing becomes conditioned by the patient's life style. It was also not clear what role femoral stem and cup positioning had on the occurrence of peripheral wear zones.

References

1. Boutin, P. Arthroplastie totale de la hanche par prothese en alumine frittee. Revue de Chirurgie Orthopedique et Reparatrice de l'Appareil Moteur 58(3):229-246, 1972.
2. Sedel, L., Kerboull, L. Christel, P., Meunier, A. and Witvoet, J. Alumina-on-Alumina Hip Replacement. J. Bone Joint Surg. (Br.) 72B(4): 658-663, 1990.
3. Nizard RS, Sedel L, Christel P, Meunier A, Soudry M, and Witvoet J. Ten-Year Survivorship of Cemented Ceramic-Ceramic Total Hip Prosthesis. Clin. Orthop. Rel. Res., 282:53-63, 1992.
4. Hamadouche M, Bizot P, Nizard RS, and Sedel L. Hybrid Alumina-Alumina Hip Replacement: A Survivorship Analysis and Results at a Minimal Five Year Follow-up. Bioceramics 10:131-134, 1997.

5. Alumina on Alumina , TKR, Patients 40 or younger. Alumina-on Alumina Total Hip Prostheses In Patients 40 years of Age or Younger. Clin. Orthop. Rel. Res. 379: 68-76, 2000.
6. Prudhommeaux, F., Hamadouche, M., Nevelos, J., Doyle, C., Meunier, A., Sedel, L. Wear of Alumina-on-Alumian total Hip Arthroplasties at a mean 11-year followup. Clin. Orthop. Rel. Res. 379:113-122, 2000.
7. Griss, P. Four- to eight-year postoperative results of the partially uncemented Lindenhof-type ceramic hip endoprosthesis. In "The Cementless Fixation of Hip Endoprostheses", Ed: E. Morscher, pub: Springer-Verlag, p220-224, 1984.
8. Mittelmeir, H. Selbsthaftende Keramik-Metall-Verbund-Endoprothesen. Medizinisch-Orthopadische-Technik. 95(6):152-159, 1975.
9. Salzer M., Zweymuller K., Locke H., Zeibig A., Stark N., Plenk H. and Punzet G. Further Experimental and Clinical Experience with Aluminum Oxide Endoprostheses. J. Biomed. Materials Res. 10:847-856, 1976.
10. Scholes, SC, Unsworth A., and Goldsmith, AAJ. A frictional study of total hip joint replacements. Phys. Med. Biol. 45:3271-3735, 2002.
11. Garino, J.P.. Modern Ceramic-on Ceramic total Hip Systems In the United States. Clin. Orthop. Rel. Res. 379:41-47, 2000.
12. D'Antonio, J., Capello, W., Manley, M and Bierbaum, B. New experience with alumina-on-alumina ceramic bearings for total hip arthroplasty. J. Arthrop. 17:390-397, 2002.
13. Dorlot, J. M. Long-Term Effects of Alumina Components in Total Hip Prostheses. Clin. Orthop. Rel. Res. 282:47-52, 1992.
14. Mittelmeier H, and Heisel J. Sixteen Years Experience with Ceramic Hip Prostheses. Clin. Orthop. Rel. Res. 282:64-72, 1992,.
15. Boehler M., Knahr, K., Plenk, H., Walter, A., Salzer M. and Schreiber, V. Long term results of uncemented alumina acetabular implants. J. Bone Jt. Surg. 76B: 53-59, 1994.
16. Walter, A. and Plitz, W. Wear mechanism of alumina-ceramic bearing surfaces of hip-joint prostheses. In "Biomaterials and Biomechanics", eds: P. Ducheyne, G. Van der Perre and A.E. Aubert. Elsevier Science Pub, Amsterdam, p55-61, 1984.
17. Sedel, L. Hamadouche, M., Bizot, P. and Nizard, R. Long-term data concerning use of alumina on alumina bearings in total hip replacement. Key Eng. Mat. vol 240-242: 769-772, 2003.
18. Walter WL, Insley G, Walter WK, Tuke M. The Mechanics of Stripe Wear Formation in a Modern Ceramic on Ceramic Bearing. In 70th Ann. Mtg. AAOS, New Orleans, p278, 2003.
19. Gustafson, GA., Shishido, T., Clarke, IC., Williams, PA., Boehler, M., Manaka, M. and Imakiire, A. Consolidation of clinical and experimental experiences with all-alumina THR. In 70th Ann. Mtg. AAOS, New Orleans, SE-211, 2003.
20. Dawihl, W., Mittelmeier, H., Dorre, E., Altmeyer, G., and Hanser, U. Zur tribologie von huftgleenk-endoprosthesen aus aluminiumoxidkeramik. Med. Orthop. Teche. 99:114-118, 1979.
21. Semlitsch M, Lehmann M, Weber H, Doerre E, and Willert G. New prospects for a prolonged functional life-span of artificial hip joints by using the material combination polyethylene/aluminum oxide ceramic / metal. J. Biomed. Mat. Res. 11:537-552, 1977.
22. Oonishi H, Ueno M, Okimatsu H, and Amino H. Investigation of the wear behavior of ceramic on ceramic combinations in total hip prostheses. Bioceramics. 9:503-506, 1996.
23. Walter, A. Investigations on the wear couple BIOLOX forte/BIOLOX forte and earlier alumina materials. In "Proc 2nd Symp on Performance of the Wear Couple Biolox-forte in Hip Arthroplasty", Stuttgart, Pub: CeramTec, Germany, p123-135, 1997.
24. Saikko, V. and Pfaff, H. G. Wear of alumina-on-alumina total replacement hip joints studied with a hip joint simulator. In "Proc 2nd Symp on Performance of the Wear Couple Biolox-forte in Hip Arthroplasty", Stuttgart, Pub: CeramTec, Germany, p117-122, 1997.

25. Kaddick, C and Pfaff, HG. Results of hip simulator testing with various wear couples. In Bioceramics in Joint Arthroplasty, Proc 7th Int. Biolox Symposium, eds: JP Garino and G. Willmann, p16-20, 2002.
26. Kaddich C. and Pfaff, HG. Wear study in the alumina-zirconia system. In Bioceramics in Hip Joint Replacement, Eds: G. Willmann and K. Zweymuller, Proc 5th International CeramTec Symp, p146-150, 2000.
27. Nevelos, J., E. Ingham, C. Doyle, & J. Fisher. Influence of acetabular cup angle on the wear of 'Biolox Forte' alumina/alumina hip joints in a physiological simulator. In 45th ORS, p 857, 1999.
28. Taylor, SK. In-vitro wear performance of a contemporary alumina:alumina bearing couple under anatomically-relevent hip joint simulation. In Reliability and long-term results of ceramics in orthopaedics, Eds. L. Sedel and G. Willmann, p85-90, 1999.
29. Clarke IC., Williams, PA., Shishido, T., Good, V., Oonishi, H. and Gustafson, GA. Hip simulator validations of alumina THR wear rates for run-in and steady-state wear phases. In Bioceramics in Joint Arthroplasty, Proc 7th Int. Biolox Symposium, eds: JP. Garino and G. Willmann, p20-26, 2002.
30. Toni A. & S. Affatato. New Wear Couples for THR- Simulator Testing. In "Reliability and Lonmg-term Results of ceramics in Orthopaedics, Ed L. Sedel and G. Willmann, pub: Geoge Thieme, New York, 1999.
31. Nevelos, J.E., Ingham, E., Doyle, C., Nevelos, A.B., Fisher, J.. Wear of HIPed and non-HIPed alumina- alumina hip joints under standard and severe simulator testing conditions. BIOMATERIALS 22: 2191-2197, (2001).
32. Clarke, IC, Oonishi, H., Good, V. and Williams, PA. Evaluation of ceramic and CoCr hips: Up to 20 million cycles in simulator studies. In Biotribology Fukuoka-2000 and Related Topics, p9-12, 2000.
33. Clarke, IC., Good, V. and Williams, PA. In Proc Int. Tribology Conference (ITC-2000) and 21st Biotribology Symposium, Nagasaki, 2000.
34. Clarke, IC. Clinical and tribological perspectives of wear in alumina-alumina THR. Key Engineering Materials. Vol. 240-242, 755-764, 2003.
35. Stewart, T., Nevelos, J., Tipper, J., Ingham, E., Streicher, R., Insley, G., Fisher, J. Long term simulator studies of alumina- alumina ceramic hip joints with swing phase micro-separation analysis of wear and wear debris Generation. Combined ORS, Rhodes, 2001.
36. Shishido,T., Clarke, I.C., Williams,P.A., Gustafson, A., Shoji, H., Boehler, M., Keggi, K., Imakiire, A.. Clinical wear and simulator study of ceramic-ceramic THR to 20 years and beyond. ORS, p1019, 2001.
37. Insley, GM., Turner, I., Fisher, J., and Streicher, RM. In-vitro testing and validation of zirconia toughened alumina (ZTA) 2002. In Bioceramics in Joint Arthroplasty, Proc 7th Int. Biolox Symposium, eds: JP. Garino and G. Willmann, p26-31, 2002.
38. Manaka, M., Clarke, I.C., Gustafson, A., and Imakiire, A. Impingement in Ceramic Hip Patient A Retrieval and Wear-Scar Analysis of Femoral Head. Key Engineering Materials,.Vol. 240-242, 847-848, 2003.
39. Manaka, M., Shishido, T., Clarke, I.C., Gustafson, A., and Imakiire, A. Wear analysis of all-alumina THR using micro-separation kinematics in orbital-type simulator (In preparation, 2003).

Rerences needed for Table-1

40. Plitz, W. and Hoss, H.V. Wear of alumina-ceramic hip joints: Some clinical and tribological aspects.. Biomaterials 1980, ed: G.D. Winter, D.F. Gibbons and H. Plenk, Jr., p187-196, 1982.
41. Frankel VH, Stuchin S, Newport ML, Shapiro I, Brinker MR, and Rice JC. The Autophor Non-Cemented Ceramic Hip System. In "Non-Cemented Total Hip Arthroplasty", ed. R. Fitzgerald, Jr., Raven Press, Ltd., New York, p381-391, 1988.

42. Kummer, F.J., Stuchin, S.A., and Frankel V.H.. Analysis of Removed Autophor Ceramic-on-Ceramic Components. J. Arthroplasty, 5(1):28-33, 1990.
43. Mahoney OM. and Dimon, JH. Unsatisfactory results with a ceramic total hip prosthesis. J. Bone Jt. Surg, 72A, 663-6711990.
44. Ivory, JP., Kershaw, CJ. Choudhry, R., Parmar, H., and Stoyle TE. Autophor cementless total hip arthroplasty for osteoarthrosis secondary to congenital hip dysplasia. J. Arthroplasty 9(4): 427- 433, 1994.
45. Huo MH, Martin RP, Zatorski LE, and Keggi KJ. Total Hip Replacements Using the Ceramic Mittlmeier Prosthesis. Clin. Orthop. Rel. Res. 332:143-150, 1996.
46. Huo MH, Martin RP, Zatorski LE, and Keggi KJ. Cementless Total Hip Arthroplasties Using Ceramic-on-Ceramic Articulation in Young Patients. J. Arthroplasty 11(6):673-678, 1996.
47. Hyder N, Nevelos AB, and Barabas TG. Cementless Ceramic Hip Arthroplasties in Patients Less Than 30 Years Old. J. Arthroplasty, 11(6):679-686, 1996.
48. Refior HJ, Plitz W, and Walter , A. Ex Vivo and In Vitro Analysis of the Alumina/Alumina Bearing System for Hip Joint Prostheses. In " Bioceramics-10":127-130, 1997.
49. Nevelos, J.E, Prudhommeaux, F.,Hamadouche, M., Doyle, C., Ingham, E., Meunier, A.. Nevelos, AB., Sedel, L., and Fisher, J. Comparative analysis of two different types of alumina-alumina hip prosthesis retrieved for aseptic loosening. J. Bone Jt. Surg. 83B(4), 598-603 2001.

1.2 Wear Behaviour of New Generation Ceramics

C. B. Rieker, G. Liebentritt and R. Schön

Introduction

The wear of ultra high molecular weight polyethylene (UHMWPE) is the major cause of aseptic loosening in total joint prostheses (6).

In Europe alternative bearing articulations, like metal-on-metal, ceramic-on-ceramic or highly cross-linked polyethylene, were developed to minimize the incidence of aseptic loosening of total hip prostheses.

With their bio-stability, high hardness and low roughness, ceramic-on-ceramic bearings are an attractive solution. The typical, current ceramic-on-ceramic solution is a bearing manufactured in alumina-on-alumina.

Since this solution has an in-vivo fracture rate of approximately 1:2,000 over a period of 10-years (5), alternative ceramic-on-ceramic bearings are now being evaluated to reduce this fracture rate. Two possible solutions are currently being investigated.

- Zirconia has a higher toughness (1) and therefore should minimize the risk of invivo failures.
- Zirconia toughened alumina (ZTA) also has a higher toughness (7) in comparison to alumina and has therefore the potential to decrease the risk of invivo failures.

The zirconia-on-zirconia bearing has already been evaluated in-vitro with contradictory results (2, 7).

The first goal of this investigation was to analyse the in-vitro wear behaviour of these two alternative ceramic-on-ceramic bearing systems in comparison to an alumina-on-alumina bearing on a modern hip simulator.

Methods

Two 28.00 mm alumina-on-alumina (Cerasul™ - Centerpulse Orthopedics - Switzerland), six 22.25 mm zirconia-on-zirconia (Prozyr™ - Saint-Gobain - France), six 28.00 mm zirconia-on-zirconia (Prozyr™ - Saint-Gobain - France), and three 28.00 mm ZTA-on-ZTA (Biolox Delta™ - CeramTec - Germany) specimens were tested up to five million cycles on an AMTI hip simulator using the ISO kinematics, described in the document ISO 14242-1 with following parameters: temperature: 37°C, frequency: 1.0 Hz.

The ISO 14242-1 kinematics requires the following motions and load:

- Flexion - extension: 25° - 18°
- Abduction - adduction: 7° - 4°
- Internal / external rotation: 10° - 2°
- Maximum load [double peak]: 3,000 N

A stabilised mixture of Ringer's solution with 33 per cent calf serum and buffered at pH 7.6 served as the lubricant for all the wear tests.

The component wear was measured with a co-ordinate measuring machine having a measurement resolution of less than one µm. A measurement was made every 7.5 degrees on 12 concentric circles, as well as on the pole of the component (total of 577 measurements for each component).

The surface dimensions of the components were measured prior to each experiment. These measurements were used as reference values and compared afterwards with the measurements made every 0.5 or 1.0 million cycles.

The linear wear was defined by the sum of the maximum positive deviations and maximum negative deviations that was obtained by comparing the measurements made after a given number of cycles with the reference values. The volumetric wear rate was calculated based on the volume change according to the ISO 14242-2 standard (dimensional change method).

To investigate the influence of the tetragonal-monoclinic phase transformation of the zirconia-on-zirconia bearings (4), three of the 22.25 mm zirconia-on-zirconia bearings were heat-treated for 24 hours at 140°C. For the same reason, three of the 28.00 mm zirconia-on-zirconia bearings had fifty steam sterilisation cycles (137°C - 30 minutes - 3 atm). The influence of the heat treatment on the tetragonal-monoclinic phase transformation was measured by standard RX diffraction techniques.

The wear patterns of the bearings were examined by scanning electron microscopy (SEM).

All results were analysed statistically with a t-test (level of significance 0.05).

Results

The two heat treatments made on the zirconia-on-zirconia bearings have a very similar influence on the tetragonal-monoclinic phase transformation, with a transformation within the range of 10-15%.

The following linear running-in wears were measured (first million cycles):

- Alumina-on-alumina 28.00 mm: 7.0 ± 0.0 µm
- Zirconia-on-zirconia 22.25 mm not heat-treated: 9.5 ± 3.7 µm
- Zirconia-on-zirconia 22.25 mm heat-treated: 8.0 ± 2.4 µm
- Zirconia-on-zirconia 28.00 mm not heat-treated: 10.3 ± 2.6 µm
- Zirconia-on-zirconia 28.00 mm heat-treated: 8.6 ± 2.5 µm
- ZTA-on-ZTA 28.00 mm: 9.4 ± 0.8 µm

No statistically significant differences were observed between the six running-in wear values.

The following linear wear rates were measured (one to five million cycles):

- Alumina-on-alumina 28.00 mm: 0.5 ± 0.1 µm/106 cycles
- Zirconia-on-zirconia 22.25 mm not heat-treated: 0.0 µm/106 cycles
- Zirconia-on-zirconia 22.25 mm heat-treated: 0.0 µm/106 cycles
- Zirconia-on-zirconia 28.00 mm not heat-treated: 0.6 ± 0.6 µm/106 cycles
- Zirconia-on-zirconia 28.00 mm heat-treated: 0.3 ± 0.2 µm/106 cycles
- ZTA-on-ZTA 28.00 mm: 0.8 ± 0.2 µm/106 cycles

No statistically significant differences were observed between the six linear wear rates.

As no differences were seen between the not heat-treated and the heat-treated zirconia bearings, no differentiation between the two zirconia groups was made for the determination of the volumetric wear rate. The following amounts of volumetric wear rates were measured:

- Alumina-on-alumina 28.00 mm: 0.09 ± 0.04 mm3/106 cycles
- Zirconia-on-zirconia 22.25 mm: 0.06 ± 0.02 mm3/106 cycles
- Zirconia-on-zirconia 28.00 mm: 0.21 ± 0.04 mm3/106 cycles
- ZTA-on-ZTA 28.00 mm: 0.28 ± 0.23 mm3/106 cycles

Figure 1 shows these four volumetric wear rates.

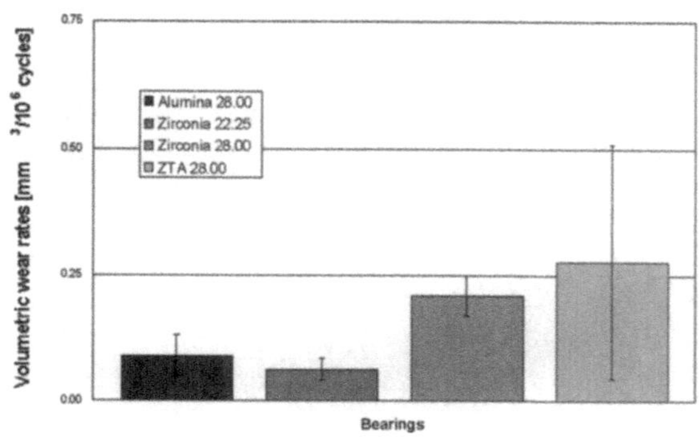

Figure 1

The statistical analysis of these four volumetric wear rates gave the following results:

- The alumina-on-alumina 28.00 mm wear rate is lower than the zirconia-on-zirconia 28.00 mm wear rate ($p = 0.01$).
- The zirconia-on-zirconia 22.25 mm wear rate is lower than the zirconia-on-zirconia 28.00 mm wear rate ($p < 0.01$).
- The other comparisons show no statistically significant differences

Figure 2 shows the wear pattern of a 28.00 mm alumina head after 5 million cycles.

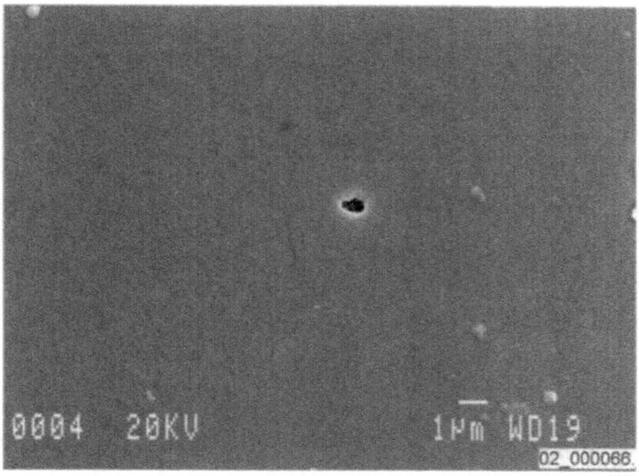

Figure 2

Fine scratches could be found on this alumina head. The grain structure of the alumina (grain size: approximately 2 µm) and a sub-micron pore are also apparent.

Figure 3 shows the wear pattern of a 28.00 mm zirconia head (without sterilisation cycles) after 5 million cycles.

Figure 3

Only fine scratches could be found on this zirconia head.

Figure 4 shows the wear pattern of a 28.00 mm zirconia head (after 50 sterilisation cycles) after 5 million cycles.

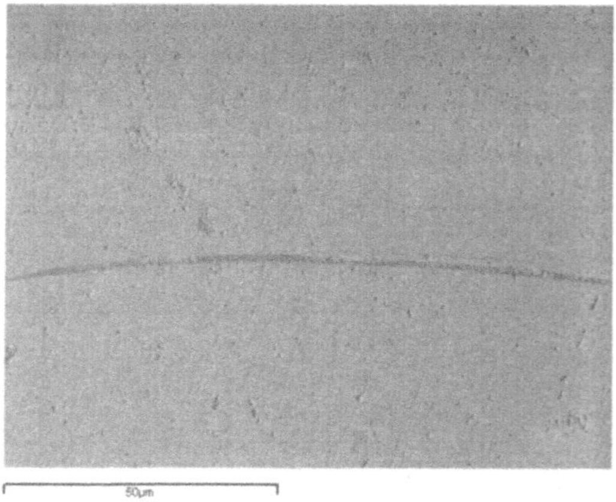

Figure 4

Fine scratches could be found on this zirconia head. The small spots apparent on this figure represent the monoclinic phase induced by the heat treatment.

Figure 5 shows the wear pattern of a 28.00 mm ZTA head after 5 million cycles.

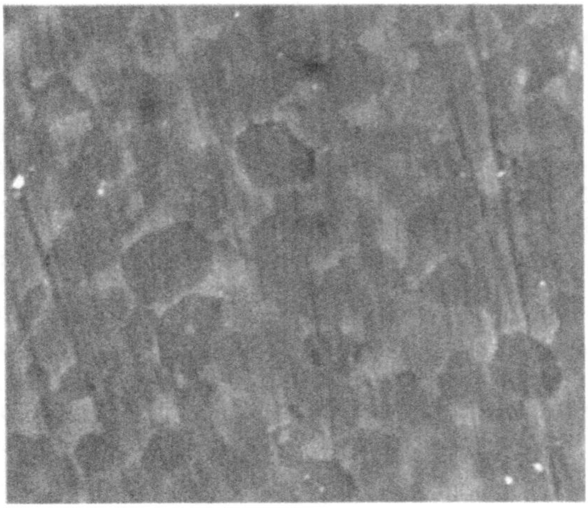

Figure 5

Fine scratches could be found on this ZTA head. The grain structure of the ZTA (grain size: approximately 1 µm) is also apparent.

The fact that only fine scratches could be observed on these four heads indicates that the wear mechanisms are mildly abrasive for these ceramic-on-ceramic bearings.

Discussion

Only mild abrasive wear could be observed on these alternative ceramic-on-ceramic bearings.

For the zirconia-on-zirconia bearings, the heat treatments (24 hours at 140°C or fifty steam sterilisation cycles) are responsible for 10 to 15% of phase transformation. This amount of monoclinic phase has no influence on the in-vitro wear behaviour of these bearings.

This experiment shows that all these ceramic-on-ceramic bearing systems have very stable wear behaviour with a low linear wear rate and a minute volumetric wear rate, and they may be considered as an alternative solution for the current alumina-on-alumina bearings. According to Delaunay (3), a hip prosthesis with a volumetric wear rate lower than 10 mm3 per year is a low wear solution, minimizing the risk of osteolysis. Assuming that a patient walks 1 million steps per year, the four ceramic-on-ceramic bearings investigated in this study are well below this threshold value and they could help to solve the problem of late aseptic loosening of hip prostheses.

Acknowledgments

The authors would like to thank F. Villermaux (CREE - Cavaillon - France) for the RX diffraction measurements and for the SEM observations.

References

1 B. Calès; Zirconia as a Sliding Material; Clinical Orthopaedics and Related Research, 2000, 379, p. 94.

2 I. Clarke, B. Calès; Zirconia-Zirconia Bearing Couple: Design and Wear Behaviour; SICOT - Paris, 2001, p. 150.

3 C. Delaunay; Couple de frottement des prothèses totales de hanche - Ce qu'un chirurgien orthopédiste devrait savoir!; Conférence d'enseignement 2001, édité par J. Duparc, Elsevier 2001, Paris, p. 64.

4 K. Haraguchi et al.; Phase Transformation of a Zirconia Ceramic Head after Total Hip Arthroplasty; Journal of Bone and Joint Surgery - British Edition, 2001, 83B, p. 996.

5 L. Sedel; Evolution of Alumina-on-Alumina Implants; Clinical Orthopaedics and Related Research, 2000, 379, p. 48.

6 H.-G. Willert; Reactions of the Articular Capsule to Wear Product of Artificial Joint Prostheses; Journal Biomedical Materials Research, 1977, 11, p. 157.

7 G. Willmann; The Evolution of Ceramics in Total hip Replacement; Hip International, 2000, 10, p. 193.

1.3 Hip Simulator Testing

G. Reinisch, K.P. Judmann and A. Pauschitz

Introduction

The development of new, highly sophisticated materials for the articulating surfaces of total hip endoprostheses has led to an increasing demand for testing and verification. This includes tests and research regarding bio-compatibility, static load bearing capacity of the prostheses as well as tribological (wear) investigations. Wear debris plays a dominant role in the osteolytic loosening of implants [19,22] and therefore wear testing becomes especially important with newly developed materials (eg composite ceramics, 2nd generation metal-on-metal bearings, cross-linked polyethylene). A reduction of wear extends the service life of endoprostheses.

The wear resistance of materials utilized for the bearing surfaces of endoprostheses has been tested by the use of wear simulators for decades at laboratories throughout the world [2,4,8,10,12,18,21]. However, as a consequence of widely diverging wear testing machines being in use (pin-on-disk, ring-on-disk, bi- and multi-axial hip simulators, orbital bearing machines), the technical committee TC150 Implants for Surgery of the ISO (International Organization for Standardization) has aimed to develop an International Standard, ISO 14242 Wear of total hip-joint prostheses on the basis of kinematics and kinetic data from gait-analysis [7]. The standard is divided into two parts: Part 1 - Loading and displacement parameters for wear testing machines and corresponding environmental conditions for tests and Part 2 - Methods of measurement. This new standard will constitute a base for the comparability of scientific data resulting from wear testing of total hip endoprostheses. New hip simulators have been developed according to the new ISO standards and tests are currently performed and published [8,16].

Model Analysis

Displacement and load data of the human gait are derived from gait analysis. Rela-tive angles of the extremities and thus displacement curves of the hip joint are col-lected through optometric gait analysis systems (Vicon, Ortho Trak, etc) and usually recorded in a co-ordinate system that is fixed to the laboratory. Forces are measured by means of ground force plates [9,14] or by implanted telemetric force transducers [1,13]. The natural lubricant between the femoral head and the acetabulum, the synovial fluid, is described by its chemical and biological composition, its viscosity and amount of soluble gases.

Co-ordinate systems

To describe the spatial movement of the femur relative to the pelvis different co-ordinate systems can be used [23,24]. The origin of most anatomic oriented co-ordinate systems is regarded as in the centre of the hip joint. It is generally acknowledged in clinical assessment to use right-handed co-ordinate systems for the right body side and left-handed co-ordinate systems for the left body side. For an anatomical description of human gait the following co-ordinate system is commonly used:

The inward/outward rotation axis (IOR) is fixed to the femur, the flexion/extension axis (FE) is fixed to the pelvis and a "floating" adduction/abduction axis (AA) stands always perpendicular to the plane originated by the FE and IOR axes. Thus flexion/extension is always accomplished about an axis that is permanent to the pelvis, regardless of the two other displacements. The IOR axis coincides to the longitudinal axis of the femur in any leg position (Fig. 1).

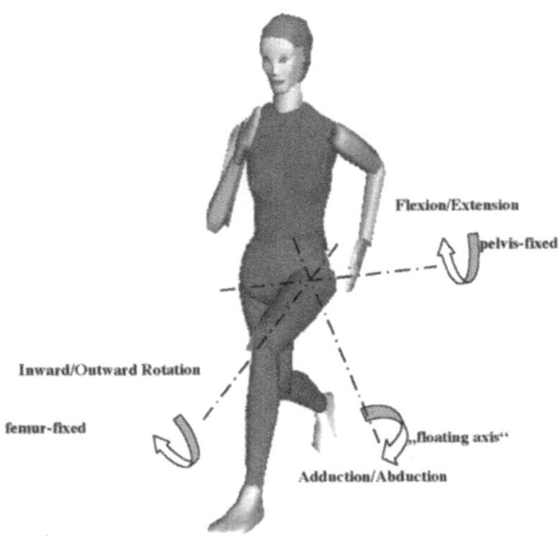

Figure1: Anatomical body-fixed rotation axes in a non-orthogonal co-ordinate system.

A non-orthogonal co-ordinate system is determined with a defined sequence of rotations as flexion/extension before adduction/abduction before inward/outward rotation.

Displacement curves of the extremities derived from gait analysis that are recorded in a laboratory co-ordinate system need to be adapted for the biomechanical model in a hip simulator. Depending on the definition of the co-ordinate system of the gait analysis, a transformation of co-ordinates might be necessary to apply the measured data to hip simulator testing. However, to simulate human walking properly, as described by the ISO standard, this demands a three axial movement of the articulating components.

A Simplified Biomechanical Model

Since the complex form and varieties of femoral ball heads cannot be replicated economically by manufacturing technologies, the natural hip joint is replaced by a sphere (ball head) with a corresponding socket (cup).

As the access to human synovial fluid is very limited, different lubricants (water, syn-thetics, calf serum, etc) have been used in wear testing of endoprostheses. The use of calf serum at 37°C, diluted with de-ionized water to achieve a protein content similar to human synovial fluid, has been acknowledged by many wear testing labo-ratories and is included to the ISO standards.

Hip Wear Testing Machines

Hip wear testing machines are generally divided into multi-axial machines and so called orbital bearing machines (OBM). Today, pin-on-disk and ring-on-disk tribome-ters are only used for screening wear parameters of new materials.

In OBM simulators [4,10,11,21] one bearing partner of the hip joint (usually the femoral ball head) is fixed and the other component (cup) is mounted eccentrically on a rotating, inclined block. Most OBM simulators run in an anatomical inverted position, ball head above acetabular cup, in a vessel containing a minimum of 300 ml lubricant, with at least three testing stations driven by one motor.

Bi-axial and three-axial hip simulators [2,8,16,18] usually perform wear testing in an anatomical position with less lubricant necessary. Depending on the mechanical setup single- or multi-station simulators are built with the possibility of choosing between different relative motions between the bearing partners. While the track of an arbitrary single point on the surface of (eg) the acetabular cup can be generated by rotation about only two axes (bi-axial movement), only a three axial motion determines the common properties of all trajectories in the articulating zone. Fig. 2-4 illustrates the differences of relative motion tracks between the three-axial ISO displacement, the OBM motions and mean of 90 patients all displayed in the same co-ordinate system.

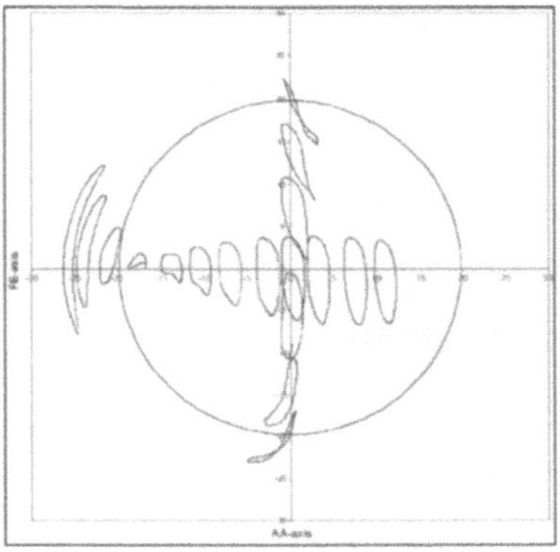

Figure 2:
Projected area of the femoral ball head viewed from the IOR axis performing the ISO 14242-1 motion showing the relative displacements between femur and acetabulum at specific locations.

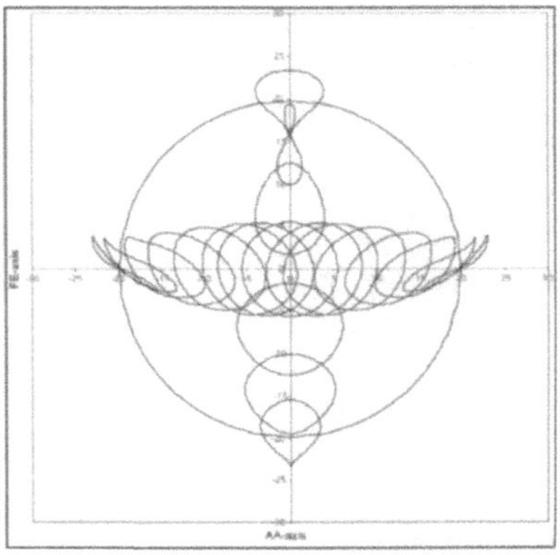

Figure 3:
Projected area of the acetabular cup viewed from the IOR axis performing the motion of an OBM-hip simulator showing the relative displacements between femur and acetabulum at specific locations.

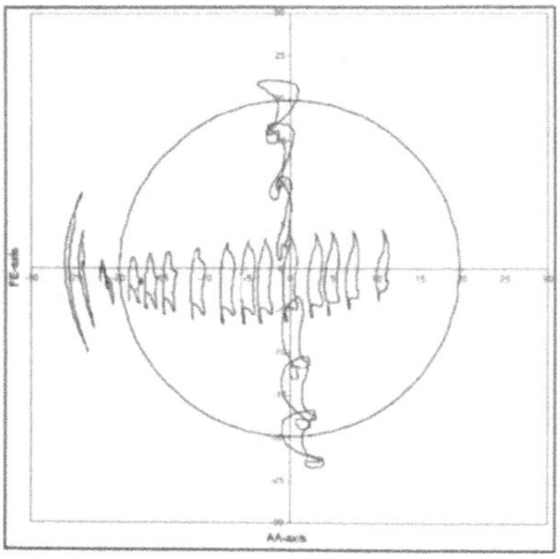

Figure 4:
Projected area of the femoral ball head viewed from the IOR axis in human gait, averaged values of 90 test subjects showing the relative displacements between femur and acetabulum at specific locations.

ISO standard 14242 Wear of hip-joint prostheses

The ISO standard defines a three-axial movement of the bearing partners with a double peak load curve according to gait analysis data [7,8,14,16]. The specimen are to be mounted in an upright, inclined position and sub-merged in calf serum lubricant. Wear testing is performed at 1 Hz up to a total duration of 5.000.000 cycles, roughly corresponding to five years service time in-vivo. At intervals of 500.000 cycles wear measurements are to be performed by means of gravimetric analysis of the bearing partners and/or the dimensional method using a co-ordinate measuring machine (CMM) to assess the contour of the worn specimen [17].

Assessment of wear

After a specified number of wear cycles the bearing partners are dismounted and the wear of each component is measured separately. There are two standard proceedings for the assessment of wear. The amount of wear can be determined by weighing of the specimen before and after the test. However, using this method there is no information on the size of the worn area and the depth of wear, expressed in the maximum linear wear. Also the fluid absorption properties of the material (eg polyethylene) has to be accounted for in gravimetric measurements. Alternatively a CMM is used to map the articulating surfaces of a total hip prosthesis relative to an initial state of sphericity. The result of the dimensional method is a wear map (Fig. 5) with information on the total volume loss, its depth and its relative position on the specimen. However, dimensional wear data are easily corrupted by creep (plastic deformation without mass loss) of the material. A combination of both measurement methods seems to provide a satisfying quantitative wear analysis.

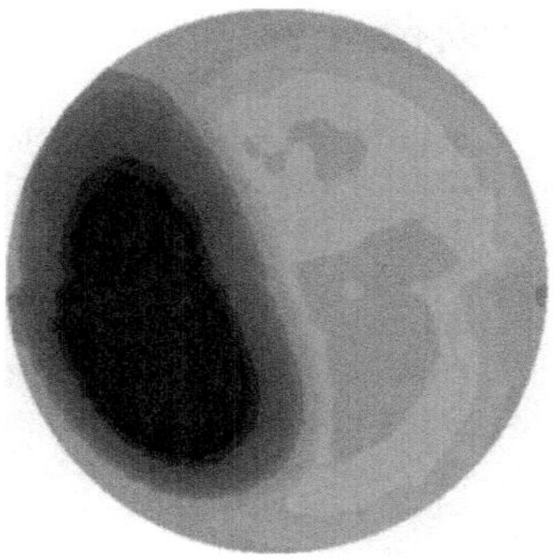

Fig. 5:
Wear map in equivalent azimuthal projection of a worn metallic femoral ball head after five years in-situ. The femoral ball head is viewed from above with the pole in the centre of the picture. Measured radius 14.005 mm, worn volume 5.363 mm³, worn area 548.9 mm³, maximum linear wear (depth) 17.3 µm.

The inspection of worn areas by means of optical and optoelectronic equipment combined with roughness measurements provides substantial data on wear modes such as abrasive, adhesive and third body wear [15,20,21]. Additionally, element determination with energy dispersive x-ray analysis (EDX) specifies impurities or foreign particles in alloys, plastics and ceramics.

Besides the amount of wear the size distribution of wear debris has a high impact on the biological response on wear particles. It has been shown that macrophage activation depends on the size of the worn particles as well as on their chemical composition [3,6]. In this respect another ISO standard DIS/17853 [5] is currently developed, describing the methods of particle extraction from retrieved peri-prosthetic tissue and calf serum used in hip simulator testing.

Results of hip simulator testing

Wear results from hip simulator testing are usually expressed by cycles (time) over amount of wear diagrams. Depending on the method of wear assessment, either volumetric, gravimetric or linear wear properties are presented (Fig. 6). As a common criterion wear rates (the amount of worn material per 1.000.000 cycles) are calculated and compared to wear rates of specimen retrieved after revision surgery.

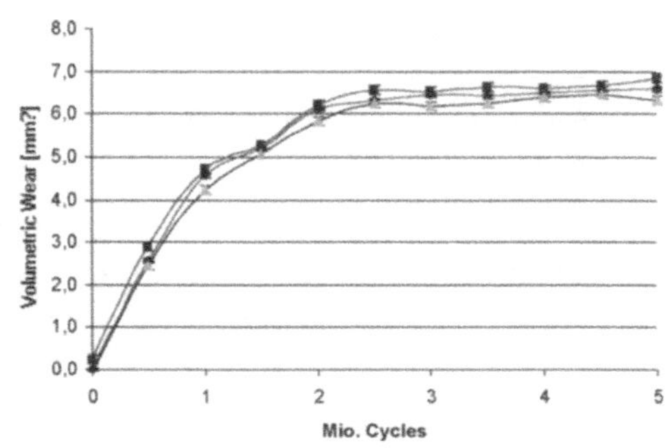

Figure 6:
Volumetric wear [mm³] over number of cycles [1·106 cycles]. Until the first 1.000.000 cycles the wear rate is higher and decreases rapidly to a steady-state wear rate ("running-in").

The formation of wear modes analysed in hip simulator testing provides important data for the development of new materials and their tribologic performance under nearly physiological conditions. Although there is an inherent possibility of failure of a new bearing system in clinical application, thorough hip simulator studies are an essential contribution of risk reduction before clinical trial.

References

1. Bergmann G, Deuretzbacher G, Heller M, Graichen F, Rohlmann A, Strauss J, Duda GN (2001) Hip contact forces and gait patterns from routine activities. J. Biomechanics, 34:859-871
2. Bragdon CR, O´Connor DO, Lowenstein JD, Jasty M and Syniuta WD (1996) The Importance of Multidirectional Motion on the Wear of Polyethylene. Pro-ceeding of the Institution of Mechanical Engineers, 210[H]:157-165
3. Catelas I, Petit A, Zukor DJ, et al. (1999) Induction of macrophage apoptosis by ceramic and polyethylene particles in vitro. Biomaterials 20:625-630
4. Clark IC (1981) Wear of artificial joint materials: IV hip joint simulator studies. Engng in Medicine, 10(4):189-198
5. Draft International Standard (2002) Wear of implant materials - Polymer and metal wear particles - Isolation, characterization and quantification. ISO/DIS 17853
6. Ingham E, Fisher J (2000) Biological reactions to wear debris in total joint re-placement. Proc Inst Mech Eng [H] 214(1):21-37
7. International Standard (2002) Implants for surgery – Wear of total hip joint prosthesis, ISO 14242 Part 1 - Loading and displacement parameters for wear testing machines and corresponding environmental conditions for tests; Part 2 - Methods of measurement
8. Kaddick C, Pfaff HG (2002) Results of Hip Simulator Testing with Various Wear Couples. In: Garino JP, Willmann G (editors) Bioceramics in Joint Ar-throplasty – Proc 7th Inter. Biolox ® Symposium. Thieme,16-20
9. Lu TW, Taylor SJ, O'Connor JJ, Walker PS (1997) Influence of muscle activity on the forces in the femur: an in vivo study. J. Biomechanics, 30(11-12):1101-1106
10. McKellop H, Lu B, Wiser H (1999) The Effect of Specimen Orientation and Lu-bricant Concentration on the Wear of Metal/Metal Hip Implants in a Wear Simulator. Trans 45th ORS:849
11. Medley JB, Krygier JJ, Bobyn JD, Chan FW, Lippincott A, Tanzer M (1997) Kinematics of the MATCO™ Hip Simulator and Issues Related to Wear Test-ing of Metal-Metal Implants. Proceeding of the Institution of Mechanical Engi-neers, 211[H]:89-99
12. Nevelos J, Ingham E, Doyle C, Fisher J (1999) Influence Of Acetabular Cup Angle On The Wear Of "Biolox®forte" (Alumina/Alumina Hip Joints In A Physiological Simulator). 45th ORS:857
13. Oh I, Harris WH (1978) Proximal Strain Distribution in the Loaded Femur. An in vitro Comparison of the Distributions in the Intact Femur and After Insertion of Different Hip-Replacement Femoral Components. J Bone Joint Surg Am 60(1):75-85
14. Paul JP (1966/67). Forces Transmitted by Joints in the Human Body. Proc. Inst. of Mech. Eng., 181:8-15
15. Reinisch G, Judmann KP, Lhotka C, Lintner F, Zweymüller KA (2003) Re-trieval study of uncemented metal-metal hip prostheses revised for early loos-ening. Biomaterials 24(6):1081-1091
16. Reinisch G, Judmann KP, Plitz W, Schörg J (2001) Ein neuer, der ISO 14242 entsprechender Hüftsimulator: E-SIM. Biomed. Technik 46:362-365
17. Reinisch G, Pfeifer N, Judmann KP, Schörg J (2001) Wear measurement of hard/hard pairings in total hip replacement using the dimensional method. Trans. 4th combined ORS, 126
18. Saikko V (1996) A Three Axis Hip Joint Simulator for Wear and Friction Stud-ies on Total Hip Prostheses. Proceeding of the Institution of Mechanical Engineers, 210[H]:175-185
19. Schmalzried TP, Jasty M, Harris WH (1992) Periprosthetic bone loss in total hip arthroplasty: The role of polyethylene and the concept of the effective joint space. J Bone Joint Surg 74-A:849-856.

20. Walter A (1997) Investigations on the Wear Couple Biolox®forte/Biolox®forte and Earlier Alumina Materials. In: Pfuhl W (editor) Performance of the Wear Couple Biolox®forte in Hip Arthroplasty – Proc 2nd Symposium on Ceramic Wear Couple. Enke:123-135
21. Wang A, Essner A, Stark C, Dumbleton JH (1996) Comparison of the size and morphology of UHMWPE wear debris produced by a hip joint simulator under serum and water lubricated conditions. Biomaterials 17(9):865-871
22. Willert, H-G (1977) Reactions of the articular capsule to wear products of arti-ficial joint prostheses. J. Biomed. Mater. Res. 11: 57-164
23. Woltring HJ (1994) 3-D Attitude Representation of Human Joints: A Standardization Proposal, J. Biomechanics, 27(12):1399-1414
24. Wu G, Cavanagh PR (1995) ISB Recommendations for a Standardization in the Reporting of Kinematic Data, J. Biomechanics, 28(10):1257-1261

1.4 The Influence of the Wear Bearing Coupling on Range of Motion and Stability against Dislocation of Total Hip Replacement

R. Bader, R. Scholz, E. Steinhauser, S. Zimmermann, G. Willmann and W. Mittelmeier

Introduction

Modular total hip replacement (THR) systems have been clinically proven and usually consist of a stem onto which a metal or ceramic femoral head is fixed. The acetabular cup is composed of a metal-back and an insert. Due to increased life expectancy of the population and a broadening of indications for hip arthroplasty a lengthening of performance life times of THR has become necessary. The most frequent reason for total hip prosthesis failure is the particle induced aseptic loosening [5], therefore low wear bearing couples like ceramic-on-ceramic are increasingly used.

An important factor for the life quality of patients and undisturbed long-term function of THR is the range of motion (ROM) of the artificial hip joint. An insufficient ROM can lead to contact between the femoral neck of the stem and the rim of the cup (= prosthetic impingement). The consequent material stress may result in deformation by creep (cold flow) and subsequent onset of higher polyethylene wear or chipping off or fracture of ceramic components [1].

Furthermore impingement may cause subluxation and dislocation of THR. The incidence of dislocation following primary total hip replacement is on average between 2% and 5% [12] and significantly higher after revision surgery. The most important risk factors related to prosthetic instability are, apart from the surgical approach itself, an inadequate implant design and unfavourable implant orientation [9].

The objective of this study was to analyse the influence of different wear couples (ceramic-on-ceramic vs. metal-on-polyethylene) on the range of motion and the stability against dislocation of THR.

Materials and Methods

With different implant designs the ROM until impingement and the ROM until dislocation of THR was determined by means of an especially developed testing device (Fig. 1).

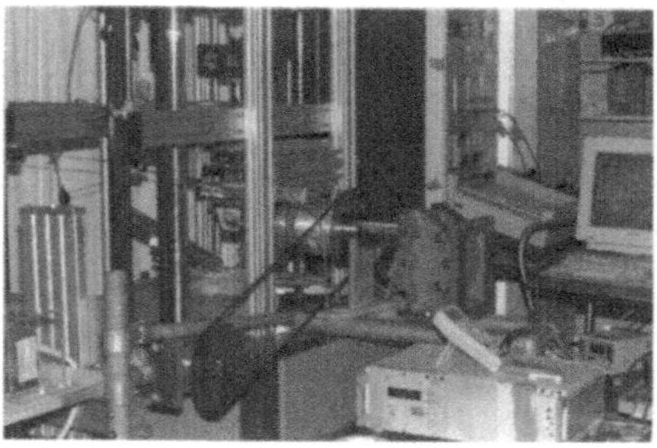

Figure 1: Dislocation testing device in the lateral view, mounted in an universal testing machine. Examined movements: maximum internal and external rotation combined with 10° extension and 15° adduction.

In addition the occuring resisting (subluxation) moments against levering the femoral head out of the acetabular cup or insert were recorded [2].
For this rotation movements of the prosthetic femoral stem (in accordance with an internal and external rotation movement of the leg) were carried out subsequently to adjusting the flexion/extension and abduction/adduction movements respectively, i.e. the influencing combined movements for dislocation of total hip replacement could be set reproducably.

In this study standard hip implants with different wear bearing couples were compared concerning their stability against dislocation. Both examined acetabular cups (CL-Metallsockel size 4, Fa. ESKA Implants, Lübeck and Plasmacup® SC size 52, Fa. Aesculap, Tuttlingen, respectively) were modular. The metal-backs were embedded in the acetabular implant fixture by means of epoxy resin (Ureol®). Due to the modular structure of the acetabular cup the inserts could be implanted or exchanged during the testings.

The stability against dislocation in dependence on the wear bearing couples metal-on-polyethylene vs. ceramic-on-ceramic was analyzed on the basis of a cup system with differing geometry of the polyethylene (PE) and ceramic insert respectively, and on the basis of a system with similar insert design.
For this a neutral polyethylene insert (Fa. ESKA) (Fig. 2) with an internal diameter of 28 mm and a slightly raised rim (displacement of the centre of the articulating femoral head towards the dome of the cup of approx. 2 mm) was implanted in the CL-socket. The inner rim was only rounded off slightly (radius of the rim about 0.5 mm). The other insert used was a neutral ESKA-Ceram® insert (composite material made of aluminium-oxide ceramic (Al_2O_3) and polyurethane [13] with an internal diameter of 28 mm) (Fig. 2). Compared to the polyethylene insert this insert showed several differences in design, e.g. an approx. 1.5 mm displacement of the centre as well as a clearly rounded off inner rim.

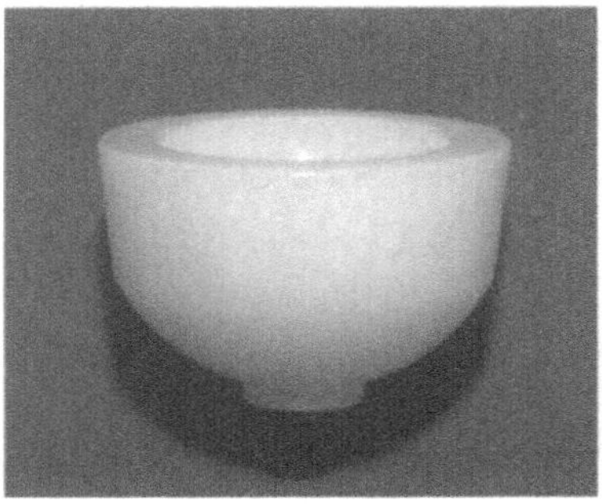

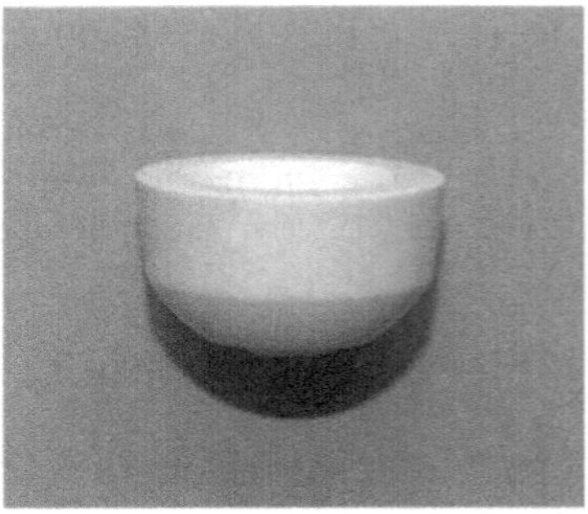

Figure 2:
Left: neutral (standard) polyethylene insert (Fa. ESKA Implants).

Right: neutral composite ceramic insert (ESKA-Ceram)

In the Plasmacup® SC a neutral polyethylene insert with an internal diameter of 28 mm (Fig. 3) and a neutral aluminium-oxide ceramic insert (Biolox® forte, Fa. CeramTec, Plochingen, with an internal diameter of 28 mm (Fig. 3) were implanted. Both insert designs showed similar geometry. In both cases the inner rim was clearly rounded off (radius approx. 2 mm) and the inset of the centre for the articulating femoral head was about 1 mm in the case of the ceramic insert and only slightly increased in the case of the polyethylene insert.

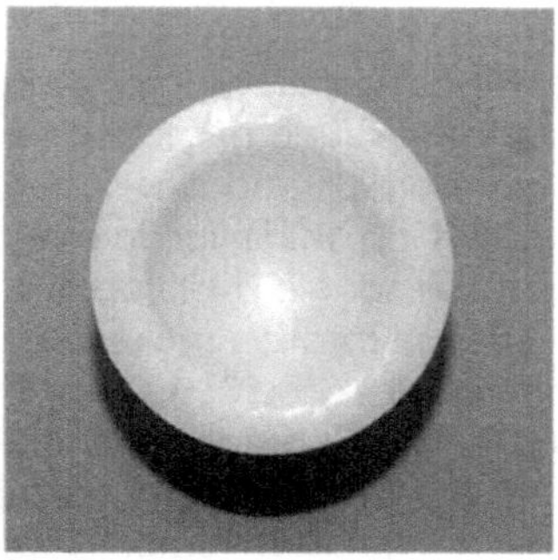

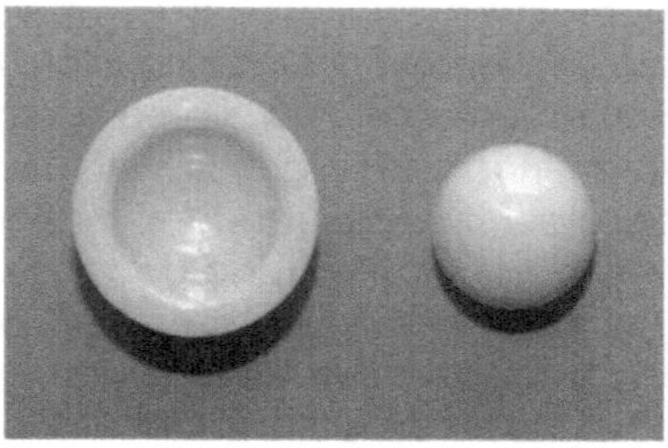

Figure 3:
Left: Tested neutral polyethylene insert (Aesculap AG).

Right: tested neutral aluminium-oxide ceramic insert and spherical head (Biolox® forte)

The opening plane of the embedded cup was non-recessed and orientated centrical towards the acetabular implant fixture. A reproducable positioning of the acetabular cup in a lateral inclination angle of 30°, 45° or 60° could be achieved by means of a form fitted link with the implant fixture. At the same time angles of the acetabular cup of -15°, 0°, +15°, +30° for retro- and anteversion respectively could be set and the centre of rotation of the cup always fell within the respective opening plane.

Matching cobalt-chromium or aluminium-oxide standard spherical heads with a diameter of 28 mm each one articulated with the corresponding insert. The femoral heads were fixed onto total hip stems (C-Hüftstiel Simplex, taper 12-14, Fa. ESKA Implants as well as Bicontact® S, taper 12-14, Fa. Aesculap, Tuttlingen) designed for cemented fixation. The femoral stems were embedded in a special fixture, which was integrated into a measurement device, by means of epoxy resin. The measurement device included a rotational angle detector (type MA 751, Fa. Megatron, Putzbrunn) and a torque detector (type 8628-5100, Fa. Burster, Gernsbach). In this study the position, i.e. rotation of the stem (ante- or retrotorsion) was not varied and held constantly in the 0°-position respectively.
In order to realize realistic stress situations, in vivo data by Bergmann et al. [4], who measured resulting hip joint forces by means of instrumented prosthetic stems telemetrically, were referred to. The examinations were carried out under dry conditions and at room temperature.

After implantation of the required implants, setting of their position and a rotation position of 0° and the subsequent application of the hip joint forces, following dislocation-associated movements were carried out on the artificial hip joint:

- Maximum internal and external rotation after 90° flexion and 0° adduction (Fig. 1), in accordance with an increased risk of posterior dislocation in low sitting position [8].
- Maximum external and internal rotation after an extension movement of 10° and 15° adduction, in accordance with an increased risk of anterior dislocation connected with hyperextension movements of the patient [8].

Results

A low inclination angle of the CL-socket (i.e. 30°) with no anteversion and no stem antetorsion respectively merely allowed an insufficient range of motion for the movement "internal rotation with flexion movement of 90° and adduction movement of 0°" until impingement (ROM_{Imp}) or allows no ROM for internal rotation at all (Fig. 4). With increasing cup inclination angle (45° or 60°) significantly larger range of motion (ROM_{Imp}) for the internal rotation movement was possible. With regard to the used wear bearing couples the ESKA-Ceram® insert showed an increased ROM of up to 5° for internal rotation compared to the ESKA neutral polyethylene insert.

The ROM until impingement is particularly influenced by the cup version. Thus e.g. a cup retroversion (at an inclination angle of 45°) always led to impingement in the whole interval of internal rotation movements with both wear bearing couples (Fig. 5). Sufficient range of motion can only be achieved through cup anteversion and stem antetorsion.

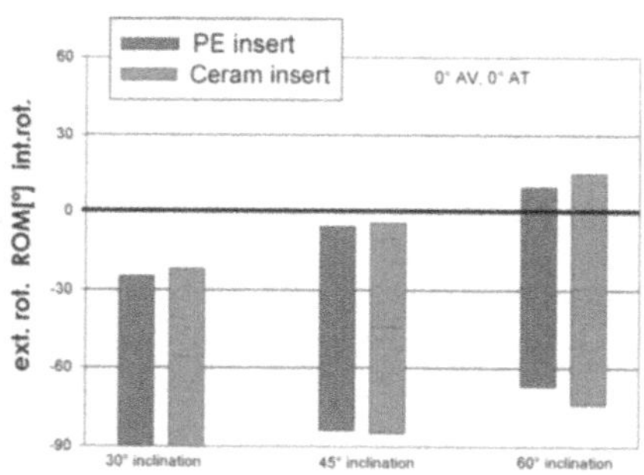

Figure 4:
Maximum range of motion until impingement (ROM_{Imp}) for interal rotation and external rotation. The columns show the impingement-free interval in the above-mentioned rotation movements for the femoral stem (up to ± 90°). Test conditions: Combination with 90° flexion and 0° adduction using the wear couples metal-on-polyethylene (PE-Insert, Fa. ESKA) and ceramic-on-composite ceramic (Ceram-Insert, ESKA-Ceram).
Different inclination angles (CL-socket version of 0° and stem torsion of 0°, neck taper always 12-14).

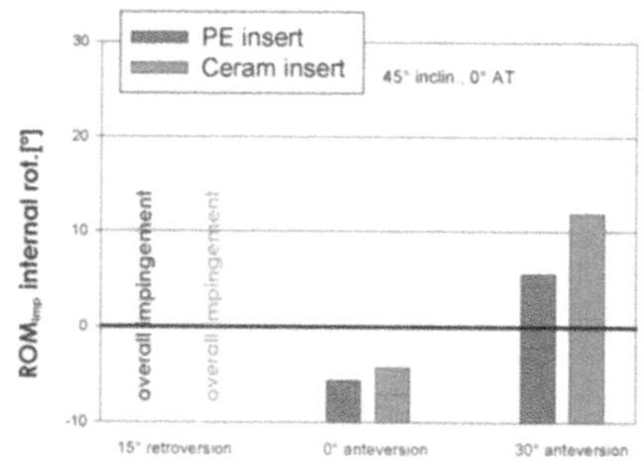

Figure 5:
Maximum range of motion until impingement (ROM_{Imp}) for interal rotation. The columns show the impingement-free interval in the internal rotation movements for the femoral stem. Test conditions: Combination with 90° flexion and 0° adduction using the wear couples metal-on-polyethylene and ceramic-on-composite ceramic. Different ante- and retroversion angles (CL-socket inclination of 45° and stem torsion of 0°, neck taper always 12-14).

Concerning the maximum subluxation (resisting) moment in the course of internal rotation movement significantly higher values were recorded for cups with a low inclination angle (Fig. 6). For example the 28 mm femoral head in combination with a neutral PE-insert at a cup inclination angle of 30° almost led to a doubling of the subluxation moment compared to an inclination angle of 60°. Additionally, clear differences in subluxation moments were recorded between metal-on-polyethylene and ceramic-on-composite ceramic (ESKA-Ceram®) wear bearing couples (Fig. 6). On average the subluxation moment at an inclination angle of 45° was 1.56 Nm for the combination of metal-on-polyethylene and 1.07 Nm for the couple with the ESKA-Ceram® insert.

Figure 6:
Maximum resisting moment (in subluxation) for interal rotation movements.
Test conditions:
Combination with 90° flexion and 0° adduction using the wear couples metal-on-polyethylene and ceramic-on-composite ceramic.
Different inclination angles (CL-socket version of 0° and stem torsion of 0°, neck taper always 12-14).

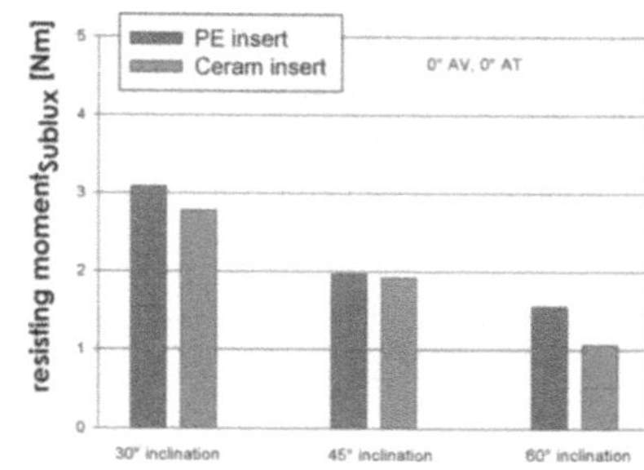

For the actual point of dislocation during the movement "internal rotation with 90° flexion and 0° adduction" a significantly delayed dislocation in posterior direction was achieved by increased anteversion of the acetabular cup with both low and high inclination angles (Fig. 7, 8). An increasingly steep positioned cup (inclination angle of 60°) caused earlier dislocation especially in combination with cup retroversion (Fig. 7). Unlike with the neutral PE-insert, no stable articulation in the artificial hip joint could be realized with the ESKA-Ceram® insert. However, during pronounced cup anteversion of a steep or flat positioned cup (inclination angle of 30°) increased range of motion until dislocation (ROM_{Lux}) was recorded for the wear bearing couple ceramic-on-composite ceramic (Fig. 7, 8).

Figure 7:
Maximum range of motion until dislocation (ROM_{Lux}) for interal rotation. The columns show the dislocation-free interval in the internal rotation movements for the femoral stem.
Test conditions:
Combination with 90° flexion and 0° adduction using the wear couples metal-on-polyethylene and ceramic-on-composite ceramic.
Different ante- and retroversion angles (CL-socket inclination of 60° and stem torsion of 0°, neck taper always 12-14).

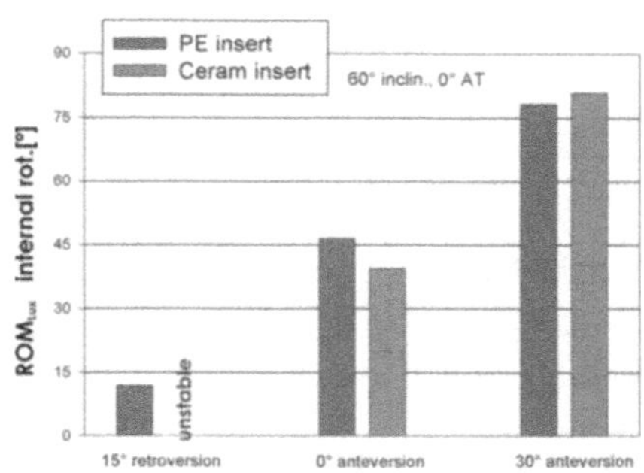

Figure 8:
Maximum range of motion until dislocation (ROM_{Lux}) for interal rotation. The columns show the dislocation-free interval in the internal rotation movements for the femoral stem.
Test conditions:
Combination with 90° flexion and 0° adduction using the wear couples metal-on-polyethylene and ceramic-on-composite ceramic.
Different ante- and retroversion angles (CL-socket inclination of 30° and stem torsion of 0°, neck taper always 12-14).

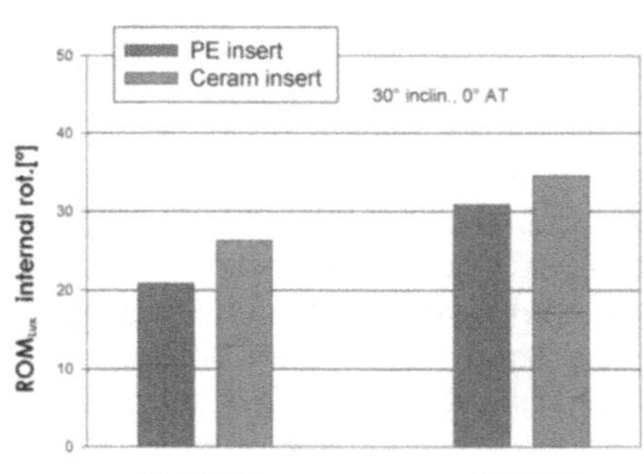

On the inner rim of the tested PE-insert significant deformations (cold flow) consequent to recurrent impingement and dislocation of the femoral head could be detected. However, minor material damage also appeared on the rim of the ESKA-Ceram® inserts.

Using the Plasmacup® SC as metal-back and inserts with similar design a decrease of overall ROM of about 5° compared to the neutral PE-insert (Fa. Aesulap) was achieved in the movement "internal and external rotation with a flexion movement of 90° and adduction movement of 0°" using the ceramic insert (Biolox® forte) (Fig. 9).

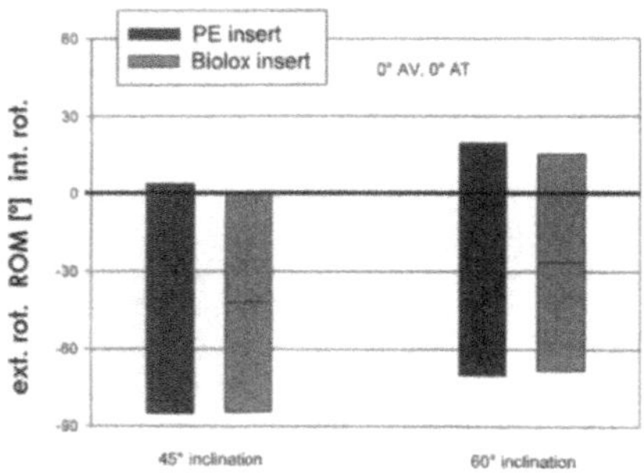

Figure 9:
Maximum range of motion until impingement (ROM_{Imp}) for interal rotation and external rotation. The columns show the impingement-free interval in the above-mentioned rotation movements for the femoral stem (up to ± 90°).
Test conditions:
Combination with 90° flexion and 0° adduction using the wear couples metal-on-polyethylene (PE-Insert, Aesculap AG) and ceramic-on-ceramic (Biolox, forte, CeramTec AG).
Different inclination angles (Plasmacup SC version of 0° and stem torsion of 0°, neck taper always 12-14).

In this case no significant differences in degree of maximum occuring subluxation moments in the course of an internal rotation movement could be observed between the wear bearing couples metal-on-polyethylene and ceramic-on-ceramic (Table 1). However, with a low inclination angle or with an anteverted cup increased moments were recorded.

		internal rotation (with 90° flexion und 0° adduction)	
		PE-insert	**ceramic insert**
45° inclination 0°AV, 0°AT	RM_{Sublux}	1,28 ± 0,1 Nm	1,30 ± 0,1 Nm
	ROM_{Lux}	42,4 ± 0,1°	48,8 ± 0,2°

Table 1:
Maximum resisting moment (in subluxation) (RM_{Sublux}) und ROM until dislocation (ROM_{Lux}) for internal rotation movement in combination with 90° flexion and 0° adduction for the wear couples metal-on-polyethylene and ceramic-on-ceramic (Biolox® forte) in case of identical metal-back (Plasmacup SC) in 45° inclination and 0° anteversion, each with 28 mm metal or ceramic head, identical femoral stem with taper 12-14 and 0° antetorsion.

In the movement "internal rotation with flexion of 90° and adduction of 0°" the range of motion until dislocation (ROM_{Lux}) was slightly higher for the ceramic-on-ceramic couple, i.e. a slightly delayed dislocation in posterior direction than with the metal-on-polyethylene couple (Table 1). Again, significant deformations (cold flow) were visible on the inner rim of the PE-insert, whereas no defects could be detected macroscopically on the ceramic insert (Biolox® forte).

In an external and internal rotational movement in combination with an extension of 10° and adduction of 15° the range of motion until impingement clearly depended on the implant position. For example between 15° retroversion and 30° anteversion of the acetabular cup the decrease in ROM for external rotation amounted to about 40° (Fig. 10). According to further investigations steep positioned cups in combination with a stem rotation in anterior direction were especially susceptible to posterior impingement. Only slight differences in

ROM existed between the wear bearing couples metal-on-polyethylene and ceramic-on-ceramic. With the use of the ceramic insert a decrease in range of motion of about 2° was recorded (Fig. 10).

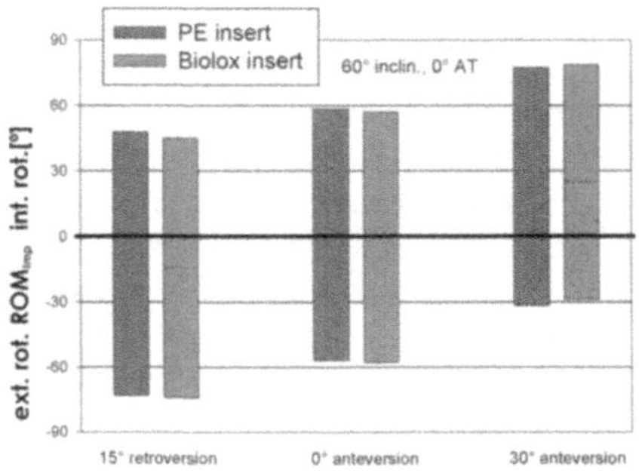

Figure 10:
Maximum range of motion until impingement (ROM_{imp}) for internal and external rotation movements. The columns show the impingement-free interval in the above-mentioned rotation movements for the femoral stem.
Test conditions:
Combination with 10° extension and 15° adduction using the wear couples metal-on-polyethylene and ceramic-on-ceramic (Biolox® forte).
Different anteversion angles (Plasmacup SC cup inclination of 45° and stem torsion of 0°, neck taper always 12-14).

Discussion

Recurrent dislocation following total hip replacement (THR) is a serious postoperative complication, which makes a revision surgery necessary in about one third of these cases [16]. Important risk factors apart from the surgical approach itself are inadequate implant design and poor implant position [10]. Increased dislocation rates have been clinically observed for high inclination angles [7]. Furthermore an increase of the cup anteversion was described as being more beneficial for the hip stability [11]. The stability of THR against dislocation is also affected by implant design variables like head-neck-ratio and cup / insert geometry [14]. Especially using smaller femoral head sizes, there is the danger of the head sliding over the rim of the cup [3]. A weak hip musculature favours dislocation as does poor tissue tension.

Furthermore, leg movements which exceed the guaranteed ROM of total hip replacement can lead to the leverage of the femoral head out of the cup consequent to contact between the femoral neck and the rim of the cup (prosthetic impingement). In this case, subluxation, dislocation, and the subsequent repositioning of the femoral head involving ceramic inserts may lead to local overstress of the implant material due to a reduced contact area with the possibility of failure (rim flaking, fracture) [6]. This is promoted by the lower damage tolerance of ceramic materials in comparison to polyethylene.

To our knowledge there are no experimental studies so far, in which the stability against dislocation of artificial hip joints in dependence on the implanted wear bearing couple was analyzed explicitly. In clinical studies no increased dislocation rate for hard-hard wear couples could be observed up to now. An exception to this is the recently presented study by Toni et al. [15] about the survival rate of various total hip arthroplasty systems with ceramic-on-ceramic and metal-on-polyethylene respectively. In a follow-up of 7 years a significantly lower total revision rate was registrated for ceramic-on-ceramic wear bearing couples compared to metal-on-polyethylene. However the revision rate for ceramic cups due to dislocation was higher (0,51% vs. 0,14%) [15], but possible reasons for this observations were not given.

In our experimental study the question was whether the implanted wear bearing couple has an influence on the range of motion and the stability against dislocation of artificial hip joints and to what extent the design and position of the implants is of importance.

Our results demonstrate the close connection between the position of the hip implants and the maximum range of motion leading to impingement (ROM_{Imp}) and to dislocation (ROM_{Lux}) as well as the maximum subluxation moment. This applies to all used wear bearing couples. In order to achieve a sufficient range of motion of the total hip replacement a horizontal position (e.g. inclination angle of 30°) and a cup retroversion respectively as well as a stem retrotorsion must be avoided in any case.

In particular, pronounced cup anteversion leads to higher subluxation (resisting) moments and increased ROM until dislocation, i.e. an enhanced stability against the posterior dislocation. However, excessive anteversion (>30°) in combination with stem antetorsion should be avoided due to increased risk of posterior impingement and anterior dislocation by combined extension, adduction and external rotation movements.

design between the ESKA polyethylene insert and the composite ceramic insert (ESKA-Ceram®). Because the centre of rotation of the femoral head is located closer to the opening plane of the cup and the inner rim is rounded off on the ESKA-Ceram® insert it lead to an increased ROM_{Imp} in all tested movements and implant positions, but also a lower subluxation moment was observed. For the time of actual joint dislocation especially in unstable joint positions, this leads to an earlier dislocation than with a PE-insert. Furthermore, no stable condition in the artificial hip joint can be achieved with a steep positioned cup and additional retroversion using the ESKA-Ceram® insert. Due to above-mentioned design features of the insert the prosthetic head can slide over the inner rim of the insert or dislocate at an early stage.

However, with adequate anteversion combined with a flat cup position (45° or 30°) larger range of motion until dislocation (ROMLux) was recorded using the ESKA-Ceram® insert compared to the wear bearing couple metal-on-polyethylene. The earlier dislocation and shorter subluxation period respectively with stable implant position is likely to be due to the elastic and/or plastic deformation of the PE-insert, which favours the femoral head sliding out of the cup.

In case of similar insert geometry in combination with the Plasmacup® SC socket no substantial difference of the ROM until impingement was observed between the couple metal-on-polyethylene and ceramic-on-ceramic. In the case of a ceramic-insert made of Biolox® forte the ROM is slightly decreased, because the inner rim was not deformed during the tests consequent to recurrent prosthetic impingement unlike the PE-insert. The maximum subluxation moments in the course of the examined rotational movements showed no significant differences between the metal-on-polyethylene and the ceramic-on-ceramic wear bearing couples. Using the Biolox® forte insert a slightly increased range of motion until dislocation (ROM_{Lux}) was recorded. The longer subluxation period is probably linked to the absent deformation of the ceramic insert and the accompanying enhanced stability.

In order to be able to completely rule out the effect of differences in design of the implants on the assessment of stability against dislocation of differing wear bearing couples, further examinations on an absolutely identical design of THR implants are in process. For this dislocation testings are carried out on the same prosthetic stem and metal-back, into which polyethylene and aluminium-oxide ceramic inserts with identical internal and external geometry are implanted.

Conclusion

Due to their effect of minimizing aseptic implant loosening caused by wear particles, hard-hard wear couples are increasingly used in young or active patients. Inadequate implant position can result in restricted range of motion and instability of THR. With implantation of ceramic components specific risks have to be considered such as intra-operative handling, implant orientation and post-operative patient behaviour. Therefore ceramic-on-ceramic couples should only be applied in case of optimized implant position to prevent impingement and dislocation with following material failure (enhanced wear or brittle fracture).

In the presented study the maximum resisting moment and the range of motion until impingement and dislocation were mostly influenced by the implant position. In addition, the stability of THR against dislocation was clearly affected by design variables of the insert like chamfer angle and inset of the head center, whereas the use of different wear couples, i.e. metal-on-polyethylene vs. ceramic-on-ceramic, had less impact.

Acknowledgements:
The authors would like to thank ESKA-Implants, Aesculap AG, and CeramTec AG for support by providing the implants.

References

1. Bader RJ, Steinhauser E, Willmann G, Gradinger R (2001) The effects of implant position, design and wear on the range of motion after total hip arthroplasty. Hip International 11: 80-90
2. Bader R, Scholz R, Steinhauser E, Gradinger R (2002) Biomechanische Untersuchungen zur Evaluierung von Einflussfaktoren auf die Luxationsstabilität von künstlichen Hüftgelenken. Z. Orthop. (140) Supplement 1: 90
3. Bader R, Scholz R, Steinhauser E, Mittelmeier W, Gradinger R (2002) Verwendung großer Prothesenköpfe bei totalem Hüftgelenkersatz: Welche Vorteile ergeben sich für Bewegungsumfang und Luxationsstabilität? Orthopädische Praxis, Sonderausgabe 165-166
4. Bergmann G (1994) In vivo Messung der Belastung von Hüftimplantaten. Habilitationsschrift, Freie Universität Berlin
5. Herberts P, Malchau H (2000) Long-term registration has improved the quality of hip replacement: a review of the Swedish THR Register comparing 160,000 cases. Acta Orthop Scand 71: 111-121
6. Klabunde R, Jäggi C (2000) What to watch out with Ceramic-on-Ceramic. In: Rieker C, Oberholzer S, Wyss U (Hrsg) World Tribology Forum in Arthroplasty. Hans Huber, Bern, S 295-304
7. Kohn D, Rührmann O, Wirth CJ (1997) Die Verrenkung der Hüfttotalendoprothese unter besonderer Beachtung verschiedener Zugangswege. Z Orthop 135: 40-44
8. Kummer FJ, Shah S, Iyer S, DiCesare PE (1999) The effect of acetabular cup orientations on limiting hip rotation. J Arthroplasty 14: 509-513
9. Lavernia C, Barrack R, Thornberry R, Tozakoglou E (1998) The effects of component position on the motion to impingement and dislocation in total hip replacement. New Orleans: Scientific Exhibit presented at AAOS Meeting
10. Morrey BF (1992) Instability after total hip arthroplasty. Orthop Clin North Am 23: 237-248
11. Robbins GM, Masri BA, Garbuz DS, Greidanus N, Duncan CP (2001) Treatment of hip instability. Orthop Clin North Am 32: 593-610.

12. Sanchez-Sotelo J, Berry DJ (2001) Epidemiology of instability after total hip replacement. Orthop Clin North Am 32: 543-552
13. Scholz J, Grundei H, Klingbeil K (2000) ESKA-Ceram--a new material in hip endoprosthetics. Biomed Tech 45: 377-379
14. Scifert CF, Noble PC, Brown TD, Bartz RL, Kadakia N, Sugano N, Johnston RC, Pedersen DR, Callaghan JJ (2001) Experimental and computational simulation of total hip arthroplasty dislocation. Orthop Clin North Am 32: 553-567
15. Toni A, Stea S, Bordini B, Sudanese A (2002) Survival analysis of ceramic-on-ceramic coupling vs. metal-on-polyethylene. The experience of implant register at Istituto Rizzoli. In: Garino J, Willmann G (Hrsg) Bioceramics in Joint Arhroplasty. Georg Thieme, Stuttgart, S 75-80
16. Woo RYG, Morrey BF (1982) Dislocations after total hip arthroplasty. J Bone Joint Surg (Am) 64: 1295-1306.

1.5 The Influence of Artificial Ageing on the Stability of Ceramic Inserts in Sandwich Acetabular Cups

H. Schmotzer, M. Simnacher, M. Zuberbühler and K. Zweymüller

Introduction

Ultrahigh molecular weight polyethylene (UHMWPE) was introduced in total hip arthroplasty by Charnley in 1962 as a bearing material articulating against a stainless steel ball head [3]. This combination proofed to be highly successful clinically in the short to medium term. However, already early on wear of UHMWPE was recognized as a potential source of problems. Attempts to improve on this issue were the introduction of ceramic ball heads made from high purity alumina ceramics or elimination of UHMWPE altogether by the use of hard-on-hard bearing, either metal-on-metal or ceramics-on-ceramics.

Boutin in France has been credited with being the first to implant a ceramic-on-ceramic bearing in 1970 followed by Mittelmeier in Germany [2,5]. These early designs utilized modular femoral components but monoblock acetabular implants. Fixation of the cup was either achieved by screw-in or cemented fixation. Although initial results were promising, radiolucency and cup migration presented a problem. The main reason for these observations were poor osseo-integration and the development of a fibrous interface [7]. Other factors included the use of skirted heads and the high stiffness gradient at the bone-implant interface.

These findings led to the development of modular designs using a titanium or CoCrMo shell for fixation to the bone and a ceramic insert for the articulation. In addition to the markedly improved potential for osseo-integration, these modular designs have several advantages including the choice of various bearing options for one shell and the possibility to exchange the insert without removal of the shell after osseo-integration has taken place.

For the modular connection between insert and shell two solutions have evolved over the last 10-15 years and have proven themselves as viable alternatives for this problem. In one design the ceramic insert is anchored directly in the metal shell by a taper connection (direct anchorage); in the other, the ceramic insert is embedded in UHMWPE which is secured in the shell by snap-lock (sandwich design).

Both designs have distinct advantages and disadvantages. Direct anchorage, for example, eliminates one interface and facilitates thereby the use of the ceramic-on-ceramic bearing even in relatively small cup sizes. On the contrary, the sandwich design is much more forgiving as far as intra-operative handling and seating is concerned. Small bone chips, remaining in the insert-shell interface become embedded in the UHMWPE; in the direct anchorage they may act as stress risers leading to premature failure of the insert. Another aspect is the stiffening of the construct, when the insert is directly anchored. This is of lesser importance for press-fit cups, which are generally thick-walled to accommodate screw heads. However, the characteristics of thin-walled, more flexible cups, which attempt to reduce the stiffness gradient from the bone to the implant, would be unduly altered. An example for this concept is the BICON-PLUS®[1] cup (Figure 1) which is approximately 1 mm thick.

BICON-PLUS® is a registered trademark of PLUS Endoprothethik AG, Rotkreuz, Switzerland

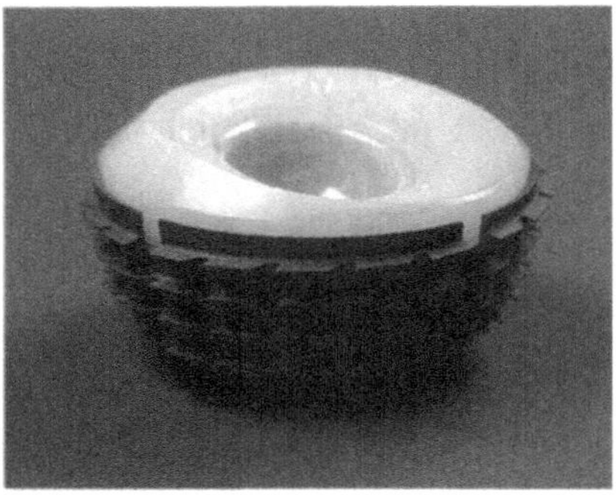

Figure 1:
BICON-PLUS® with ceramic-on-ceramic antiluxation insert. In order to preserve the flexibility of the system a sandwich design for the insert is used.

Another advantage of sandwich designs is the possibility to develop antiluxation inlays (hooded, raised lip liner) as shown in Figure 1. The ceramic insert can be tilted relative to the cup axis without decrease in range of motion, loss of support and the risk of fracture of the insert. However, the major cause of concern is the ageing of the UHMWPE resulting in a loss of support and loosening of the ceramics in its backing [8].

It was therefore the goal of this study to compare the strength of standard and antiluxation inlays and determine the loss of stability of the insert after artificial ageing.

Materials and Methods

This study was conducted in two parts. In the first part the lever-out strength of the antiluxation design was compared to the standard (neutral) version of the implant system. In the second part neutral liners were artificially aged in accordance with ASTM F2003-00 test method B [1] and then fatigue tested using a modified lever-out protocol. After fatigue testing the static lever-out test was performed to determine whether any weakening of the construct has occurred. Testing was performed on a materials test system (858 Bionix MTS Systems, Minneapolis, MN). Of the shelf inserts were pressed into the shell using the MTS machine applying three times an axial force of 2000 N at a rate of 500 N/sec.

The set-up for the lever-out test is shown schematically in Figure 2. Testing was done under displacement control with a head speed of 2 mm/min. The tests were terminated either at failure or a maximum load of 5000 N to avoid damage

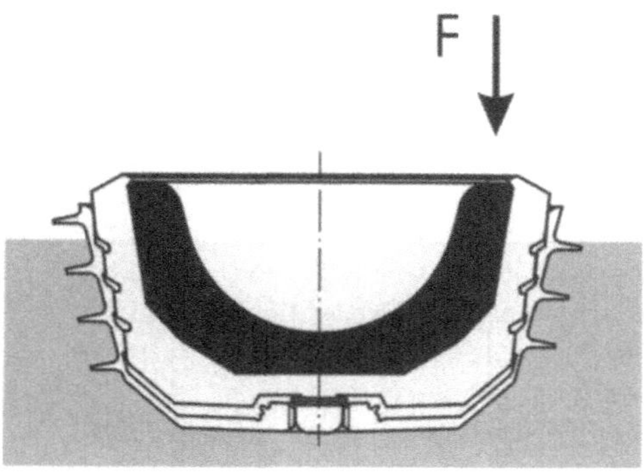

Figure 2:
Schematic representation of the test set-up used in this study. The lever-out test was chosen in order to model rim loading as it may occur during subluxations

to the test set-up. Prior to testing the specimens were tempered at 37 °C for one hour in water. These tests are semi-standardised and part of the regular CE approval process of the product.

For part 2 new of the shelf insert were divided in two groups. The first group was tested as is while the second group was placed in a pressure vessel filled with pure oxygen at a pressure of 503 kbar. The vessel was kept at a constant temperature of 70 °C for 2 weeks. Details for this protocol can be found in ASTM F2003-00 Method B [1].

For fatigue testing an identical set-up was chosen as in Part 1 and shown in Figure 2. The load was applied cyclically with an R-ratio of 0.1 and a maximum load of 3000 N at a frequency of 10 Hz for a total of 5 million cycles. Testing was conducted in a saline bath at a temperature of 37°C. Loading the rim simulated a recurrent subluxation and was modelled in analogy of the micro-separation test design described by Nevelos et al. for their hip simulator studies [6]. Clearly, this represents a worst case situation unlikely to occur in a clinical situation. After fatigue testing, semi-static loading was repeated.

Results

No failure – neither during the semi-static nor the fatigue test – occurred. All static tests were terminated at the pre-defined upper limit of 5000N without dislodgement of the ceramic insert in the UHMWPE backing. Also, no visible separation occurred during cyclic loading.

In order to compare the different tests quantitatively two parameters were determined. For the static test the total deformation as measured by the LVDT of the materials test system at a load of 800N was established. This load equals approximately body weight and may be applied to the rim during a subluxation occurring prior to at heel strike. Figure 3 summarizes the findings for the four testing conditions; i.e. for the standard and antiluxation insert as well as the standard insert after cyclic testing with and without artificial ageing.

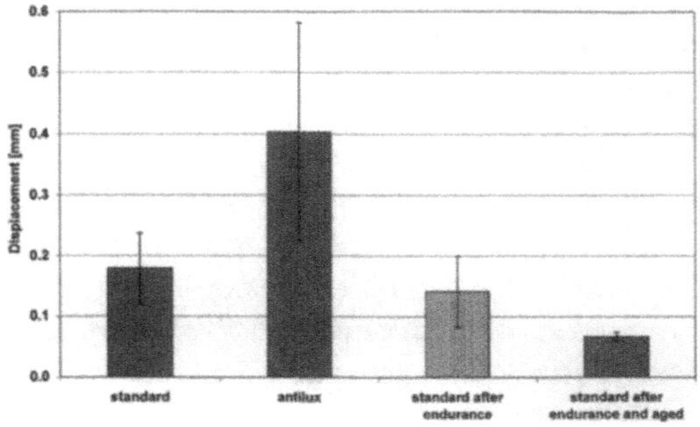

Figure 3:
Total displacement at a load of 800N applied to the rim of the ceramic insert. The smaller displacement observed after cyclic loading may be due to settling of the ceramic insert as well as the effect of the artificial ageing method

Also, the subsidence of the standard insert during cyclic loading with and without artificial ageing was determined. In order to compare the steady-state migration readings were taken after 20 000 cycles (after settling) and at the end of the test; i.e. 5 Mio. cycles. The results are shown in Figure 4.

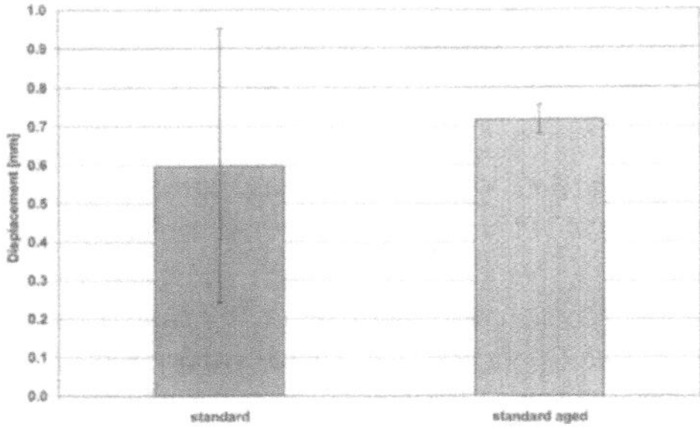

Figure 4:
Steady state migration of the ceramic insert between 20 000 and 5 million load cycles during fatigue testing. The applied load of 3000N exceeds the anticipated physiological loading by 3.5 times.

Discussion

The lever-out test has been chosen for this study as it combines several parameters which are critical for the longevity of the pairing. Unilateral, asymmetrical loading increases local stresses in the ceramic and polyethylene backing. Any degradation of the assembly is more likely to result in significant changes in the stability and lead to early failure. Also, rim loading may occur during micro-separation. Although this has not been demonstrated clinically by fluoroscopic examination [4], a comparison between clinical retrievals and hip joint simulation modelling micro-separation suggested that this phenomenon may indeed occur at least in some of the patients [6]. In such a case the question of loosening and dislodgement of the ceramic insert from the UHMWPE backing needs to be carefully examined. For this issue not only mechanical fatigue of the polymer is of interest. More importantly, chemical ageing in form of oxidative degradation of the UHMWPE needs to be included in a model designed to study this matter.

This study demonstrated that the sandwich design for the ceramic-on-ceramic bearing is a viable alternative to the direct anchorage. All of the specimens tested by far exceeded the "minimum requirement" of 3000N. This minimum requirement was defined based on the assumption that this load level would give a safety factor of more than 3 compared to a more realistic load level of body weight (800N) which may act on the rim during a subluxation. Furthermore, ageing of the UHMWPE did not influence the fixation strength of the ceramic liner in its backing. In fact, our data suggested, that the stability improved with time. This may be an artefact of the ageing process together with the stiffening of the PE due to its oxidation. The elevated temperature used to accelerate the ageing of the components will not be encountered in a clinical situation. It may, however, reduce residual stresses in the UHMWPE introduced during assembly of the components and improve the fit between insert and backing. Nevertheless, it has been shown previously that this methods produces levels and pattern of oxidation seen in clinical retrievals and is, therefore, a valid representation of the clinical reality.

Oxidation results in a severe degradation of the material including a decreased resistance against crack propagation, an increase in the modulus of elasticity and a decrease in the deformation at failure. It is, therefore, important to note that no cracks could be observed even after 5 million cycles although the applied load of 3000N by far exceeded the anticipated in vivo loading. Also, no failure occurred during the subsequent quasi-static test. This demonstrated that the quality of the anchorage had not degraded during the ageing process and subsequent fatigue testing.

Our tests also confirmed that it is possible to design and manufacture standard (neutral) and antiluxation (hooded or lipped liner) inserts. Both exceeded by far the requirements set at 3000N. This unique option of the BICON-PLUS® cup gives the surgeon the possibility to add a supplementary protection against dislocation. Clearly, this option is not designed to compensate for a mal-aligned cup, in particular placement of the cup in abduction, but it can give additional posterior coverage and more anteversion as needed. Both of these factors are important in preventing impingement and dislocation.

Conclusions

- UHMWPE backing (sandwich design) is a reliable alternative to direct anchorage of the ceramic liner in the metal acetabular shell
- This technology allows the design of antiluxation liners, an essential addition to a hip cup system
- Accelerated ageing does not reduce the stability and strength of the anchorage of the ceramics in its backing.
- Therefore, long term degradation of the UHMWPE is not a concern for sandwich designs in hard-on-hard pairings

Literature

1. ASTM F2003-00: Standard guide for accelerated aging of ultra-high molecular weight polyethylene
2. Boutin P (1972) Arthroplastie totale de hanche par prothèse en alumine frittée. Rev Chir Orthop 58 :229-246
3. Charnley J (1979) Low friction arthroplasty of the hip – Theory and practise, Springer-Verlag, Berlin Heidelberg New York
4. Komistek R, Sedel L, Hammill C, Northcut E, Walker S and Bizot P (2002) In vivo determination of hip joint separation in subjects having variable bearing surfaces. Trans. 48th Annual Meeting of the ORS:0127
5. Mittelmeier H (1975) Selbsthaftende Keramik-Metall-Verbund-Endoprothese. Med Orthop Technik 95:152-159
6. Nevelos J, Ingham E, Doyle C, Streicher R, Nevelos A, Walter W and Fisher J (2000) Microseparation of the centers of alumina-alumina artificial hip joints during simulator testing produces clinically relevant wear rates and patterns. J Arthroplasty 15(6):793-795
7. Willmann G, Kramer U. (1998) Keramische Pfannen für Hüftprothesen Teil 5: Konzeptionelle Überlegungen. Biomed. Technik 43:342-349
8. Zweymüller K (2000)Indikation und Kontraindikation für unterschiedliche Gleitpaarungen bei modularen Hüftpfannen. In: WillmannG, Zweymüller K (eds.) Bioceramics in hip joint replacement – Proceedings 5th international Ceramtec Symposium. Georg Thieme Verlag, Stuttgart, pp 2-8

1.6 Role of Ceramic Components in the Era of Crosslinked Polyethylene for THR

A. Wang, J. H. Dumbleton, M. T. Manley and P. Serekian

Abstract

This paper presents a summary of 10 years experience of the authors in the search of advanced wear reduction bearing technologies for total hip replacement. By adhering to the principles of anatomical testing, cross-shear motion and biological lubrication in in-vitro hip simulator testing, the authors successfully reproduced the clinical wear- mechanisms, wear-debris, wear-rates and wear-rankings of past successful and unsuccessful bearing materials. This validated hip simulator test protocol was used to evaluate the wear performance of various next genetation bearing materials including metal-on-crosslinked polyethylene, ceramic-on-crosslinked polyethylene, metal-on-metal and ceramic-on-ceramic. A key criterion in determining the efficacy of the next generation bearing surface was that it show superior wear performance over predicate devices consistently and predictably in the laboratory. Metal-on-crosslinked polyethylene showed superior wear performance over metal-on-conventional polyethylene. However, this combination was still susceptible to 3rd-body wear. Ceramic-on-crosslinked polyethylene significantly reduced the susceptibility to 3rd-body wear while ceramic-on-ceramic articulation completely eliminated the 3rd-body wear problem. In contrast, precision made metal-on-metal devices failed the basic criteria test due to erratic and unpredictable wear behavior under carefully controlled laboratory conditions.

1. Introduction

Total hip replacements are being performed on younger and higher demand patients with increased life expectancies. As a result, the orthopaedic community is continually seeking new methods and materials that may extend the useful life of hip implants. A major challenge for total hip arthroplasty is to minimize wear and osteolysis in young, active patients. Research activities have focused on understanding the biological consequences of wear debris as well as the underlying mechanisms governing the generation of wear particles. Significant advances have been achieved on all fronts. Two potential solutions have been investigated for improving the wear performance of hip bearing surfaces. These investigations include:

1. research and development of highly crosslinked polyethylenes to provide intrinsic resistance to abrasive and adhesive wear due to cross-shear motion
2. the resurgence of interest in alternative hard-on-hard bearings such as metal-on-metal and ceramic-on-ceramic

This paper presents a scientific evaluation of wear reduction technologies and wear testing methodologies developed in the authors' laboratory during the past 10 years. The objectives are to provide answers to the following two fundamental questions. First, how close are we in developing hip joint simulator test methodology in reproducing as well as predicting clinical wear performance of past and present bearing surfaces? What is the role of ceramic components in the era of crosslinked polyethylene and metal-on-metal articulation for total hip replacement?

2. Hip Joint Simulator Validation

The Howmedica Osteonics hip simulators (MTS, Eden Prairie, MN) were designed to simulate the anatomical positioning, physiological loading, cross-shear motion and biological environment (lubricant) of the human hip joint (see Figure 1). In the hip simulator, an acetabular component is positioned superiorly to a femoral head component while a physiologic load (with a peak load of 2450N) [1] is applied to the acetabular component via the moving head. Both

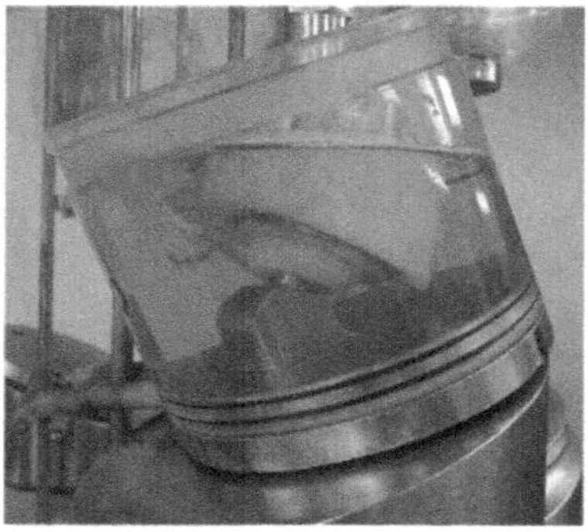

Figure 1:
Hip joint simulator configuration showing anatomical positioning of components immersed in a diluted serum lubricant.

the acetabular and femoral head components are fully immersed in a diluted serum lubricant. To reduce potential artifacts associated with serum protein degradation, a large quantity of lubricant (500 ml) is used per test chamber and this lubricant is changed frequently at every 250,000 cycles of testing [2,3]. Before arriving at this optimized set of test parameters, a comprehensive series of studies comparing various bearing materials that had demonstrated undisputed clinical records was conducted, i.e., UHMWPE vs. PTFE and UHMWPE vs. Hylamer. The following validation criteria were applied:

1. the wear rates produced by the hip simulator must agree with those reported clinically;
2. the wear rate rankings must agree both qualitatively and quantitatively with those reported clinically;
3. the wear debris size and morphology produced by the hip simulator must agree with those reported clinically.

All validation test results are presented below.

2.1. UHMWPE vs. PTFE

Charnley's early clinical experience with Polytetrafluoroethlene (PTFE) Low-Friction Arthroplasty was disastrous [4]. Linear wear rates for his clinical series of PTFE cups ranged from 2.0 mm/year to 3.5 mm/year. His later series of UHMWPE cups were a tremendous success with reported clinical wear rates varying from

0.07 mm/year to 0.22 mm/year [5,6]. Therefore, the known clinical wear rate ratios between PTFE and UHMWPE ranged between 10 and 50 with a mean ratio of 30. To reproduce Charnley's clinical results, both UHMWPE and PTFE cups were tested in the MTS hip simulator with different serum-based lubricants containing various levels of protein concentration. Fig. 2 shows the hip simulator wear rate ratios between PTFE and UHMWPE. Only those low-protein containing lubricants (5-20 g/l) produced the Charnley ratios.

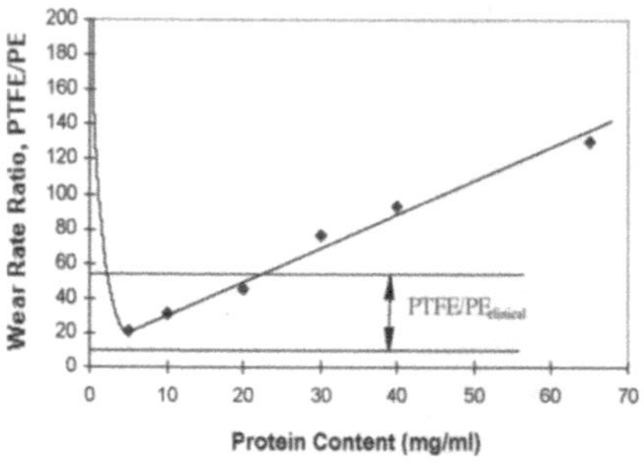

Figure 2:
PTFE/UHMWPE wear rate ratio vs. lubricant protein concentration (5-20g/l) produced the Charnley ratios).

2.2. UHMWPE vs. Hylamer

Hylamer UHMWPE was another example of clinical failures in THR. Clinically Hylamer acetabular cups were shown to wear significantly faster than conventional polyethylene [7,8]. In 1995, Howmedica Osteonics conducted a validation test comparing commercially available Hylamer liners with conventional UHMWPE liners (GUR4150 gamma sterilized in air). The results are shown in Figure 3. The gamma-in-air sterilized Hylamer liners had an average wear rate more than twice that of the conventional UHMWPE liners while the gamma-in-vacuum sterilized Hylamer was 40% higher. To date, this is the only hip simulator test that has successfully reproduced the higher clinical wear rate reported for Hylamer cups [9]. This was done without artificial treatment of the liners.

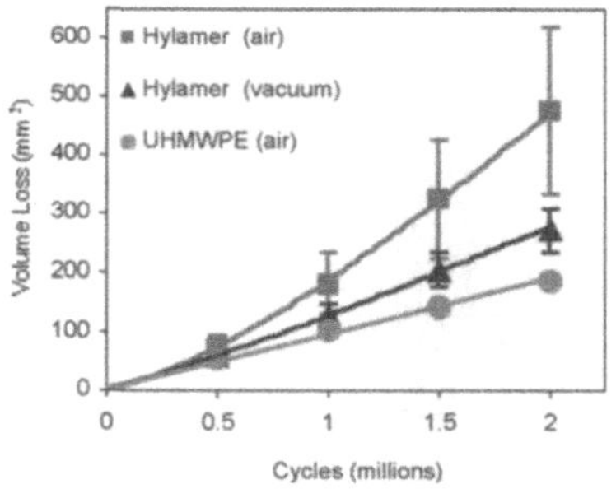

Figure 3:
Hip simulator wear comparison of Hylamer and conventional UHMWPE liners.

2.3. Duration® Stabilized UHMWPE vs. Gamma-in-Air Sterilized UHMWPE

In 1996, Howmedica Osteonics launched Duration® Stabilized UHMWPE for THR after rigorous laboratory tests. A multi-center randomized clinical study demonstrated a 45% wear reduction for Duration® liners in comparison with gamma-in-air sterilized liners [10]. This clinical finding was in agreement with and confirmed hip simulator predictions [11]. Figure 4 shows the in-vitro and in-vivo

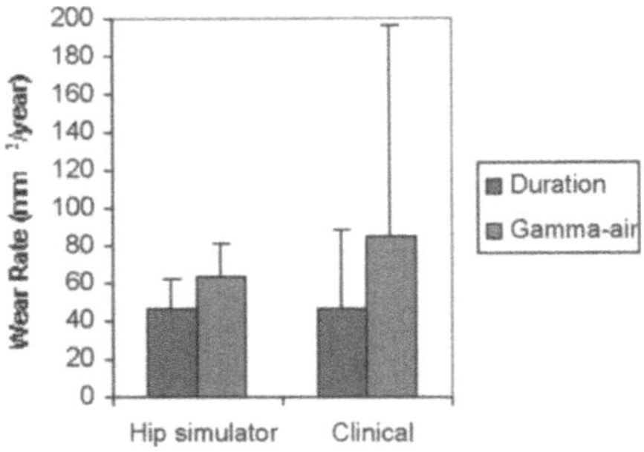

Figure 4:
hip simulator and clinical wear comparisons for Duration and gamma-air UHMWPE liners.

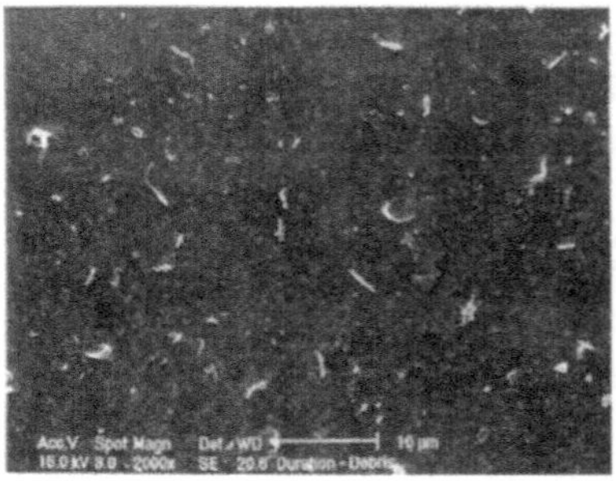

Figure 5:
Micron and submicron sized PE particles produced by the hip simulator.

wear comparisons. In addition, polyethylene wear particles produced from the hip simulator were similar to those isolated from periprosthetic tissues of failed hip implants, Figure 5.

3. Metal-on-Metal

3.1. 40 mm McKee-Farrar vs. 28 mm Metasul

Our first Metal-on-Metal (M/M) experience began with a hip simulator test comparison of the first generation M/M (McKee-Farrar) and the second-generation M/M bearings (Sulzer Metasul). Eight pairs of M/M bearings of the McKee-Farrar design (40 mm) were tested against four pairs of 28 mm Sulzer Metasul design using the MTS hip simulator that had been previously validated. Four McKee-Farrar pairs were tested in the as-cast condition and the other four pairs were tested after heat-treatment (solution anneal to eliminate large carbides). Manufacturing records showed that both as-cast and solution treated CoCr alloys were used clinically in the McKee-Farrar design (Howmedica). Figure 6 shows the comparison.

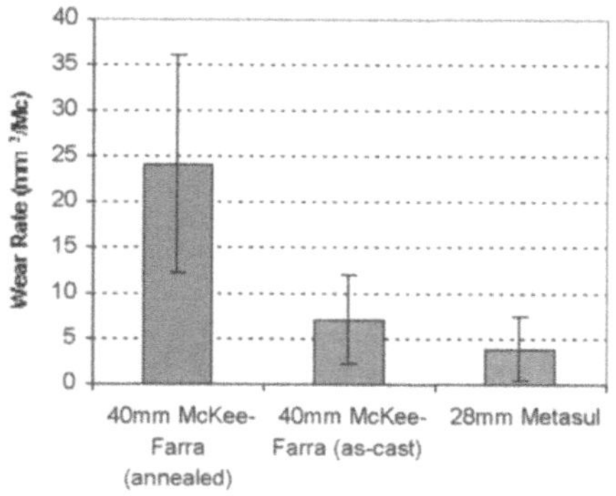

Figure 6:
Hip simulator wear rate comparison of McKee-Farra and Metasul at 1 million cycles.

The average wear rate at 1 million cycles for the solution treated McKee-Farrar bearings was about four times that of the as-cast McKee-Farrar, indicating that the presence of carbides played a significant role in wear performance of M/M joints. Interestingly, the second generation Metasul M/M (28 mm) exhibited comparable wear to the first generation as-cast McKee-Farrar (P=0.29) despite the fact that the Metasul bearings were significantly smaller than the McKee bearings. Compared to the early hip simulator wear rate of a conventional UHMWPE/metal articulation, both the as-cast McKee-Farrar and Metasul bearings showed an order of magnitude lower wear rate.

3.2. 40 mm Metal-on-Metal (As-Cast CoCrMo)

Encouraged by the positive short-term wear performance of the 40 mm as-cast McKee-Farrar bearings, Howmedica Osteonics conducted a second hip simulator test of eight pairs of precision-manufactured 40 mm as-cast CoCrMo M/M bearings for 5 million cycles. All bearings had a radial clearance of 50-90 microns, a sphericity better than 10 microns and a surface finish better than 0.01 microns R_a. Figure 7 shows the accumulative volume wear loss of the cups as a function of test cycles. While five of the eight bearings showed a steady-state wear rate less than 1 mm^3/million cycles, three of the eight bearings (38%) showed excessive wear with two bearings exhibiting a runaway wear pattern after 1 and 4 million cycles, respectively. The runaway wear rates were 40 and 30 mm^3/million cycles, respectively.

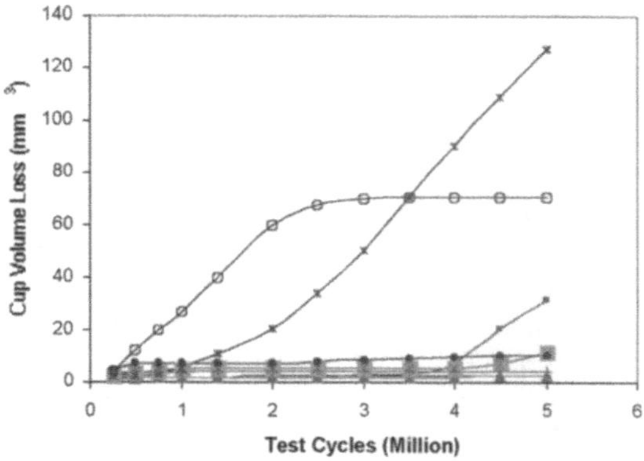

Figure 7:
Hip simulator results of 8 pairs of precision-made as-cast CoCrMo bearings (40mm McKee-Farrar design) showing erratic wear behavior of the M/M.

3.3. 40 mm Metal-on-Metal (As-Cast CoCrMo) with Reduced Radical Clearances

Disappointed by the erratic wear behavior of the 40 mm M/M bearings, Howmedica Osteonics began a third round of testing using components precision-manufactured with tighter tolerances. Four pairs of 40 mm M/M (as-cast CoCrMo) bearings were produced with a radial clearance of 25-50 microns (similar to the 28 mm Metasul bearings). The results were once again disappointing. While three of the four bearings showed excellent wear performance (wear rate < 1mm3/million cycles), one pair exhibited a run-away wear pattern (wear rate = 45 mm3/million cycles), Figure 8(a). For the run-away wear pair, the 500cc-lubricant was completely darkened throughout the duration of the test, Figure 8(b).

3.3. 40 mm Metal-on-Metal (As-Cast CoCrMo) with Reduced Radical Clearances

Disappointed by the erratic wear behavior of the 40 mm M/M bearings, Howmedica Osteonics began a third round of testing using components precision-manufactured with tighter tolerances. Four pairs of 40 mm M/M (as-cast CoCrMo) bearings were produced with a radial clearance of 25-50 microns (similar to the 28 mm Metasul bearings). The results were once again disappointing. While three of the four bearings showed excellent wear performance (wear rate < 1mm³/million cycles), one pair exhibited a run-away wear pattern (wear rate = 45 mm³/million cycles), Figure 8(a). For the run-away wear pair, the 500cc-lubricant was completely darkened throughout the duration of the test, Figure 8(b).

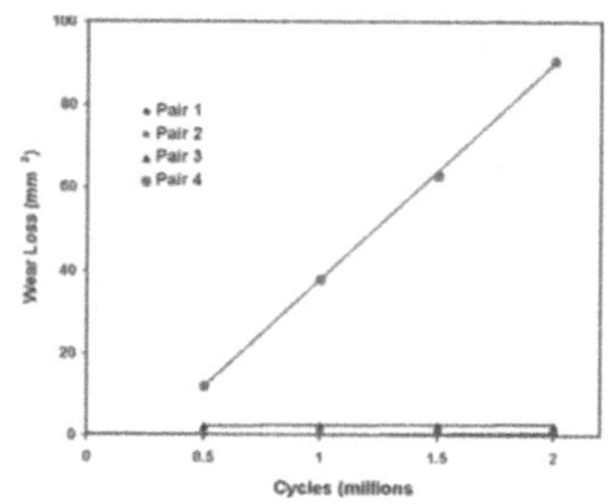

Figure 8a:
Hip simulator wear of four pairs M/M bearings (40 mm) with one pair showing a run-away wear pattern.

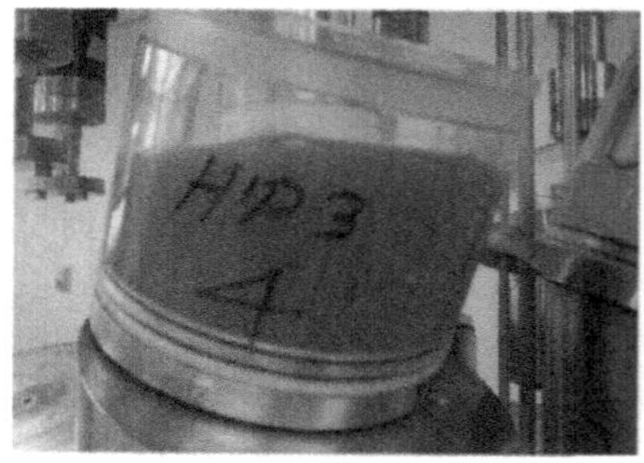

Figure 8b:
Lubricant darkening for the run-away wear pair (pair 4).

4. Metal-on-Polyethylene and Ceramic-on-Polyethylene

4.1. Metal-on-polyethylene vs. Radiation Dose

In 1995, we hypothesized that the wear rate of UHMWPE acetabular components could be significantly reduced by radiation crosslinking at elevated doses followed by thermal stabilization [12]. In a hip simulator test, it was demonstrated for the first time that the wear rate of polyethylene cups decreased exponentially with increasing the total dose of gamma irradiation, Figure 9. At a radiation dose of 10 MRads, the wear rate was only 1/20ᵗʰ that of the unirradiated cup and 1/10ᵗʰ that of the conventional 3 MRads gamma-in-nitrogen sterilized cup. This finding eventually led to the development of Crossfire® Highly Crosslinked UHMWPE for acetabular bearing applications.

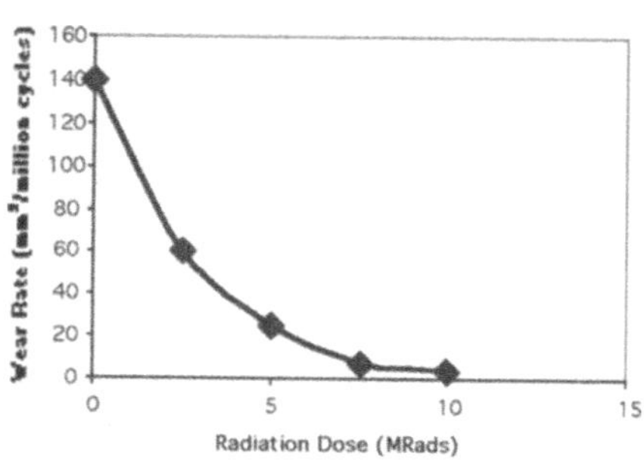

Figure 9:
Wear rate of UHMWPE acetabular cup as a function of radiation dose.

4.2. Metal-on-Conventional Polyethylene vs. Metal-on-Highly Crosslinked Polyethylene

Crossfire highly crosslinked polyethylene was processed by first irradiating ram-extruded GUR1050 bars by Co^{60} gamma rays at 7.5MRads, then subjecting the irradiated bars to a below-melt annealing cycle at 130°C, machining the irradiated/annealed bars into acetabular cups, and finally sterilizing the cups with an additional 3.0MRads gamma-irradiation in air-impermeable packages filled with nitrogen. Initial hip simulator evaluations of Crossfire® highly crosslinked cups were conducted on the hip joint simulator against undamaged CoCr femoral heads. Both the System-12® and Trident® liner designs (Howmedica Osteonics, Mahwah, NJ) were tested. For the System-12 design, Duration® Stabilized UHMWPE liners were used as the control. For the Trident® design, N_2Vac™ liners were the control. Figures 10(a) and (b) show the test results. For both designs, the Crossfire® liners showed 90% wear reduction compared to the controls.

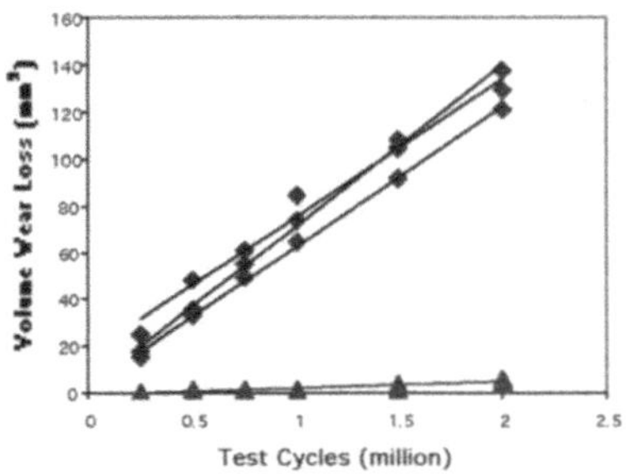

Figure 10a:
Duration/CoCr vs. Crossfire®/CoCr (System-12® design)

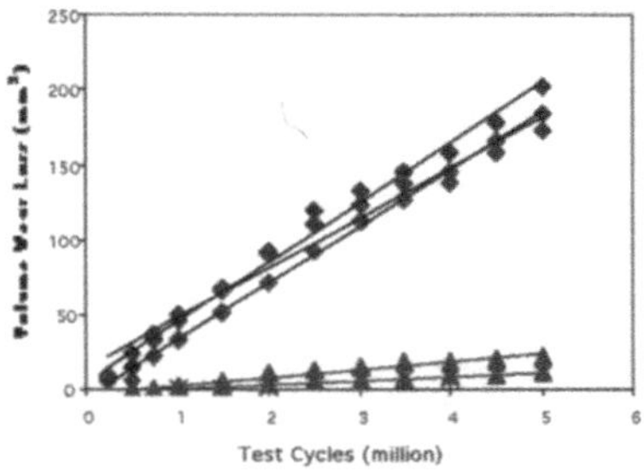

Figure10b:
Fig. 10b: N2Vac™/CoCr vs. Crossfire®/CoCr (Trident® design)

4.3. Ceramic-on-Crossfire® Polyethylene vs. Head Size

Trident® Crossfire® liners of 32 mm and 36 mm internal diameters were tested in the hip simulator against matching alumina ceramic heads for 5 million cycles. Trident® N_2Vac™ liners matched with 28 mm alumina heads were used as the control. Four duplicate samples for each bearing combination were used in the test. Figure 11 shows the accumulative volume wear loss for each cup as a function of test cycles. All liners showed a linear relationship between wear and test duration. Both the 32 mm and 36 mm Crossfire® liners had 87% lower wear rate than the 28 mm N_2Vac™ liners. No lubricant darkening was seen in any Crossfire® test chamber against metal or ceramic.

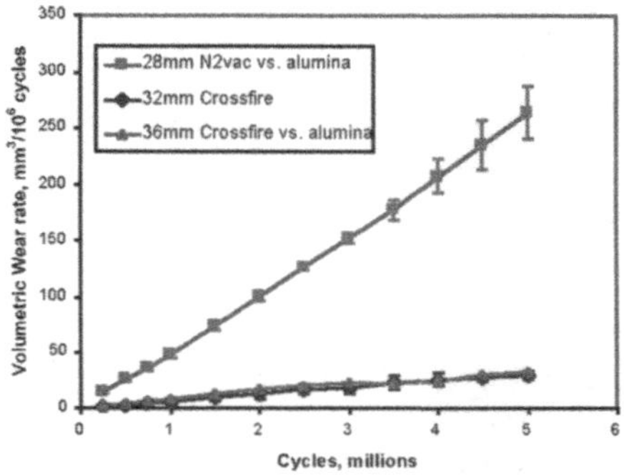

Figure 11:
Duration/CoCr vs. Crossfire®/CoCr (System-12® design)

4.4. Third-Body Wear: Metal-on-Crossfire vs. Ceramic-on-Crossfire

4.4.1. Wear By Damaged CoCr Femoral Head

To simulate 3rd-body wear by damaged CoCr femoral heads, both Crossfire® and N_2Vac™ cups were tested against damaged heads with a wide range of surface roughness. Significant wear rate increases were found for both Crossfire® and N_2Vac™ cups with increases in the peak-to-valley roughness of the CoCr femoral heads, Figure 12. It is clear that both the conventional N_2Vac™ and the Crossfire® cups are not immune to 3rd-body wear. To protect Crossfire® cups against 3rd-body wear under adverse conditions, the matching femoral head components must be kept smooth and immune to 3rd-body scratching. Since an alumina ceramic head is immune to 3rd-body damage, its combination with Crossfire® represents a superior choice to CoCr/Crossfire® [13].

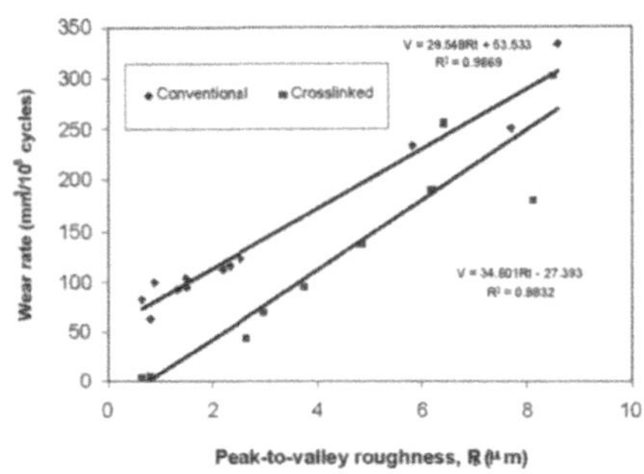

Figure 12:
Volumetric wear rate as a function of CoCr head roughness (Peak-to-valley) for both the highly crosslinked (Crossfire) and the control cups (N2vac).

4.4.2. Wear By PMMA Bone Cement Particles

Undamaged CoCr and alumina ceramic heads of 32 mm diameter (Howmedica Osteonics, Mahwah, NJ) were coupled with the Crossfire highly crosslinked cups. The test was conducted in two phases. During the 1st phase, which lasted 1.5 million cycles, clean serum lubricant was used. During the 2nd phase, which lasted from 1.5 to 3.5 million cycles, pre-polymerized PMMA bone cement (Simplex, Howmedica Osteonics) particles with an average size of 150 um were mixed with the serum lubricant at a concentration of 5 g/L. Wear was determined by weight loss measurement after soak-correction. Four duplicate cups were tested against each head material. Students'-t test was used to measure statistical significance at the 95% confidence level ($P<0.05$).

Fig. 13 shows the volumetric wear loss as a function of test cycles for the highly

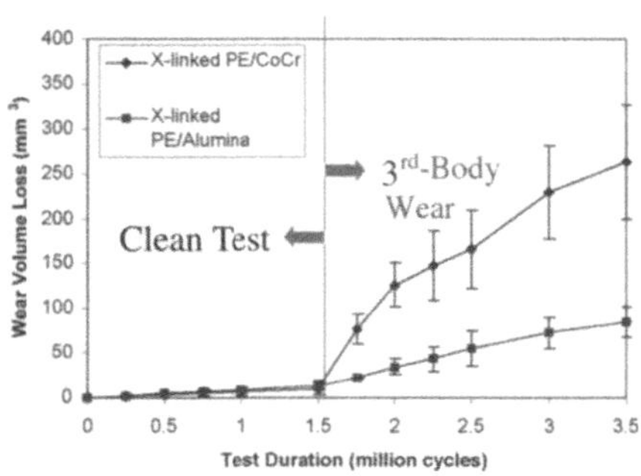

Figure 13:
Waer of Crossfire highly crosslinked cups against CoCr and alumina heads under clean and 3rd-body conditions.

crosslinked cups against CoCr and alumina heads. During the initial 1.5 million cycles of testing in which no PMMA particles were added to the lubricant, the cups against CoCr and alumina heads showed comparable wear rates (P=0.3). During the 2nd phase of testing in which 5g/L PMMA cement particles were mixed into the lubricant, the cup wear rate against CoCr head was increased from 6.1 mm^3/Mc to 118 mm^3/Mc, whereas the cup wear rate against the alumina heads was increased to 35 mm^3/Mc, respectively. Under this severe 3rd-body environment, the use of ceramic heads prevented run-away wear for the crosslinked cups. In fact, the wear rate of the crosslinked cups against the alumina head under the 3rd-body conditions is still only 60% that of the 30kGy cups against undamaged CoCr head in a clean lubricant.

5. Ceramic-on-Ceramic

Nine pairs of alumina-on-alumina bearings were evaluated by the hip simulator under clean conditions and three pairs were tested under 3rd-body conditions (5 g/L PMMA particles added to lubricant). Under the clean test conditions, all nine pairs of the alumina-on-alumina bearings showed extremely low wear rates (0.10 mm^3/million cycles) and very tight variations (+/- 0.05 mm^3/million cycles). Under the 3rd-body conditions, the wear rate was hardly measurable (<0.05 mm^3/million cycles), see Fig. 14. These results indicate that alumina-on-alumina bearings are immune to 3rd-body wear by loose bone cement particles.

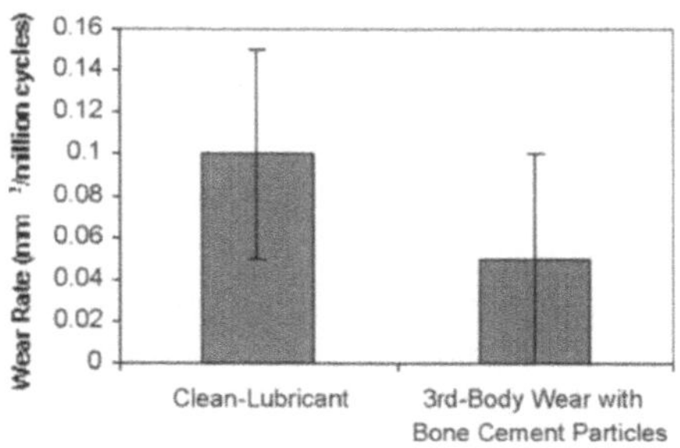

Figure 14: Hip simulator wear of alumina-on-alumina bearings under clean and 3rd-body conditions.

6. Metal-on-Metal vs. Ceramic-on-Polyethylene vs. Ceramic-on-Ceramic

Figure 15 summarizes the wear rate data of 50 pairs of bearing surfaces tested in the MTS hip simulator including 10 ceramic/N_2Vac™ pairs, 10 ceramic/Crossfire® pairs, 21 M/M pairs (2nd generation M/M) and 9 ceramic-on-ceramic pairs. The mean wear rates and ranges for each combination were as follows:

Alumina/N2Vac™ - 50.96 mm^3/million cycles (33.7 – 69.1)
Alumina/Crossfire® - 5.62 mm^3/million cycles (4.7 – 11.7)
M/M - 7.40 mm^3/million cycles (0.14 – 45.67)
C/C – 0.10 mm^3/million cycles (0.05 – 0.15)

The mean wear rates between alumina/N_2Vac™ and M/M and between alumina/N_2Vac™ and alumina/Crossfire® are statistically significantly different (P<0.0001 for both). However, there is no difference in the mean wear rate between M/M and alumina/Crossfire® (P=0.50). In fact, 4 out of 21 M/M pairs (18%) show higher wear rates than the highest wear pair of alumina/Crossfire®. In addition, the maximum to minimum wear rate variation for the M/M group is more than 300,000% whereas it is only 120% for both the alumina/N_2Vac™ and alumina/Crossfire® groups. The wear rate for the C/C group was significantly lower than each of the other groups ($P<0.05$). The data is self-evident and shows that M/M articulations are intrinsically unpredictable while alumina/Crossfire® and alumina/alumina bearings offer a consistent and predictable improvement over conventional alumina/UHMWPE surfaces for total hip replacement.

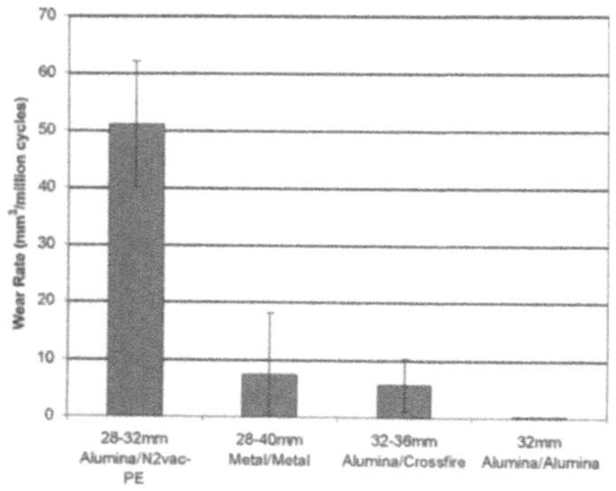

Figure 15:
Wear rate comparisons of alumina/ N_2Vac™, metal/metal, alumina/Crossfire® and alumina/alumina bearings.

7. Biological Considerations

Basic research and scientific review are important considerations in evaluating implant performance criteria. Equally important is an analysis of the potential clinical benefits and consequences from the surgeon and patient's perspectives. A methodical review of the scientific body of evidence is provided to allow the surgeon to consider biological implications that may impact their bearing material decision.

7.1. Metal-on-Metal

Concern has been expressed in the literature regarding the unknown biological effects of metal-on-metal bearings as they relate to wear particles, metal ion release, toxicity and hypersensitivity [14-26]. It has been estimated from retrieval analysis that metal-on-metal hip prosthesis generate up to 500 times the number of particles as a metal on polyethylene hip [14]. While most of these particles have a similar composition to that of the alloy, studies of tissue indicate these particles may have a higher chromium content to that expected from the alloy composition which may be due to corrosion of wear particles [15]. In addition it has been demonstrated that cobalt-chromium alloy particles are toxic to macrophages [16]. The particles can modulate the growth of osteoblast cells in vitro [17] and have been shown to interfere with bone formation in a bone harvest chamber model [18].

Metal ion levels have been reported to be elevated in patients with metal-on-metal hip prostheses [19]. The small size of metallic debris leads to their clearance from around the joint into the lymphatic circulation and thus to the blood and organs. The observed higher serum levels are probably associated with elevated rates of metal storage in organs such as the liver and kidneys and patients with compromised kidney function may experience even higher concentrations and storage rates [20].

Finally, the literature has raised the issue of an immune response with metal-on-metal hip prostheses. Metals such as cobalt and chromium can induce hypersensitivity reactions in humans on the skin and it may also develop in the tissue next to hip implants that release a number of metal ions [21].

7.2. Ceramic-on-Crosslinked Polyethylene

The biological response to conventional Ultra-High Molecular Weight Polyethylene (UHMWPE) is reasonably well understood [22]. Polyethylene debris is cleared from around the joint and can be found in remote tissue. However, adverse systemic effects have not been reported. The main effect of polyethylene debris is local to the implant. In sufficient quantity, polyethylene debris cannot be entirely cleared from the joint and the debris accumulation results in osteolytic reactions mediated via macrophages. This leads to loss of bone stock via osteoclast resorption. The macrophage response is greatest for particles in the size range 0.2 – 0.8 mm [23]. Polyethylene debris falls in this size range (range: 0.1 – 1 mm with mean: 0.5 mm). However, there appears to be a wear rate threshold for osteolysis due to polyethylene wear debris. The literature indicates that osteolysis is uncommon provided the wear rate is <0.1 mm/year and that osteolysis should be avoided if the wear rate is <0.05 mm/year [27].

Hip simulator studies have demonstrated that ceramic-on-Crossfire® highly crosslinked polyethylene bearings generate polyethylene debris that is in the size range found with conventional UHMWPE i.e. 0.1 – 1 mm [25]. Therefore, the biological mechanisms of response of Crossfire® polyethylene should be the same as with conventional polyethylene. From hip simulator studies and early clinical measurements [28,29], crosslinked polyethylenes such as Crossfire® polyethylene are expected to have a wear rate in the range 0.01 – 0.02 mm/year. This range of wear is well below the osteolysis threshold.

7.3. Ceramic-on-Ceramic

Ceramic-on-ceramic bearings not only generate far fewer wear particles than polyethylene and metal-on-metal bearings, ceramic debris is also less stimulating biologically than polyethylene and metal debris [14,24,30]. The combination of a lower particle generation rate and a less biological response makes ceramic-on-ceramic joints the most favorable choice in the fight against osteolysis.

8. Discussion and Conclusions

The art and science of hip joint simulator wear testing has been advanced significantly in the past decade. In the authors' laboratory, we have successfully reproduced the wear performance and wear rankings of clinically disproven and proven bearing materials. By adhering to the principles of anatomical testing, cross-shear motion and biological lubrication, we have correctly predicted the higher wear rate of Hylamer enhanced polyethylene compared to conventional polyethylene. This validated test protocol was used to evaluate modern bearing surfaces. Both metal-on-highly crosslinked polyethylene and metal-on-metal articulations exhibited an order of magnitude wear reduction over conventional metal or ceramic-on-polyethylene under ideal conditions. However, both bearing couples showed limitations. Metal-on-crosslinked polyethylene was susceptible to 3rd-body wear while metal-on-metal was unpredictable in performance.

In the era of highly crosslinked polyethylene, metal-on-metal articulation, given its inherent unpredictable nature, cannot be considered a superior bearing option for total hip replacement. Clinically, the first generation M/M joints

(McKee-Farrar) performed poorly compared to the first generation M/PE joints (Charnley). Even the 2nd generation M/M joints have failed to demonstrate superior clinical performance over 2nd generation ceramic-on-polyethylene joints.

The limitations of metal-on-crosslinked polyethylene against 3rd-body wear can be overcome by the use of ceramic-on-crosslinked polyethylene articulation. A five-fold wear reduction was obtained by the use of alumina ceramic heads under severe 3rd-body conditions compared to the use of metal heads. The use of ceramic-on-ceramic articulation completely eliminated the 3rd-body wear problem associated with polyethylene joints.

The biological response to metallic debris is not well understood. The concerns are systemic rather than local. Although there is over 30 years experience with metal-one-metal hip prostheses, these issues have not been resolved. Concern has been expressed in the literature regarding the unknown biological effects associated with metal-on-metal bearing debris as it relates to metal ion release, hypersensitivity, wear particle dissemination, and runaway wear. The biological response to polyethylene, on the other hand, is reasonably well understood. There do not appear to be systemic concerns. The literature indicates that osteolysis is uncommon provided the wear rate is <0.1 mm/year and that osteolysis should be avoided if the wear rate is <0.05 mm/year. From hip simulator studies and early clinical measurements, crosslinked polyethylenes such as Crossfire are expected to have a wear rate in the range 0.01-0.02 mm/year. This range of wear is well below the osteolysis threshold. The use of ceramic-on-crosslinked polyethylene and ceramic-on-ceramic bearings would further reduce the likelihood of runaway wear by 3rd-body particles.

While industry must continually evaluate the theoretical versus clinical advantages and disadvantages of these technologies, the physician must ultimately determine the potential patient benefits and risks after weighing the scientific evidence.

Acknowledgements: the authors acknowledge Ash Chopra, Aaron Essner, Gregg Schmidig and Shi-Shen Yau for experimental support.

References:

1. Paul J, Force Actions Transmitted by Joints in the Human Body. Proc. R. Soc. Lond. B, 192 (1976) 163-172.
2. Wang A, et. al., The Impact of Lubricant Protein Concentration on the Outcome of Hip Joint Simulator Testing. 45th ORS, 1999, p. 52.
3. Wang A, et. al., Quantitative Analysis of Serum Degradation and its Effect on the Outcome of Hip Joint Simulator Wear Testing of UHMWPE. 45th ORS, 1999, p. 73.
4. Charnley J, Kamangar A, and Longfield MD. The Optimum Size of Prosthetic Heads in Relation to the Wear of Plastic Sockets in Total Replacement of the Hip. Med. & Biol. Engng. 7:31-39, 1969.
5. Griffith MJ, Seidenstein MK, Williams D, Charnley J: Socket Wear in Charnley Low Friction Arthroplasty of the Hip. Clin Orthop 137 (1978) 37.
6. Charnley J, Halley DK: Rate of Wear in Total Hip Replacement. Clin Orthop 112 (1975) 170.
7. Livingston BJ, Chmell MJ, Spector M, Poss R: Complications of Total Hip Arthroplasty Associated with the Use of an Acetabular Component with a Hylamer Liner. JBJS 79A (1997) 1529.

8. Graeter JH, Nevins R: Early Osteolysis with Hylamer Acetabular Liners. J. Arthroplasty 14 (1999) 464.
9. Essner A, et. al., Hip Simulator Wear of "Enhanced" UHMWPE Acetabular Inserts, 44th Ann. Mtng ORS, New Orleans, Mar. 16-19, 1998: 774.
10. Martell J, et. al., Preclinical Evaluation Followed by Randomized Clinical Study of a Crosslinked Polyethylene for Total Hip Arthroplasty at Two Year Follow-up, 47th Ann. Mtng, ORS, San Francisco, Feb. 25-28, 2001: 163.
11. Essner A, et. al., In Vitro and In Vivo Acetabular Cup Wear Corroboration, 47th Ann. Mtng, ORS, San Francisco, Feb. 25-28, 2001: 1007.
12. Wang A, Essner A, Polineni VK, Stark C and Dumbleton JH. Lubrication and Wear of Ultra-High Molecular Weight Polyethylene in Total Joint Replacements. Tribology International, Vol. 31, No. 1-3: 17-33, 1998.
13. Wang A and Schmidig G, Ceramic Heads Prevent Runaway Wear for Crosslinked UHMWPE Against 3rd-body Damage. 49th ORS, 2003 (accepted).
14. Doorn PF, PA Campbell, J Worrall, PD Benya, HA McKellop and HC Amstutz, Metal Wear Particle Characterization From Metal-on-Metal Total Hip Replacements: Transmission Electron Microscopy Study of Periprosthetic Tissues and Isolated Particles, J Biomed Mater Res, 42, 103-111, 1998.
15. Jacobs JJ, NJ Hallab, AK Skipor, RM Urban, K Mikecz and TT Glant, Metallic Wear and Corrosion Products: Biological Implications, in Metasul: A Metal-on-Metal Bearing, Rieker C, M Wyndler and U Wyss (eds), Hans Huber, Bern, 1999, pp 125-132.
16. Haynes Dr, SD Rogers, S Hay, MJ Pearcy and DW Howie, The Differences in Toxicity and Release of Bone-Resorbing Mediators Induced by Titanium and Cobalt-Chromium-Alloy Wear Particles, JBJS, 75A, 825-834, 1993.
17. Allen MJ, BJ Myer, PJ Millet and N Rushton, The Effects of Particulate Cobalt, Chromium and Cobalt-Chromium Alloy in Human Osteoblast-like Cells In Vitro, JBJS, 79B, 475-482, 1997.
18. Goodman S, P Aspenberg, Y Song, G Knoblich, P Huie, D Regula and L Lidgren, Tissue Ingrowth and Differentiation in the Bone-Harvest Chamber in the Presence of Cobalt-Chromium-Alloy and High-Density-Polyethylene Particles, JBJS, 77A, 1025-1035, 1995.
19. MacDonald SJ, RW McCalden, DG Chess, RB Bourne, CH Rorabeck, D Cleland and F Leung, Metal-on-Metal Versus Polyethylene in Hip Arthroplasty: A Randomized Clinical Trial, CORR, in press.
20. Brodner W, P Bitzan, V Meisinger, A Kaider, F Gottsauner-Wolf and R Kotz, Elevated Serum Cobalt with Metal-on-Metal Articulating Surfaces, JBJS, 79B, 316-321.
21. Willert H-G, GH Buchhorn, A Fayyazi and CH Lohmann, Histopathological Changes in Tissues Surrounding Metal/Metal Joints – Signs of Delayed Type Hypersensitivity? (DTH), in World Tribology Forum in Arthroplasty, Rieker C, S Oberholzer and U Wyss (Eds), Hans Huber, Bern, 2001, pp 147-166.
22. Iida H, E Kaneda, H Takada, K Uchida, K Kawanabe and T Nakamura, Metallosis Due to Impingement Between the Socket and the Femoral Neck in a Metal-on-Metal Bearing Total Hip Prosthesis, JBJS, 81A, 400-403, 1999.
23. Implant Wear in Total Joint Replacement, TM Wright and SB Goodman (eds), AAOS, Rosemont, Illinois, 2001.
24. Ingham E and J Fisher, Biological Reactions to Wear Debris in Total Joint Replacement, Proc Instn Mech Engrs, 214, 21-37, 2000.
25. Lee JM, et. Al., Size of Metallic and Polyethylene Debris Particles in Failed Cemented Total Hip Replacement, JBJS, 74B, 1992, p. 380-384.
26. Urban, Robert M, Jacobs, Joshua J. et. al., Dissemination of Wear Particles to the Liver, Spleen an Abdominal Lymph Nodes of Patients with Hip or Knee Replacement. Journal of Bone and Joint Surgery, Vol. 82-A, No. 4, April 2000.

27. Dumbleton JH, Manley MT, Edidin A, A literature review of the association between wear rate and osteolysis in total hip arthroplasty, J. Arthroplasty Vol. 17 No 5 (2002) 649-661.
28. Martell J, Incavo S, Clinical Performance of a Highly Crosslinked Polyethylene at 2 Years in THA. A Randomized Prospective Trial, 49th ORS, 2003 (accepted).
29. Nivbrant B, Roerhl S, Hewitt BJ, In Vivo Wear and Performance of Highly Crosslinked Polyethylene Cups – a RSA Study of 30 Hips. 49th ORS, 2003 (accepted).
30. Williams PA, Clarke IC, Ceramic wear debris in total joint replacements: review of debris morphology and biological response, Key Engineering Materials Vols 218-220 (2002) 591-594.

SESSION 2

Adverse Reactions in Total Joint Replacement: Infections, Allergic Reactions and others

2.1 Hypersensitivity to Wear Products in Metal-on-metal Articulation

H.-G. Willert, G. H. Buchhorn and A. Fayyazi

Abstract

The good experience with low articular wear was the reason to reintroduce the Co-Cr-metal-metal pairing for artificial hip joints. Midterm clinical results of this second generation of all-metal joints confirmed the expectation of a reduced wear.

The estimated revision rate ranges about 0,15 % per year, which may double by the number of unknown cases. If metal/metal articulations of the second generation cause problems, clinical symptoms like hip or thigh pain, (re)appear mostly within the first 2 years after primary implantation, increase in intensity and finally call for revision. X-rays show radiolucent lines and progressive osteolyses. At revision surgery often massive serous and fibrin containing joint effusion, sometimes in connection with bursa – formation, are to be found, while the implants may be loose or still fixed.

Histomorphologically, the periprosthetic tissues contain only very small amounts of metal debris but show distinct aseptic inflammatory changes with extended infiltration of lymphocytes and plasmacells, high endothelial venules, pronounced macrophage reaction and massive fibrin exudation. These changes were absent in periprosthetic tissues from the control group of endoprostheses not containing cobalt, chromium or nickel.

Both, clinical course and morphological findings give reason to assume a possible hypersensitivity reaction as cause for failure of the second generation of metal-metal hip joints.

Introduction

Low articular wear was the reason to reintroduce the Co-Cr-metal/metal pairing for artificial hip joints [29]. The early and mid-term results of this new generation of all-metal joints have been reported to be satisfying after 4 – 10 years [2, 6, 7, 8, 13, 15, 16, 18, 19, 27, 28, 30, 31]. The amount of metal abrasion from the articulating surfaces of the femoral head and the cup, measured on retrieved components, was similar to the results from hip simulator tests [21, 22, 24, 25]. Compared to ceramic-polyethylene articulations, the debris volume of the metal/metal joints was up to 60-fold reduced.

The estimated revision rate at present ranges around 0.15% per year [20] this may double by the number of unknown cases.

Material and Methods

We received in 1995 for the first time periprosthetic tissue, taken at revision from a metal/metal hip joint. This was when SULZER Medica (now Centerpulse

Orthopedics) Winterthur launched a comprehensive retrieval program. In the course of this program we obtained tissue samples for investigation from more than hundred revised hip endoprostheses with metal/metal articulations of various types and from different manufacturers so far. This material came from several centres in Australia, Austria, Belgium, France, Germany, New Zealand and Switzerland.

Data regarding the patients' complaints, the course after the primary implantation of the metal-metal hip joint, the revision surgery and the final outcome, were asked for and collected by means of a special questionnaire.

The material originated from the joint capsule, the bone-implant interface, and the bony implant bed of revised hip endoprostheses with metal/metal articulations. We received the tissues mostly fixed in formalin, some as blocks, already embedded in paraffin. The formalin fixed tissues were decalcified, if necessary, and also imbedded in paraffin. 5 –10µm sections were made and routinely stained with haematoxylin– eosin (HE), Giemsa, van-Gieson, Prussian-Blue, and PAS. Immunohistochemistry was performed on selected cases with the following markers:

CD68 (Macrophages), 25F9 ("old" Macrophages), MRP8, MRP14 ("young" Macrophages) CD20 (B – Lymphocytes), CD3 (T – Lymphocytes), Ki67 (T – Lymphocytes expressing proliferation associated antigen) [10, 23]. The sections were examined microscopically under normal light and with polarization (BX 50, Olympus, Hamburg, Germany).

Tissues from the surrounding of noncemented hip endoprostheses, free of Cobalt, Chromium, Molybdenum and Nickel served as controls. The components of these endoprostheses consisted of Titanium – alloy stems (Type Zweymüller, AlloPro GmbH, Germany), Al2O3 ball heads (Biolox, Ceramtec, Germany) and noncemented UHMW-Polyethylene screw cups (Type Endler, AlloPro GmbH, Germany).and revision became necessary between 3 and 16 (average 10.9) years after primary implantation because of loosening of the cups, accompanied by more ore less extended osteolyses [34]). The re-examined periprosthetic tissues had consecutively been taken at revision surgery in the Dept. of Orthopaedics, University of Göttingen, during the years 1998 and 1999.

Results

In the following communication we report by way of summarizing on the most important clinical and histomorphological findings. More details may be found in our recent publications [35, 36].

The **clinical course** of the cases which required revision was characterized mainly by persistence or early reoccurrence of complaints like hip or thigh pain at start up and weight bearing and often by a pronounced hip joint effusion.

In the majority of cases, patients' complaints about increasing pain (Table 1) and the appearance of osteolyses gave rise for revision. The average term of function between primary implantation and revision is mostly less than 3 years. X-rays often show the development of radiolucent lines and progressive osteolyses; one or all implants may be loose or still fixed. Revision surgery revealed effusion and large fibrin masses in the joint cavity, sometimes in connection with bursa –formation in several patients.

Patient's complaints

- **Pain** in the hip joint and in the thigh, especially at weight bearing, in some cases also at rest
- **Limping**
- **Noise** emerging of during joint movement
- Multiple **subluxation** or **dislocation** respectively

A certain correlation between **patients' complaints, x-ray– and intraoperative findings** could not be established.

At revision, most of the patients had an exchange of the primary metal – metal articulation against alumina on polyethylene or metal on (crosslinked) polyethylene respectively and reported that their complaints disappeared more or less completely. In contrast to this, those patients who received a second metal/metal articulation at revision did not experience relief of symptoms.

The **histomorphology** of the periprosthetic tissues shows aseptic inflammatory changes with diffuse and perivascular infiltrates of lymphocytes and plasmacells, occurring also within the walls of the post-capillary vessels. In addition, high endothelial venules, massive fluid – and fibrin exudation (Fig.1 and 2), necroses and, last but not least, accumulation of macrophages with drop-like inclusions are further typical findings (Fig.3, Table 2).

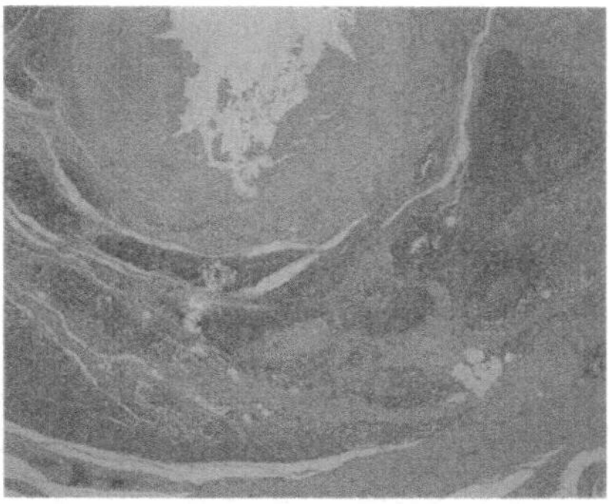

Figure 1:
Fibrin exudation at the surface and perivascular follicular lymphocytic infiltrates in the intermediate vascular layer of the joint capsule of a metal/metal – articulation. HE staining. Mikrophotograph. Case 47.99

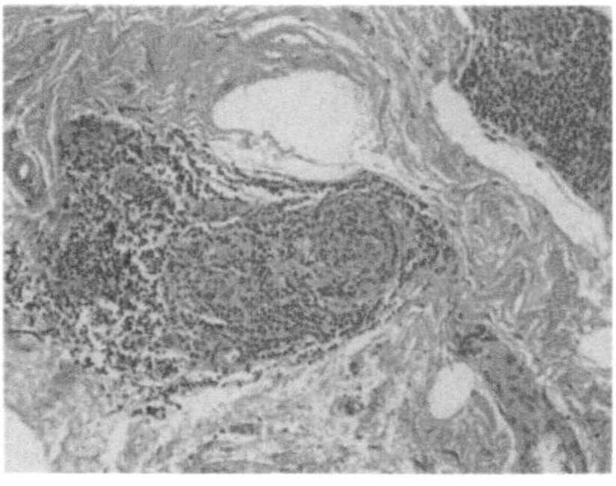

Figure 2:
Perivascular follicular lymphocytic infiltrates with "High Endothelial Venules" in the intermediate vascular layer of the joint capsule of a metal/metal – articulation. HE staining. Microphotograph. Case 16506.00

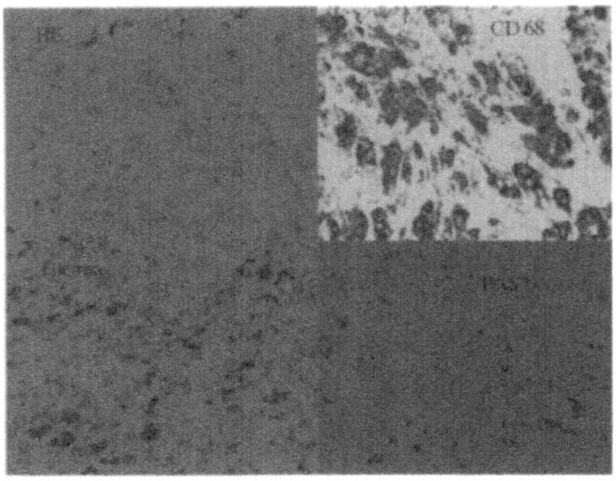

Figure 3:
Macrophages with ‚drop – like' inclusions
Top left: HE staining
Top right: CD68 staining identifies macrophages
Bottom left: Giemsa staining
Bottom right: PAS staining
Microphotographs. Case 15255.00

Characteristic histomorphological findings

- Diffuse and perivascular **infiltrates of lymphocytes and plasmacells** (+ intramural infiltration of the postcapillary vessels)
- **High endothelial venules** (HEV)
- Massive **fibrin exudation**
- Accumulation of **macrophages with drop-like inclusions**
- Sometimes **eosinophilic granulocytes** and **mast cells**

In general, the foreign body reaction to wear particles from the implant materials is relatively mild. At the light microscopic level, metal particles from the articulating surfaces can be detected only in small amounts. They are very small and measure from submicron to 5µm in diameter. Their sharp edges light up in polarised light due to refraction and shatter of light [32], (Fig.4). In addition to metal particles, also polyethylene debris and, around cemented implants, constituents of the bone cement (polymethylmethacrylate and X-ray contrast medium like Zirconium Oxide) can be found.

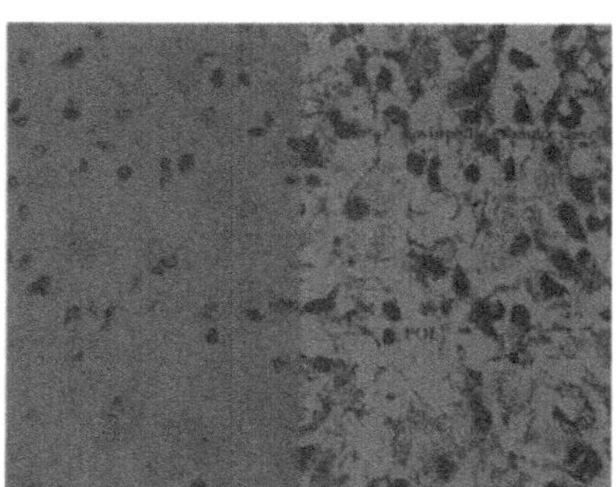

Figure 4:
Macrophages store tiny black metal particles (left: regular light).
The sharp edges of the metal particles light up in polarised light due to refraction and shatter of light (right: polarized light)
Giemsa staining, Microphotographs,
Case 17776.00

Small particles were mainly stored in mono – or multinuclear macrophages, larger ones in or surrounded by giant cells. Often the macrophages accumulate in the vicinity of vessels, very likely within the perivascular lymph spaces. In about half of the cases, macrophages contain also small drop-like inclusions within the cytoplasm. The size of the inclusions ranges from detection limit of 0.5 up to 15 µm. They are PAS positive and turn light-yellow or greenish with HE–, deep-blue with Giemsa–, and changing pale-blue with Prussian blue staining. The material is not birefringent and appears to be amorphous. The morphological characteristics preclude that the inclusions directly originate from any of the known implant materials (Fig.3).

In areas of fibrin exudation, the synovial cellular lining is mostly lacking (Fig.1).

Immunohistochemistry provides additional information:

The lymphocytic infiltrates (diffusely distributed or perivascularly aggregated) consist of CD20 – positive B – lymphocytes and CD3 – positive T – lymphocytes. 5-10% of the lymphocytes express the antigen Ki-67 which is associated with proliferation and indicates that the cellular reaction is still active [11] (Fig.5).

Figure 5:
Follicular lymphocytic infiltrate in the intermediate vascular layer of the joint capsule of a metal/metal – articulation. Histochemical stainings were used to differentiate between B - and T- lymphocytes and to identify activated T – lymphocytes.
Top left: Giemsa staining shows all lymphocytes.
Top right: B - lymphocytes identified by L26
Bottom left: T- lymphocytes identified by CD3
Bottom right: Activated T- lymphocytes identified by Ki67
Microphotographs. Case 56.99

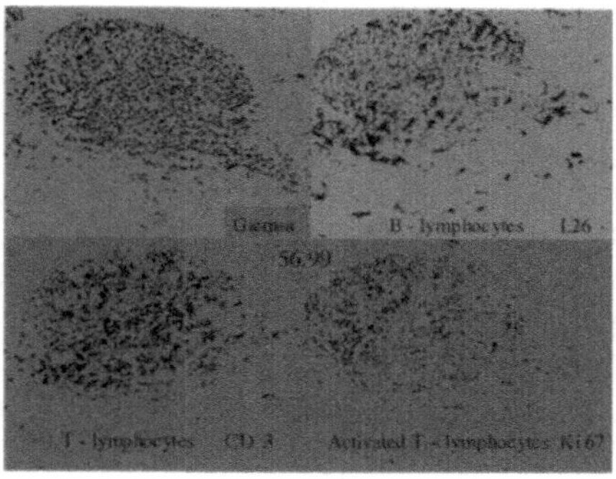

Mono- and multinuclear macrophages are generally CD68 – positive. To characterize subtypes of macrophages, further immunohistochemical studies with monoclonal antibodies against the non-clustered antigens 25F9, MRP8, and MRP14 were performed. While 25F9 - positive cells are considered mature macrophages, the MRP8 / MRP14 - positive mononuclear cells represent recently invaded, inflammatory, and active macrophages [17, 37]. Both types, mature as well as recently invaded, inflammatory and active macrophages were regularly present in the tissues surrounding the investigated new generation metal/metal joints [35]. The drop shaped inclusions in the cytoplasm of the macrophages seem to be located in the phagosomes, enveloped by a CD68 - positive membrane (Fig 3).

The **control tissues** from implants without cobalt, chromium, or nickel contained, almost exclusively, large amounts of polyethylene –, but no metallic wear particles. The size of the polyethylene particles varied between 0.5µm and 20µm, but reached sometimes more than 100µm up to 300µm [33]. The smaller particles were stored in mono– and polynuclear macrophages, the larger ones either incorporated into or surrounded by foreign body giant cells. On the whole, the foreign body reaction was much stronger than in the tissue from metal / metal joints. There were extended phagocytic granulomas with large numbers of giant cells and a marked tendency to necrosis. Four cases showed slight fibrin exudation. One single perivascular lymphocytic infiltrate could be detected in only one case. Diffuse lymphocytic infiltration and HEV were absent.

Discussion

So far, only a relatively small number of hip endoprostheses with metal/metal joints of the new generation have failed. The most important features observed with such cases are either persistence of complaints or reoccurrence within the first two to three years after implantation and specific histomorphological changes of the periprosthetic tissues.

The most characteristic histomorphological findings are infiltrates of lymphocytes and plasmacells, often forming perivascular cuffs, "High Endothelial Venules", fibrin exudation and accumulation of macrophages containing inclusions of yet unknown origin. By means of immunohistochemistry it could be shown that the lymphocytic infiltrates consist of B – and T – lymphocytes and, in addition, that the lymphocytes are still active. The presence of recently invaded active macrophages emphasizes the activity of the process.

Since several findings like the presence of B – lymphocytes, plasma cells and massive fibrin exudation are considered as not being characteristics of type IV delayed type hypersensitivity reactions (DTH) [1, 3, 4, 5, 14, 12], the observed phenomena could not be classified as DTH. Nevertheless, the histomorphological changes suggest a kind of hypersensitivity reaction to elements like Co and Cr from the all metal joint as has been suspected already in the seventies [9, 26]. This hypothesis is supported by the clinical course of early failure and the fact that patients who received a second metal/metal articulation at revision did not experience relief of symptoms.

In the control group of endoprostheses not containing cobalt, chromium or nickel, signs of immune reactions were missing.

Although local hypersensitivity in patients with an artificial metal / metal hip joint is quite a rare incident, it seems to be advisable in case of an early failure of such implants to take the possibility of an immunologic reaction into account. This is important since only an early recognition of the underlying process, followed by appropriate measures can prevent broader implications such as loosening of the endoprosthetic components. At present, the most effective therapeutic procedure seems to be to replace the metallic by a non –or only partly – metallic articulation. A second metal/metal articulation, however, should not be inserted after the first one has failed!

References

1. Abbas AK, Lichman AH, Pober JS. (2000) Cellular and Molecular Immunology. 4th ed., WB Saunders Company, Philadelphia,: 34-36.
2. Böhler N. (1997) Experiences with metal on metal components in THR. Acta Orthop Belg. 63 Suppl 1:96-7
3. Black, J. (1992) Biological Performance of Materials, Chapter 11: Allergic Foreign-Body Response, Marcel Decker Inc., New York, 184-99.
4. Brown SA, Merritt K. (1981) Metal allergy and metallurgy. In: Weinstein A, Gibbons D, Brown S, Ruff W. (eds.) Implant Retrieval: Material and Biological Analysis. Special Publ. No.601, Washington, DC, NBS, 299-322.
5. Cupps TR, Fauci A. (1981) The Vasculitides. Chapter 5: Hypersensitivity Vasculitis. In: Smith LH Jr (ed.) Major Problems in Internal Medicine, Vol. XXI, Philadelphia, Saunders Comp. 50-70.
6. Doerig MF, Odstrcilik E, Jovanovic M, Badulescu M (1999) Metal/metal cementless total hip replacement. Paper No. SYM 46-04, SICOT Sidney
7. Doerig MF, Ostrcilik E, Jovanovic M, Krattler R (1999) Uncemented metal on metal (Metasul) total hip arthroplasty early results after 2 - 6 years. Paper No 0-147, EFORT Brussels
8. Dorr LD, Wan Z, Longjohn DB, Dubois B, Murken R (2000) Total Hip arthroplasty with use of the Metasul metal-on-metal articulation. J Bone Joint Surg (Am.) 82:789-98
9. Evans EM, Freeman MAR, Miller AJ, Vernon-Roberts B. (1974) Metal sensitivity as a cause of bone necrosis and loosening of the prosthesis in total joint replacement. J Bone Joint SurgBr. 56: 625-42.
10. Fayyazi A, Schweyer S, Eichmeyer B, Herms J, Hemmerlein B, Radzun HJ, Berger H. (2000) Expression of IFN gamma, coexpression of TNF alpha and matrix metalloproteinases and apoptosis of T lymphocytes and macrophages in granuloma annulare. Arch Dermatol Res. 292:384-90
11. Gerdes J, Li L, Schlueter C, Duchrow M, Wohlenberg C, Gerlach C, Stahmer I, Kloth S, Brandt E, Flad HD. (1991) Immunobiochemical and molecular biologic characterization of the cell proliferation-associated nuclear antigen that is defined by monoclonal antibody Ki-67. Am J Pathol. 138:867-73.
12. Hallab N, Merritt K, Jacobs JJ. (2001) Metal sensitivity in patients with orthopaedic implants. J Bone Joint Surg Am. 83:428-36.
13. Hilton KR, Dorr LD, Wan Z, McPherson EJ (1996) Contemporary total hip replacement with metal on metal articulation. Clin Orthop. 329S: 99-S10
14. Keller R. (1981) Immunologie und Immunpathologie. Thieme Verlag, Stuttgart
15. Kim Y, Park M, Park T, Choi I (1999) Hydroxyapatite rough – blasted CLS hip prosthesis associated with metal on metal articulation. Paper No. OP52-02, SICOT Sidney
16. McMinn DJW, De Cook CAM, Treacy RBC, Isbister ES (1999) Metal on metal resurfacing of the hip with hybrid fixation, our first 100 consecutive cases. Paper No. OP26-01, SICOT Sidney
17. Odink K, Cerletti N, Bruggen J, Clerc RG, Tarcsay L, Zwadlo G, Gerhards G, Schlegel R, Sorg C. (1987) Two calcium-binding proteins in infiltrate macrophages of rheumatoid arthritis. Nature 330:80-2.
18. Randelli G, Romano CL, Visentin O (1999) Six years clinical experience with metal on metal coupling in total hip prosthesis. Paper No PDS15 04, SICOT Sydney
19. Randelli G, Visentin O, Lonati F, Romano C (1999) The experience with the total alloclassic prosthesis and the metal/metal Metasul coupling. Paper No 0-218, EFORT Brussels
20. Rieker C (2001) personal communication

21. Sieber HP, Rieker CB, Köttig P (1999) Analysis of 118 second - generation metal - on - metal retrieved hip implants. J Bone Joint Surg (B) 80:46-50.
22. Schmidt M, Weber H, Schön R (1996) Cobalt chromium molybdenum metal combination for modular hip prostheses. Clin Orthop 329S:S35-47.
23. Schweyer S, Hemmerlein B, Radzun HJ, Fayyazi A. (2000) Continuous recruitment, co-expression of tumour necrosis factor-alpha and matrix metalloproteinases, and apoptosis of macrophages in gout tophi. Virchows Arch. 437:534-9.
24. Streicher RM, Schön R, Semlitsch M (1990) Untersuchung des tribologischen Verhaltens von Metall/Metall - Kombinationen für künstliche Hüftgelenke. Biomed Technik 35:107-11
25. Streicher RM, Semlitsch M, Schön R, Weber H (1996) Metal - on - metal articulation for artificial hip joints: Laboratory study and clinical results. Proc Inst Mech Eng [H] 210:223-32
26. Vernon-Roberts B, Freeman MAR. (1976) Morphological and analytical studies of the tissues adjacent to joint prostheses: investigation into causes of loosening of prostheses. In: Schaldach M, Hohmann D (eds.) Engineering in Medicine, Vol 1. Advances in Artificial Hip and Knee Joint Technology. Springer Verlag, Stuttgart, 148-186.
27. Wagner M, Wagner H (1996) Preliminary results of uncemented metal on metal stemmed and resurfacing hip replacement arthroplasty. Clin Orthop 329S:S78-88.
28. Wagner M, Wagner H (1999) Mid term results of modern metal - metal articulations in total hip arthroplasty. Paper No OP26 - 02, SICOT Sydney
29. Weber BG (1992) Metall - Metall - Totalprothese des Hüftgelenkes: Zurück in die Zukunft. Z. Orthop. 130:306-9
30. Weber BG. (1996) Experience with the Metasul hip bearing system. Clin Orthop. 329S:S69-77
31. Weber BG (1999) Ten year experience with cemented and uncemented metal/meta devices. Paper No. SYM46-01, SICOT Sidney
32. Willert HG, Buchhorn GH (1999) The biology of the loosening of implants. In: Jacob R Fulford P Horan F (Eds.) European Instructional Course Lectures Vol.4. The British Society of Bone and Joint Surgery, London; 58-82
33. Willert HG, Buchhorn GH, Hess T. (1989) Die Bedeutung von Abrieb und Materialermüdung bei der Prothesenlockerung an der Hüfte. Orthopäde. 18:350-69.
34. Willert HG, Bertram H, Buchhorn GH. (1990) Osteolysis in Alloarthroplasty of the Hip - The Role of Bone Cement Fragmentation. Clin Orthop. 258:108-21.
35. Willert HG, Buchhorn GH, Fayyazi A, Lohmann CH (2000) Histopathologische Veränderungen bei Metall / Metall – Gelenken geben Hinweise auf eine zellvermittelte Überempfindlichkeit - vorläufige Untersuchungsergebnisse von 14 Fällen. Osteologie 9:165-79
36. Willert HG, Buchhorn GH, Fayyazi A, Lohmann CH (2001) Histopathological Changes in Tissues Surrounding Metal/Metal Joints – Signs of Delayed Type Hypersensitivity? (DTH) In: Rieker C, Oberholzer S, Wyss U (Eds.) World Tribology Forum in Arthroplasty, Hans Huber, Bern Göttingen Toronto Seattle, S 147 - 166
37. Zwadlo G, Broker EB, von Bassewitz DB, Feige U, Sorg C. (1985) A monoclonal antibody to a differentiation antigen present on mature human macrophages and absent from monocytes. J Immunol. 134: 487-92.

2.2 Histological and Electron Microscopic Identification and Analysis of Corrosion Products in Periprosthetic Tissue after Total Hip Replacement

M. Huber, G. Reinisch, F. Lintner and K. Zweymüller

Introduction:

In orthopedic surgery one of the most significant complications is the septic or aseptic loosening of cemented or uncemented articular implants. After aseptic loss of implants histologically investigated periprosthetic tissue may contain wear particles such as metals, ceramics or polymers. Wear particle related tissue reactions such as the development of foreign-body granulation tissue with or without inflammation may occur. Furthermore, due to various metabolic diseases endogenously produced deposits with simultaneously induced foreign-body tissue reactions are often observed in synovial tissue.

Our study comprises cases of aseptic loosening of cementless hip-implants consisting of cups made of pure titanium (Ti) and stems made of titanium-alloy (Ti6Al7Nb) with metal-on-metal (CoCrMo-alloy) and metal (CoCrMo-alloy)-on-polyethylene (UHMWPE) bearing components. In some cases the histological investigation of periprosthetic tissue revealed uncommon green or yellow to golden colored foreign bodies. By the use of electron scanning microscopy and energy dispersive x-ray analysis, these particles were identified as deposits rich in chromium, phosphorous and oxygen. This detection indicates the presence of solid corrosion products.

Particles produced by wear or corrosion are associated with an alteration of the environment and the development of periprosthetic osteolysis which may result into the loss of the implant.

Material and Methods:

Periprosthetic tissue including joint pseudocapsule, femoral and acetabular interface membranes of 62 cases of aseptic loosened cementless total hip replacements was histologically investigated.The prosthesis components consisted of cups made of pure titanium (Ti), stems made of titanium-alloy (Ti6Al7Nb) (PlusEndoprothetikAG, Switzerland) [15] with cobalt-chromium molybdenum (Co28Cr6Mo ASTM F 799, Sikomet®) (Plus EndoprothetikAG, Mödling, Austria) [16] metal-on-metal or metal (CoCrMo-alloy)-on-polyethylene (UHMWPE) (from the same manufacturer) bearing components. The investigated tissue was removed at the time of revision operation. The tissue was fixed in 10 per cent buffered formalin, embedded in paraffin, sectioned to a thickness of two micrometers and stained with hematoxylin and eosin. In one case (case 3) iron staining were additionally performed. At least two tissue blocks from each pseudocapsule and tissue blocks from the entire material of acetabular and femoral interface membranes (one to three blocks each) were prepared for investigation. The stained sections were examined by the use of conventional and polarized light microscopy. After the histological screening of 62 cases 4

cases with present uncommon particles were selected for electron microscope analysis and unstained sections were performed. The unstained slides were sputtered with gold prior to investigation and were inspected by the use of a scanning electron microscope (SEM, Philips XL40, Netherlands). In order to identify the elements energy dispersive x-ray analysis (EDX) (EDAX, Netherlands) was used on spots and in a two dimensional area mapping mode.
The clinical data of the four selected cases is summarized in table I.
In one case (case 1) the surfaces of all prosthesis components including ball head and stem with head-neck junction were inspected for the presence of a corrosive attack by the use of a SEM at 15 to 25 keV acceleration voltage with a secondary electron detector. In all cases clinical and microbial investigation was performed in order to avoid infection.

Results:

Tissue of two women and two men (table I), with ages ranging from 50 to 64 years and implantation periods ranging from 13 to 74 months (were found among sixty investigated cases of metal-metal bearing components of CoCrMo and two case of metal (CoCrMo-alloy)-polyethylene(UHMWPE) bearing components) revealed numerous irregularly shaped green and yellow to golden

Case No	Pat/Sex/Age	Side	Diagnosis	Implantation period/months	Material bearing surface	Reason for removal
1	B.S./m/50	Right	Osteoarthritis	13	Metal/metal	Stem-loosening
2	D.H./f/64	Left	Osteoarthritis	52	Metal/metal	Stem/cup-loosening
3	H.A./m/56	Left	Osteoarthritis	60	Metal/polyethylene	Stem-loosening
4	F.M./f/61	Right	Osteoarthritis	74	Metal/metal	Stem/cup-loosening

Table 1

colored, translucent and unstained particles and deposits which ranged in size from sub-micron to 400 µm (figs. 1 and 2). These foreign bodies were present at various amounts in all investigated tissues of these four cases including pseudocapsules as well as femoral and acetabular interface membranes. Some of these deposits of a larger size showed evidence of calcification and were surrounded by dense fibrous tissue (figs. 1 and 2). Other and commonly smaller

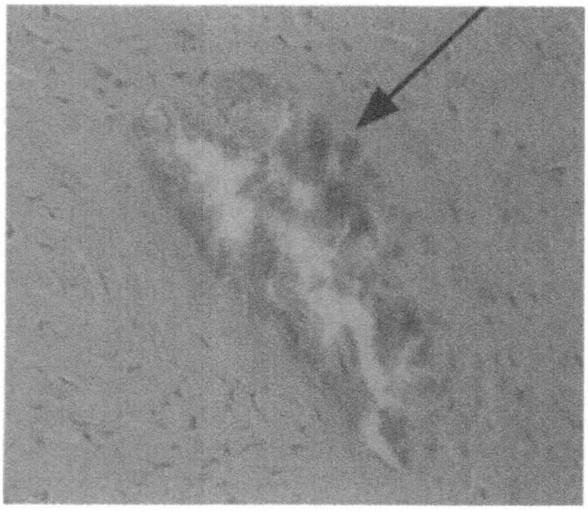

Figure 1:
Histological photograph of dense fibrous tissue surrounding a deposit of [yellow coloured] particles with small calcified area (arrow) (hematoxylin and eosin, x 500).

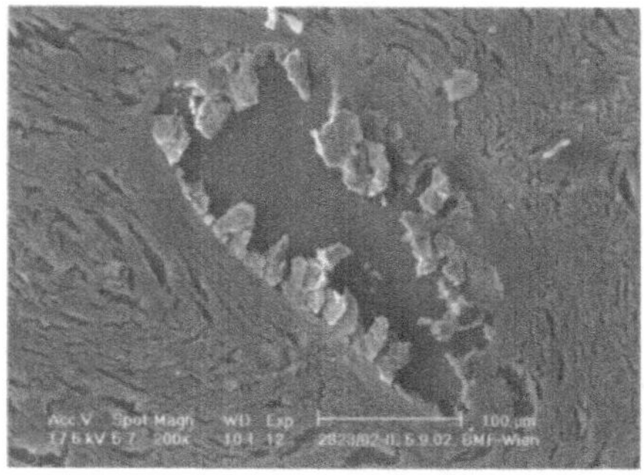

Figure 2:
Scanning electron microscope photograph of the same area of figure 1 (gold-coated, unstained paraffin section).

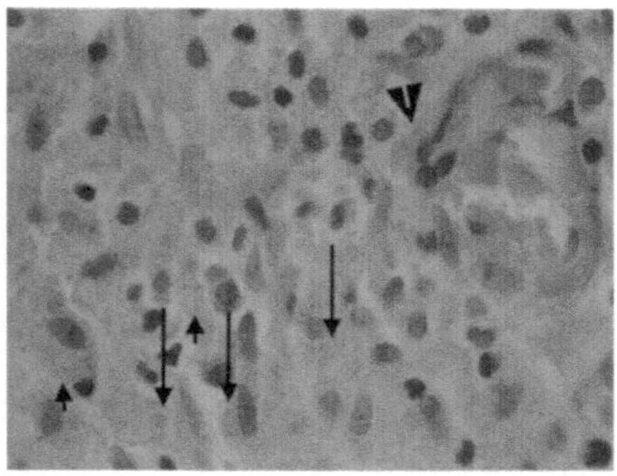

Figure 3:
Aggregate of corrosion products surrounded by foreign body giant cells (arrowhead) and corrosion particles (short arrows) and metal debris (long arrows) within the cytoplasma of mononuclear macrophages. Disseminated infiltrate of lymphocytes and plasma cells (hematoxylin and eosin x 750).

particles however, were surrounded by foreign body granulation tissue with giant cells (fig. 3). The largest deposits were observed within the pseudocapsule itself. In full-colored pictures, focally, small green and yellow particles as well as black pigmented small metallic particles were observed within the cytoplasma of mononuclear macrophages (fig. 3). This was mainly the case in acetabular and femoral interface membranes. Two cases (cases 1 and 3) revealed inflammatory cells in some areas such as lymphocytes and plasma-cells of variable density (fig. 3). In
case one a few eosinophilic granulocytes as well as mast cells were additionally observed. In one case (case 3) some particles presented as irregularly shaped flakes exhibited a birefrigence at examination under polarized light indicating polyethylene wear particles. Periprosthethic tissue including pseudocapsule, femoral and acetabular interface membranes (cases 1, 2 and 3) showed focally necrotic areas and layers of cell debris on the surfaces. Case three revealed a dark blue stained meshed area (fig. 4) which showed iron positivity in special staining. This finding was confirmed by energy-dispersive x-ray revealing iron-rich material. Energy-dispersive x-ray spectra of defined deposits in periprosthetic tissue showed Cr, P and O peaks (fig. 5). This observation indicates the presence of solid corrosion products. Various investigated aggregates of macrophages revealed material rich in Cr, P and also Ti peaks.
There was no evidence of a corrosive attack on the investigated surfaces of all prosthesis components of case one by using a SEM [9].

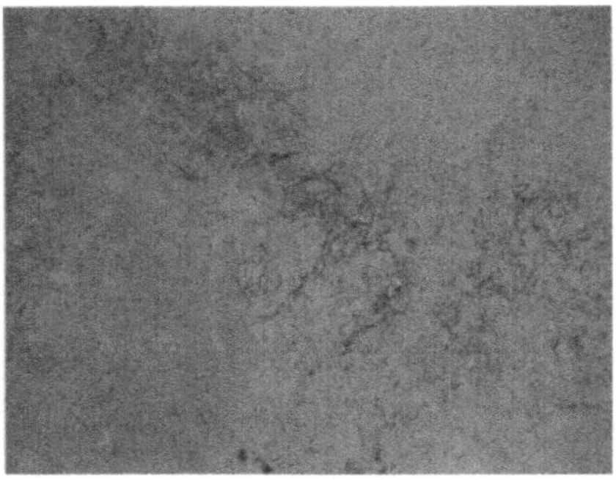

Figure 4:
Moderately lymphoid infiltrated fibrous tissue with mesh-like dark blue area (hematoxylin and eosin x 500).

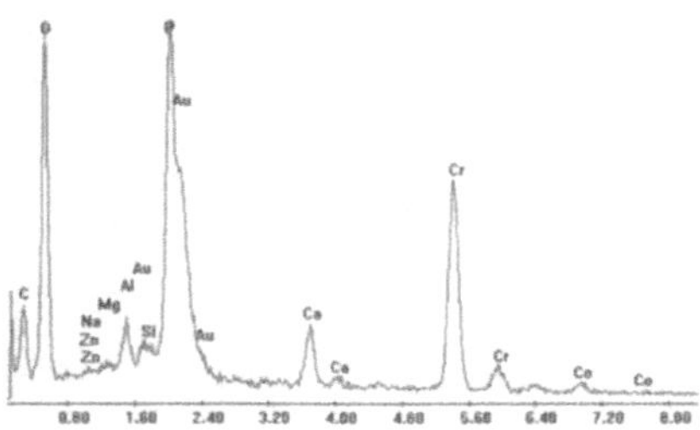

Figure 5:
Energy dispersive x-ray spectrum of corrosion product of figure 2. The photograph is showing a deposit rich in chromium, phosphorous, and oxygen. The peaks indicate the relative proportion of the individual elements.

Discussion:

Deposits of solid products occur widely in tissue either from exogenous sources, for instance after inhalation or surgery, or from endogenous sources due to aging or pathological changes. In synovial fluid of arthritic patients material such as monosodium urate monohydrate, calcium pyrophospate dihydrate, and other crystals have been found [8]. Calcifications may be seen as a consequence not only of osteoarthritis but also of various diseases including metabolic diseases [6].

Particles produced by wear of implants are commonly recognizable and identifiable by routine histological examination [3]. In rare cases electron microscopy and spectroscopic techniques may be required in oder to identify uncommon and rare particles.

Metal is predominantly released by abrasive or third body wear or is affected by chemical corrosion. The exposure of patients with a total hip or knee replacement to metal is significant [1]. Elevated levels of metals have been detected at the implant site, in various organs, in blood and in urine [12]. The systemic distribution of wear particles has shown to be greater in patients with a previously failed implant [12]. The clinical relevance of local and distant distributed wear and corrosion products has been described and discussed previously by several authors [1, 2, 10, 11, 12, 14].

In our study we identified metallic wear products from CoCrMo-alloy and Ti in all investigated cases. As in case one illustrated titanium metallosis may be found even in cases with no visible corrosion of the implant [7]. The yellow and green colored particles lying in part in between the metal laden macrophages as well as within the cytoplasma of macrophages were identified as chromium-phosphate-oxygen rich material indicating solid corrosion products. The cobalt-

chromium molybdenum bearing components were the only source in these implants. Chromium orthophosphate corrosion product has shown to activate macrophages/monocytes. The subsequent release of inflammatory mediators such as cytokines may contribute to periprosthetic osteolysis [5].
In our study, two cases showed additional tissue reactions with severe inflammatory response resembling immunologically determined or somehow metal-induced hypersensitivity reaction [4, 13]. These reactions may be caused by the presence of wear debris. The iron-rich dark blue stained area in case three also reveals an uncommon feature of periprosthetic tissue. To our knowledge, this phenomenon is unclear and has not yet been described in the literature.

In the present study, we are not able to enclose clinical histories of the patients regarding metabolic diseases or data on elevated levels of metals and corrosion products in blood or urine. Nevertheless, we were able to prove that corrosion products were also present in cases of aseptic loosened uncemented stems made of Ti6Al7Nb-alloy which is regarded to be less toxic than Ti6Al4V-alloy. Moreover, we were able to identify corrosion products in four cases of sixty-two investigated cases of aseptic loosening, representing 6.5 per cent. Obviously the occurrence of corrosion products is limited to a small number of patients having received metal articulating surfaces made of CoCrMo-alloy. These findings indicate that corrosion products may develope due to multiple factors such as underlying metabolic changes similar to other mechanism which may result into the endogenous production of deposits with foreign-body tissue reaction such as calcium pyrophosphate.
Particles produced by wear or corrosion may migrate along prosthesis components and reach the articulating surfaces serving as third body wear with consequently increased production of wear debris. These processes are associated with an alteration of the environment and the development of periprosthetic osteolysis which may result into the loss of the implant.

References:

1. Black J (1988). Does corrosion matter? [editorial] (1988). J Bone Joint Surg 70-B (4): 517-520.
2. Jacobs JJ, Gilbert JL, Urban RM (1998). Corrosion of Metal Orthopaedic Implants. J Bone Joint Surg [Am] 80-A (2): 268-282.
3. Lintner F, Zweymüller K, Böhm G, Brand G (1988). Reactions of surrounding tissues to the cementless implant Ti6Al4V after an implantation period of several years. Arch Orthop Trauma Surg 107:357-363.
4. Lintner F, Böhm G, Huber M, Zweymüller K. Synovial tissue following revision total hip replacement with metal-on-metal joints. Histologic, immunohistologic, morphometric and bacteriologic evaluation. Submitted for publication.
5. Lee S-H, Brennan FR, Jacobs JJ, Urban RM, Ragasa DR, Glant TT (1997). Human Monocyte/Macrophage Response to Cobalt-Chromium Corrosion Products and Titanium Particles in Patients with Total Joint Replacements. J Orthop Res 15(1):40-49.
6. Mohr W (2000). Stoffwechselkrankheiten in: Gelenkpathologie. Historische Grundlagen, Ursachen und Entwicklungen von Gelenkleiden und ihre Pathomorphologie, Springer Verlag ISBN 3-540-65971-4, pp: 159-214.
7. Nasser S, Campell PA, Kilgus D, Kossovsky N, Amstutz HC (1990). Cementless total joint arthroplasty prostheses with titanium-alloy articular surfaces. A human retrieval analysis. Clin Orthop 261:171-185.

8. Reginate AJ. Calcium Oxalate and Other Crystals or Particles Associated with Arthritis (1993) Arthritis and Allied Conditions, Volume 2, twelfth edition, McCarty, Koopman, Eds., pp. 1873-1893 Lea & Felbiger Philadelphia London.
9. Reinisch G, Judmann KP, Lhotka C, Lintner F, Zweymüller K (2003). Retrieval study of uncemented metal-metal hip prostheses revised for early loosening. Accepted for Biomaterials 24:1081-1091.
10. Sulzer Medizinaltechnik 0811 (1990). Mitteilung - Nr. M 4800.
11. Urban RM, Jacobs JJ, Gilbert JL, Galante JO (1994). Migration of Corrosion Products from Modular Hip Prostheses. J Bone Joint Surg [Am] 76-A, 9:1345-59.
12. Urban RM, Jacobs JJ, Tomlinson MJ, Gavrilovic J, Black J, Peoc´h M (2000). Dissemination of wear particles to the liver, spleen, and abdominal lymph nodes of patients with hip or knee replacement. J Bone Joint Surg [Am] 82(4):455-6.
13. Willert HG, Buchhorn GH, Fayyazi A, Lohmann CH (2000). Histopathologische Veränderungen bei Metall/Metall-Gelenken geben Hinweise auf eine zellvermittelte Überempfindlichkeit. Osteologie 9(3):165-179.
14. Winter GD (1974). Tissue reactions to metallic wear and corrosion products in human patients. J Biomed Mater Res 8:11-26.
15. Zweymüller K (ed.) (2002). 20 Years of Zweymüller Hip Endoprosthesis. Verlag Hans Huber ISBN 3-456-83431-4.
16. Zweymüller K (ed.) (1997). Die Metall-Metall-Paarung SIKOMET. Verlag Hans Huber ISBN 3-456-82781-4.

2.3 Analysis of Serum Cobalt levels and kinetics in 282 Patients with a Metal-Metal Friction Hip Prosthesis

J.-Y. Lazennec

Introduction

Serum cobalt, chromium and titanium levels and kinetics are studied to evaluate evolution of metal-metal hip prosthesis .

Material and Methods

282 patients with metal-metal T.H.P.(titanium stem, CrCoMo friction couple) were included through a prospective study (follow-up 24 - 72 months). Serum cobalt and chromium levels were determined by electrothermal atomic absorption spectrometry (detection limit: 1 nmol/L ~ 0.05 µg/l). Titanium levels were simultaneously studied by inductively-coupled plasma atomic emission spectrometry (detection limit : 30 nmol/l ; 1.4 µg/l).

Results

Mean and median values of cobalt chromium and titanium levels showed variation with follow-up.
Four patterns of serum cobalt and chromium kinetics were seen (decreasing frequency):

- type I, low short-term levels (<50nmol/l) ; unvarying long-term levels
- type II, high short-term levels (> 50nmol/l) ; decreasing long-term levels
- type III, low short-term levels ; increasing long-term levels
- type IV, very high short-term levels and even higher long-term levels.

Bilateral THP present specific evolution with increased levels after second implantation. Abnormal titanium levels could be correlated with femoral problems.

Discussion and conclusion

Correlation of serum cobalt levels with wear of the friction couple is difficult. Serum cobalt kinetics identified four patterns with possible prognostic significance: types I through III indicate favorable outcomes. Type IV is of concern and should prompt a search for a cause of premature wear or other biological problems. Simultaneous evaluation of cobalt and titanium levels are important for assessing head-neck interface mechanical evolution and/or femoral loosening .

Summary and conclusion

Serum cobalt, chromium and titanium kinetics identified 4 patterns with possible significance for wear and femoral loosening in 282 metal metal THP.

2.4 Tissue Reactions to Ceramic Wear Debris: Clinical Cases vs. Animal Model

G. Maccauro, C. Piconi, F. Muratori, V. De Santis and W. Burger

1. Foreword

Wear is the main limiting factor to artroprostheses' lifetime: at local level the cascade of events induced by reactions to wear debris is still the most frequent cause of implant failure and revision, while the ions released by wear debris originate systemic reactions, depending on their transport by the blood flow to peripheral organs, thanks to the vascularization of the reactive membrane surrounding the implant. (Schmalzried and Callaghan 1999, Urban et al. 2000, Archimbeck et al. 2000, Fisher et al 2001, Sedel 2001, Dumbleton et al. 2002).

Few papers are dealing with the local and systemic toxicity of load bearing ceramics, and very few are dealing with the chronic reactions including carcinogenesys (Ryu et al. 1987, Ito et al.1993, Catelas et al.1999, Mebouta et al. 2000, Lohmann et al.2002). Namely, load-bearing ceramics are characterised by a fine structure, made by micron- or sub micron-size grains. This feature is a key factor in improving mechanical properties, but concerns were raised about the toxicity of fine wear debris. As ceramic joints are intended for use in younger patient (Black J 1997, Schmalzried 2001), hence the ones with longer life expectations, the study of the chronic effects of small particles becomes more and more relevant (Archimbeck et al. 2000).

In this paper we compare the observation of biological reactions made in an animal model of chronic release of ceramic particles with the observations made in case of release of ceramic particles from THR joints due to wear or fracture.

The in-vivo model of particle release that we used is based on the implant of porous pellets formed by low cohesion grains in the patellar tendon of rabbits. Due to their poor cohesion, when rubbing against an articular cartilage, grains can be easily and progressively detached from the surface of the pellet and released to the joint space all along the nursing time of the animals. In this paper we would like to present the first results obtained, in comparison with observations made in cases of clinical failure of ceramic devices.

2. Materials and Methods

2.1 In-vivo experiments

Ceramic pellets (Ø 8 x 2 mm) were manufactured from Alumina and Y-TZP (Tetragonal Zirconia Polycrystal) precursors by cold pressing followed by pressure less sintering route. The stating powders were selected according to ISO 6474 and ISO 13536 standards.

Pellets are characterised by high porosity (44 ± 4 %) obtained stopping the sintering process during the development phase of the necks between the grains of the starting powder. In such a way, the cohesion among grains in the pellets is very low. Alumina pellets had average grain size 0.3 mm, density 2.4 g/cm3 (60% T.D), while Y-TZP pellets had average grain size 0.03 mm, density 3.2 g/cm3 (52% T.D.)

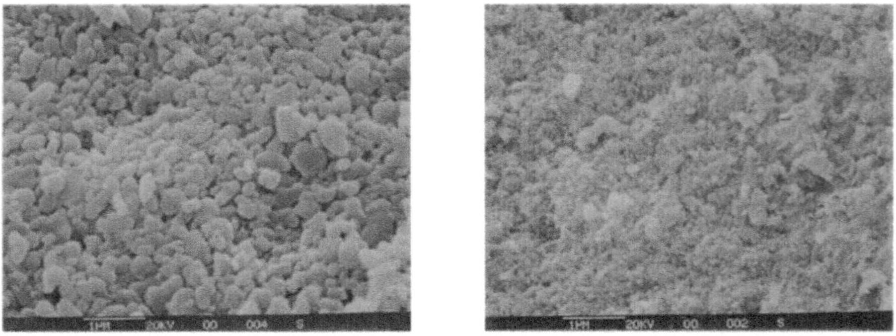

a) b)

Figure 1:
Typical fracture surface of porous pellets: a) Alumina; b) Y-TZP.

Sixteen New Zealand White adult rabbits of both sex, minimum weight 3.3 Kg were used for the experiment. 12 Y- TZP pellets were inserted into surgically created defects under both the patellar tendons of 6 rabbits of the first group. The same procedure was performed on either group of 6 rabbits, using 12 Alumina plates. Two rabbits underwent the surgical procedure without the implant of ceramics, and were used as controls. Animals were maintained in a pathogen-free environment.
Two and six months after surgery the animals were killed. Knee joints were harvested and submitted to macroscopic and x-rays examinations. Retrieved knees were divided in 2 groups: specimens of the first group were decalcified with EDTA, dehydrated and embedded in paraffin, sectioned and stained with hematoxylin-eosin, and observed with transmitted and polarised light microscopy. Pellets of the second group were removed, fixed in Karnosky's solution dehydrated with alcohol, and examined by SEM (Philips 515).
One animal of each group (Alumina, Y-TZP) for each implantation time, was submitted to autopsy. Lungs, liver, kidney, spleen and hearth were harvested, and the external and internal surfaces of these organs underwent macroscopic examinations. Lungs were injected with China ink for detecting tumours. Histological analysis was carried out on specimens of the organs fixed in 10% formalin, embedded in paraffin, cut in 3-5 mm thin sections, stained with haematoxylin-eosin and resorcin-fuchsin.

2.2 Retrieved tissues

The results obtained in-vivo were put in comparison with the observations made in periprosthetic tissues collected during three THR revision surgeries, related to the fracture of the ball head in an alumina-PE coupling (case 1), to the fracture of the zirconia-ball head in a zirconia-PE coupling (case 2) and to the failure of an alumina-alumina coupling due to wear (case 3).
Periprosthetic tissues were analysed according to a specific protocol of retrieved implants previously reported (Maccauro et al. 1998, 2000). Briefly, tissue specimens were divided in 3 groups: the first was fixed in 10% formalin, decalcified in ethylenediaminetetracetate (EDTA), dehydrated and embedded in paraffin, sectioned and stained with hematoxylin-eosin, and observed with transmitted and polarised light microscopy; the second was embedded in epoxy resin cut in thin sections and stained with toluidine blue; the third was fixed in Karnosky's solution dehydrated with alcohol, covered with colloidal palladium,

stuck onto a metal support and observed to SEM (Philips 515) coupled with energy-dispersive X-ray analysis (EDAX) to identify shape and size and chemical composition of particles observed.

3. RESULTS

3.1 In-vivo experiments

Macroscopic analysis of the retrieved rabbit knees showed the presence of large fibrosis around the joint at 2 weeks after operation. After 8 weeks knees appeared ankilotic in flexion. X-ray showed the presence of ceramic fragments in the articular spaces. Histologic sections showed ceramic particles within histiocyte-like cells as finely dispersed intracytoplasmatic granules or as yellow-brown bigger granules in extracellular matrix of a synovial-like tissue. Zirconia grains appeared or as dark structure in the intercellular space, or as microscopic yellow amber grains found in intra or in extra cellular sites, scattered in areas of cell reaction containing mononuclear histiocyte-like cells. Giant cells containing bigger ceramic fragments were rarely seen. Membranes were characterised by avascular fibrous tissue. The peripheral organs did not show pathological changes neither tumours (Figure 2 a,b,c,d).

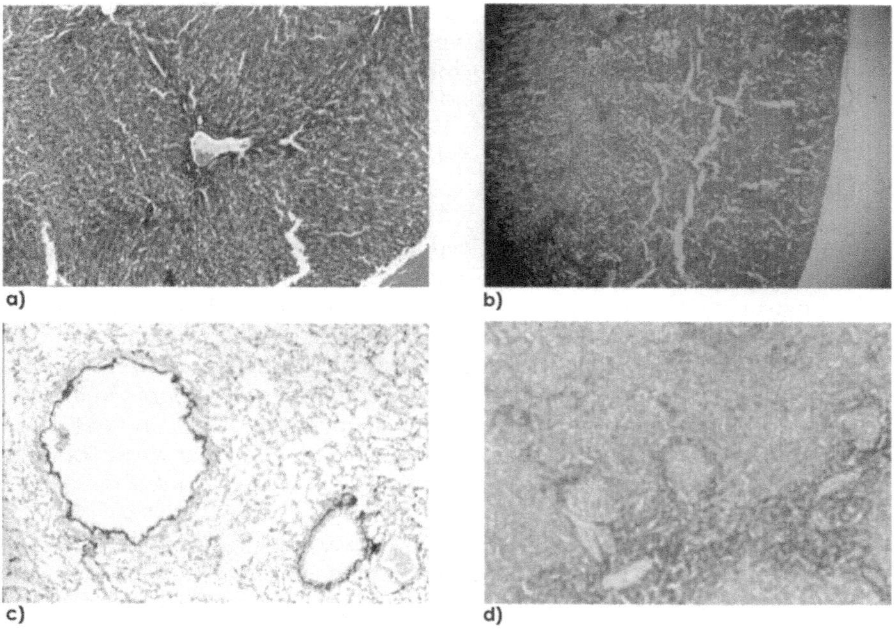

Figure 2:
Histologic sections of internal organs: a) liver; b) kidney; c) lung; d) spleen.

3.2 Retrieved tissues

3.2.1 Case 1

Histologic sections showed a large amount of debris from different sources in a pseudovillous membrane. At higher magnification oligonuclear cells contacting metal particles in a stroma poor in vessel were observed. PE debris characterised by typical birifrangent aspect in polarised light were contained into polynuclear giant cells. Ceramic debris were observed within histiocyte-like cells as finely dispersed intracytoplasmatic granules or as yellow-brown bigger granules in extracellular matrix of synovial-like tissue. SEM put in evidence that alumina particle could be alone or aggregated when in submicron size, probably due electrostatic reactions. EDAX confirmed the presence of alumina and of titanium.

3.2.2 Case 2

A wide metallosis was seen in the periprosthetic membrane. A pseudovillous membrane with many mononuclear cells phagocyting metal particles in a stroma rich in fibres was put in evidence in histological sections. Few vessels containing metal particles were also seen. Large areas of necrobiosis were visible. Zirconia grains appeared or as dark structure in the intercellular space or as microscopic yellow amber grain found in intra or in extra cellular sites scattered in areas of cell reaction containing mononuclear histiocyte-like cells. No giant cells were seen. Fragments were birifrangent at polarised light microscopy, but this polarisation was different from the PE one.

3.2.3 Case 3

Histologic sections showed a pseudovillous periprosthetic tissue membrane. At higher magnification ceramic debris were observed within histiocyte-like cells as finely dispersed intracytoplasmatic granules or as yellow-brown bigger granules in extracellular matrix of a sinovial-like tissue. In this case also SEM confirmed that alumina particles may occur alone and/or as aggregates.

4. Discussion

The method usually followed to investigate tissue reactions to particulate consists in injecting powder samples of the material under examination into the articular joints or in other sites of animals (Rae et al 1986). This situation is very different from the clinical one, as the production of debris take place along all the prosthesis lifetime, and in the case of ceramics, at a very low wear rate. As the crucial point is to investigate the chronic reactions to wear debris (metals, or ceramics) that are more and more relevant in younger patients, that will make use of the implant for longer times (e.g. thirty years, or more), many injections with a very low grains concentration may be the solution able to model the clinical situation.

Another method for evaluating the in vivo biological response to particles consists in packing the powders on a suitable carrier, like e.g. into the groove in a PMMA cylinder, and in implanting the carrier into the joint (Kubo et al 1999). Particles are released into the joint space during the joint motion, but this may imply the risk of contamination due the wear of the material of the powder carrier.

The method that we used has the advantage of the absence of contamination, but has limits depending on the animal activity, because the particle release is originated by the joint motion. The reaction to the ceramic particles in the articular joints was the formation of fibrous tissue, characterized by the absence of blood vessels, and by a cellular reaction depending on the size of the particles released. We observed in our specimens the presence of few giant cells, clearly related to ceramics only. The presence of foreign body cells in the periprosthetic membranes is considered characteristic of implant failure. Foreign body cells are typically associated to polyethylene, PMMA, and large metal particles, and rarely to ceramics: in this latter case, the presence of giant cells was depending on the presence of alumina than to zirconia debris (Lerouge et al, 1995). In our model, we did not observe differences in the response to the two materials, notwithstanding the differences in grain size between the two ceramics implanted, while rare giant cells in association to PE debris were observed in tissues retrieved in the three clinical cases reported.

The use as reference of tissue collected in cases of failures may constitute a limit in our study, but it must be observed that well performing ceramic-PE joints will likely contain mostly PE-debris, while well performing ceramic-on-ceramic joints will contain only little particles, not useful for comparison: to perform serial biopsies on well doing patients will be not feasible for many reasons (e.g. ethic and legal).

The periprosthetic membranes were poorly vascularized. Vascularization has a critical role in the transport of debris from the site of production into the peripheral organs (Willert 1977). The presence of many vessels in the periprosthetic membrane containing debris may be considered an inflammatory aspect of the tissue response, related to the cytotoxicity of the particles and to the release of humoral factors after phagocitosis by macrophages. More recently the same Author confirmed these findings, showing that vessels in the periprosthetic membrane are typical of reaction to metals (Willert et al. 1996). It is remarkable the agreement of these results with the ones reported by Sedel (Sedel 1992), that measured significant lower level of PGE 2 in membranes containing ceramics debris than in membranes surrounding metal or polyethylene debris. In previous works, some of the Authors of the present paper reported results in agreement with the Willert's ones: they observed the absence of vessels in the pseudovillous membrane in case of massive release of PE wear debris (Nizegorodcew et al 1997) in absence of metals , as well as in the periprosthetic tissue surrounding alumina particles in alumina-alumina joints (De Santis et al 2001). This latter paper hypothesize that ceramics induce less inflammatory reaction than metals, and that ceramic debris did not migrate from the production site due to the absence of vessels.

The few vessels observed in the three clinical cases taken into account in this work were containing metal particles, likely due to rubbing of the ceramic fragments against the metallic taper.

On the basis of our results, and according to paper reported in above, we consider that vessels observed may be specific of a reaction to metals, as e.g. is the necrobiosis observed in periprosthetic tissue, that according to Willert (1977) is also related to metals.

Histologic sections of the periprosthetic tissue showed that reaction to ceramic particles is dependent on their size. A threshold was observed for diameter 8 μm: the wear debris having diameter lower than the threshold being intracellular, while bigger ones were extracellular. These observations are in agreement with the ones reported previously on other materials, e.g. metals (Maccauro et al., 1998) and PE (Nizegodorcew et al. 1997).

5. Conclusions

Accepting limits due to animal activity, the method used, consisting in implanting low-cohesion pellets made out the material under test in a joint, in such a way that the pellet may loose grains simulating wear debris by rubbing against, e.g. a cartilage, may be a useful tool in screening the in vivo biological response to wear debris.

We found a good correspondence between the characteristics of the tissue reactions to debris observed in the in-vivo model in rabbits and the tissue reaction observed in clinical cases, e.g. the lack of vascularization of the tissue, and to cellular population.

In absence of metals, we did not observe vascularization of the tissue: this is well in agreement with data reported in our previous papers, and with the results published by other Authors, leading us to conclude that vascularization of the granulation tissue is a reaction typical of the presence of metal debris. This finding shows that the use of ceramics in arthroprosthes joints leads to reduce the equivalent joint space accessible to debris, a significant advantage for the joints making use of ceramics on the ones making use of metals.

References

1. Archibeck MJ, Jacobs JJ, Black J (2000) Alternate bearing surfaces in total joint arthroplasty: biologic considerations. Clin Orthop 379:12-21
2. Black J (1997) Prospects for alternate Bearing surfaces in total hip replacement arthroplasty of the hip. In: Puhl W (ed) Performance of the wear couple BIOLOX Forte in hip arthroplasty, Enke Verlag, Stuttgart, pp 2-10
3. Catelas I, Petit A, Zukor DJ, Marchand R, Yahia LH, Huk OL(1999) Induction of macrophage apoptosis by ceramic and polyethylene particles in vitro. Biomaterials 20:625-630
4. De Santis E, Maccauro G, Proietti L, et al. (2001) Histologic and ultrastructural analysis of Alumina wear debris. In: Giannini S, Moroni A (eds) Bioceramics 13, TransTech Publ, Zurich, 995-998
5. Dumbleton JH, Manley MT, Edidin AA (2002) A literature review of the association between wear rate and osteolysis in total hip arthroplasty. J Arthroplasty 17:649-661
6. Fisher J, Stone MH, Tipper JL, Ingham E. (2001) Wear debris generation with metal-on-polyethilene, Metal-on Metal, Ceramic-on-Ceramic hip prostheses. In: Rieker C, Oberholzer S, Wyss U (eds) World Tribology Forum in Arthroplasty. Hans Huber, Bern, pp 25-30
7. ISO 6474 (1994) Implants for surgery - Ceramic materials based on high purity alumina. International Standard Organization
8. ISO 13536 (1997) Implants for surgery - Ceramic materials based on yttria-stabilized tetragonal zirconia (Y-TZP). International Standard Organization
9. Ito A, Tateishi T, Niwa S, et al. (1993) In vitro evaluation of the cytocompatibility of wear particles generated by UHMWPE-zirconia friction. Clin Mater 12:203-209
10. Kubo T, Sawada K, Hirakava K, et al (1999) Histiocite reaction in rabbit femurs to UHMWPE, metal, and ceramic particles in different sizes. J Biomed Mater Res 45:363-369

11. Lerouge S, Yahia L'H, Huk O, et al. (1995) Wear debris and inflammatory response in tissues around failed alumina ceramic-on-ceramic hip prostheses. Bioceramics 8, Wilson J, Hench LL, Greenspan D (eds), Elsevier Publ., Oxford, UK, pp 145-150
12. Lohmann CH, Dean DD, Koster G, et al. (2002) Ceramic and PMMA particles differentially affect osteoblast phenotype. Biomaterials 23:1855-1863.
13. Maccauro G, Romanini E, Dall'Acqua D, et al (1998) Una scheda di valutazione degli impianti protesici rimossi GIOT 24:375-381
14. Maccauro G, Romano G, Nizegorodcew T, et al (1998) Considerazioni sull'influenza della dimensione delle particelle nella patologia da detriti metallici e plastici GIOT 24: 579-583
15. Maccauro G, Piconi C, Pilloni L, et al. (2000) Surface analysis of a femoral stem after failure of total hip replacement. Int Orthop (SICOT) 24:231-233
16. Mebouta Nkamgueu E, Adnet JJ, Bernard J, et al.(2000) In vitro effects of zirconia and alumina particles on human blood monocyte-derived macrophages: X-ray microanalysis and flow cytometric studies. J Biomed Mater Res 52: 587-594
17. Nizegorodcew T, Gasparini G, Maccauro G, et al. Massive osteolysis induced by high molecular weigh polyethylene debris (1997). Int Orthop (SICOT) 21:14-18.
18. Rae T (1986) The macrophage to implant materials with special reference to those used in Orthopaedics. CRC Crit Rev Biocomp 2: 97
19. Ryu RK, Bovill E G, Skinner HB, et al (1987) Soft tissue sarcoma associated with aluminum oxide ceramic total hip arthroplasty. A case report. Clin Orthop 216: 207-212
20. Schmalzried TP, Callaghan JJ (1999) Current Concepts Review: Wear in total hip and knee replacements. J Bone Joint Surg 81-A:115-136
21. Schmalzried TP (2001) Patient activity and wear. In: Rieker C, Oberholzer S, Wyss U (eds) World Tribology Forum in Arthroplasty. Hans Huber, Bern, pp 31-34
22. Sedel L, Simeon J, Meunier A, Villette JM, Launay SM b(1992) Prostaglandin E2 level in tissue surrounding aseptic failed total hips. Effects of materials Arch Orthop Trauma Surg 111: 225-258
23. Sedel L (2001) Tribology of hip joint replacement. In: Surgical techniques in Orthopedics and Traumatology, Edition Scientifiques et Medicales Elsevier SAS, Paris, 55-430-E-10
24. Urban RM, Jacobs JJ, Tomlinson MJ, et al (2000) Dissemination of wear particles to the liver, spleen, and abdominal lymph nodes of patients with hip or knee replacement. J Bone Joint Surg 82-A: 457-477
25. Willert MG (1977) Reactions of the articular capsule to wear products of artificial joint prostheses. J Biomed Mat Res 11:157-164
26. Willert MG, Broback LG, Buchan GM, et al (1996) Crevice corrosion of cemented titanium alloy stems in total hip replacement. Clin Orthop 333:51-75

2.5 Immuno-allergological Aspects of Adverse Reactions in Total Joint Replacement

P. Thomas and B. Summer

Introduction

Apart from the inflammatory reaction upon surgery itself, the immunological biocompatibility of a given material varies with factors like the site of implantation, immunogenicity of implant components, and the individual reactivity of the host [1, 2, 3, 4]. A number of investigations have focused on cytotoxic, genotoxic and allergological effects of wear debris and metal ions [1, 5, 6, 7, 8], but it is still controversal to which extent adverse reactions to metallic implants are due to a specific immune response. In some cases localized or generalized eczema, local swelling, recurrent urticaria or even implant loosening have been attributed to hypersensitivity to implant components [2, 4, 9, 10, 11, 12, 13]. However, the number of those patients seems to be lower than the nickel, cobalt or chromium sensitisation rates in the general population ranging between 2 – 10% [14, 15, 16]. The specific inflammatory immune response largely depends on T-lymphocytes activated by T cell receptor interaction with antigens, e.g. peptide-associated metal ions. Thus, lymphocyte reactivity is studied in vivo by patch testing and in vitro with regard to delayed type hypersensitivity associated Thelper1 (Th1) phenotype and mediator production. For example, in a patient with osteosynthesis and impaired fracture healing a dichromate allergy was proven with concomitant periimplantar oligoclonal (antigen driven) T-cell infiltrate and Th1 characteristic interferon-g production [17]. In this article potential mechanisms of hypersensitivity reactions and methods to prove the link between intolerance of implanted devices and contact allergy to one of their components are discussed.

Components of hypersensitivity reactions

Hypersensitivity reactions were classified into four types by Coombs and Gell : Type I to III reactions are antibody mediated and distinguished by the different types of antigens recognized and the different classes of antibody involved. Immediate type (type I) allergic reactions are mediated by IgE, which induces mast-cell/basophil activation and leads to urticaria/anaphylaxis, allergic rhinoconjunctivitis or asthma. Type II and III reactions are mediated by IgG, which can engage cytotoxic and complement-driven, phagocytic mechanisms. Type IV reactions (delayed type hypersensitivity, DTH) to low molecular weight substances are T-cell mediated coinvolving macrophages or eosinophils in the inflammatory response. They include tuberculin reaction, contact dermatitis or pseudolymphoma formation due to Nickel or chromium / cobalt.

Favoring factors for hypersensitivity reactions

The immunogenic / allergenic potency of a given substance

This is often linked with its capacity to provoke irritation or to penetrate the (muco)cutaneous barrier, as shown by the enzymatic properties of the major house dust mite allergen Der p 1. With regard to ceramic (Al_2O_3) surface no such effect was found in coculture studies with human peripheral blood cells [18] (Tab.1).
Concerning arthroplasty, irritative properties can be found for example for not polymerized acrylates, additives like benzoyl peroxide or some metal ions. In contrast to high levels of nickel, chromium and cobalt being rather immunosuppressive or toxic, low exposure may directly induce expression of adhesion molecules on vascular endothelium. Thus recruitment of proinflammatory cells into the tissue is favored [19]. In addition nickel ions may influence the phenotype of dendritic cells and thereby alter/favor the immune response to it [20]. With regard to metal recognition by T-cells it has been speculated that nickel (hapten) modified proteins are "seen" by the T-cell receptor (TCR) in the context of MHC class II molecules [21]. In the case of particular phenotype e.g. accessory molecule expression of antigen presenting cells a preferential induction of DTH-characteristic TH1-responses with production of IFN-γ and TNF-α may result.

Contact allergen	number of reactors / 250 individuals	(%)
Nickel(II)-sulfate x 6 H_2O	43	17,2
Fragrance mix	38	15,2
Balsam of Peru	33	13,2
Thiomersal	26	10,4
Lanolin alcohol	20	8,0
Mercury (II)-amide-chloride	17	6,8
p-Phenylendiamine	15	6,0
Dibromdicyanobutan, Phenoxyethanol	11	4,4
Colophonium	10	4,0
Potassium Dichromate	6	2,4

Table 1:
Most frequent contact allergens in a comparative serie of 250 patients of a dermatology clinic.

Properties of implant materials

The release of potential allergens like nickel, chromium or cobalt depends on composition, surface modification, chemical and physical corrosion factors. Low pH and low oxygenation of adjacent tissue may influence metallic surface – even leading to titanium release in surrounding tissue [22]. "Hidden" contamination of titanium materials by nickel may result from manufacturing processes. Formation of particulate debris may greatly enhance the contact surface to metals contained in it and phagocytosis will favor the persistance in the tissue [6]. Whereas the tribological behaviour of bioceramics is reported to minimize the wear rate [23], articulating surfaces depending on different other material combinations are linked with more or less wear formation. Amount, composition and size of different particulate species will lead to a varying degree of macrophage, fibroblast and osteoblast response [1, 8, 24, 25, 26, 27, 28]. The macrophage reaction to the particle load includes production of IL-6, TNF-α and PGE_2, creating an inflammatory bone-resorbing environment. In addition potential antigens are processed by tissue macrophages and stimulate T-cells.

The tissue environment
In a non sensitized individual antigen presenting cells (APC) in the tissue first need to be activated by "alarm" signals or proinflammatory mediators in order to then take up the potential antigen and transport it to regional lymph nodes. Then activation of T-lymphocytes, recirculation and reentry into inflamed tissue by preferential expression of homing receptors will follow. The ease of sensitisation seems to differ between various organs, the skin and subcutaneous range being most susceptible. With regard to periimplantar tissue, it is only partly known which signals induce local APC-activation for primary sensitisation of T-lymphocytes: "Pseudo-lymph follicles" have been observed in periimplantar tissue; particle-loaded macrophages have been found in regional lymph nodes; denseT-lymphocytic infiltrates in perimplantar tissue have been observed. With regard to already metal-allergic patients, the attraction of circulating specific T-cells into the tissue is speculated – however, at this point important factors like specific homing receptors and chemoattractants still need to be identified.

Adjuvans factors
Proinflammatory effects are mediated by particles or microbial constituents like lipopolysaccharide or DNA fragments, macrophages being one of the target cells [29]. Due to other preexisting allergic sensitisations peri-/postoperative inflammation may develop and facilitate sensitisation to implant constituents. Examples are allergic reactions to disinfectants, to antibiotics or natural rubber latex.

Patient derived factors
Atopic individuals are characterized by a genetically determined tendency to develop diseases like allergic rhinoconjunctivitis, asthma or atopic eczema. The irritable skin is often a typical feature. A genetical susceptibility for metal allergy or for development of delayed type or granulomatous foreign body reactions is discussed by some authors [30, 31]. Interindividual differences in the apoptotic threshold of T-Lymphocytes upon exposure to metal ions, e.g. nickel, have been reported recently [32].

Clinical examples and diagnostics

Internal or "hematogenous" exposure to the relevant allergen may provoke relapse of dermatitis in about 10% of individuals with proven metal contact allergy. The existance of this so called systemically induced contact dermatitis has been reproducibly proven by oral challenge studies [33, 34]. In nickel allergic patients reacting to oral provocation test with nickel, a higher frequency of circulating specific T-cells has been found [35]. A source of exposure may not only be alimentary uptake but also metal release from implanted devices. There are several clinical reports of eczema reactions, both local and remote, to metallic implants [10, 36, 37, 38, 39].

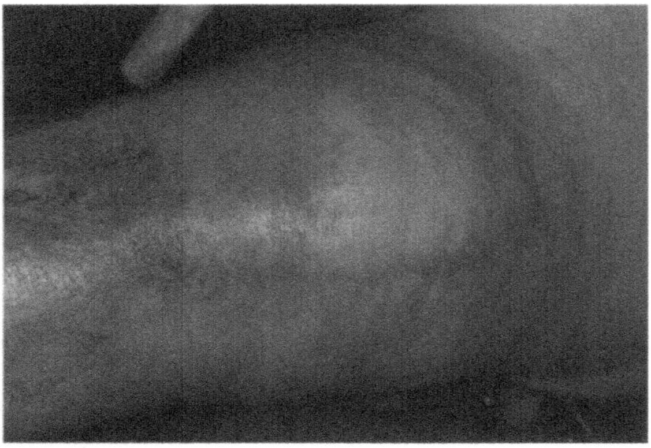

Figure 1:
Recurrent local swelling and eczema upon knee arthroplasty. Delayed type hypersensitivity to molybdenum and Benzoyl-peroxide was found.

Figure 1 shows a patient with recurrent swelling, local eczema and pain upon knee arthroplasty. Allergological diagnostics revealed a contact allergy to benzoyl peroxide (component of the bone cement) and to molybdenum.

It is difficult to estimate the actual incidence of allergic responses to implanted metallic devices that contribute to patient morbidity and to impairment of the implant function. A first step to improve available information is actually done by the authors of this article by establishing in Munich a central documentation office for implant related allergic reactions in association with the German Contact Allergy Society (DKG). Up to now, case reports show patients with local or systemic intolerance reactions [40] and in larger study populations rather low incidence of allergy-mediated cutaneous or orthopedic complications are reported [10, 12, 41]. Carlsson and Möller for example retrospectively examined patients with contact allergy to metals proven before implantation of metallic devices [11] Out of the 39 patients one had developed exzema of the feet and papular itching eruption of the trunk, both subsiding only after removal of the osteosynthesis material used to treat an ankle fracture. Being deceased at the time of retrospective analysis, this patient like others could not be included. Out of the 18 remaining patients three had developed eczema reactions, but also had preexisting eczema. In two patients mechanical loosening of the implanted devices was seen. Some patients even showed no more cutaneous reactivity upon renewed skin testing at the time of follow-up. Thus, as conclusion, an overall good implant tolerance was reported.

However open questions remain, since: Unusual manifestations of allergic reactions may not always be recognized as such [13, 42]; substances available for skin testing do not always cover all implant components; additional analysis of the periimplantar tissue or peripheral blood cell reactivity can not always be performed. In the case of a patient with implant loosening and local discomfort, the demonstration of periimplantar oligoclonal (antigen-driven) T-cell infiltrate together with Th1-type mediator production helped to link the intolerance to a proven dichromate allergy [17]. With regard to clinical allergological diagnostics, history and clinical picture are supplemented by epicutaneous testing. Actually, a new panel of test substances is prepared by the German Contact Allergy Society. The use of aliquots of implant material for skin testing is under investigation by th author of this article.

The testwise subcutaneous implantation of aliquots of the material in question is however still under discussion. In vitro methods like lymphocyte activation assays do not prove an allergy but rather indicate "sensitisation" and thus have to be interpreted with caution. However, lymphocyte transformation assays using peripheral blood mononuclear cells (PBMC) of nickel-allergic individuals can demonstrate specific in vitro reactivity to nickel [43]. Despite no preferential association with HLA-DR, -DQ or –DP specificity has been proven, a restricted use of T-cell-receptor (TCR) phenotype has been shown in nickel reactive lymphocytes [44, 45].

Outlook

It is evident, that components of most implants can be released into the tissue [6, 46, 47, 48]. In some conditions a specific immune response may arise against these components and create clinically apparent intolerance reactions. An interdisciplinary approach including cellular and molecular biology in vitro and clinical follow up will help to optimize implant materials and to identify patient derived predisposing conditions. With regard to allergological diagnostics, a new panel of test substances is prepared by the German Contact Allergy Society (DKG) and a centralized data collection office regarding "implant allergy" is established in Munich in association with the DKG.

Literature

1. Rodgers K, Klykken P, Jacobs J, Frondoza C, Tomazic V, Zelikoff J. Immunotoxicity of medical devices. Fundam Appl Toxicol 1997; 36: 1-14
2. Black J. Allergic foreign body response In: Biological performance of materials – fundamentals of biocompatibility, 3d ed., Marcel Dekker New York, Basel: 1999; 215-232
3. Janeway CA, Travers P, Walport M, Capra JD (eds.). Immunobiology: the immune system in health and disease, 4th ed., Elsevier Science Ltd. London: 1999; 461-488
4. Thomas P. Allergological aspects of implant biocompatibility. In: Bioceramics in hip joint replacement (eds. Willmann G, Zweymüller K), Thieme Stuttgart New York: 2000; 117-121
5. Büdinger L, Hertl M. Immunologic mechanisms in hypersensitivity reactions to metal ions: an overview. Allergy 2000; 55: 108-115
6. Merritt K, Brown S. Distribution of cobalt chromium wear and corrosion products and biologic reactions. Clin Orthop Rel Res 1996; 329: S233-S243
7. Wever DJ, Veldhuizen AG, Sanders MM, Schakenraad JM, van Horn JR. Cytotoxic, allergic and genotoxic activity of a nickel-titanium alloy. Biomaterials 1997; 18: 1115-1120
8. Willert HG, Semlitsch M. Tissue reactions to plastic and metallic wear products. Clin Orthop Rel Res 1996; 333: 4-14
9. Carlsson A, Magnussen B, Möller H (1980) Metal sensitivity in patients with metal to plastic total hip arthroplasties. Acta Orthop Scand 51: 57-62
10. Kubba R, Taylor JS, Marks KE (1981) Cutaneous complications of orthopedic implants. Arch Dermatol 117: 554-560
11. Carlsson A, Möller H. Implantation of orthopaedic devices in patients with metal allergy. Acta Derm Venereol 1989; 69: 62-66
12. Duchna HW, Nowack U, Merget R, Muhr G, Schultze-Werninghaus G. Prospektive Untersuchung zur Bedeutung der Kontaktsensibilisierung durch Metallimplantate. Zentralbl Chir 1998;123: 1271-1276
13. Hayashi K, Kaneko H, Kawachi S, Saida T. Allergic contact dermatitis and osteomyelitis due to sternal stainless steel wire. Contact Dermatitis 1999; 41: 115-116
14. Goh CL (1985) Prevalence of contact allergy by sex, race and age. Contact Dermatitis 14: 237-240
15. Möller H (1990) Nickel dermatitis: problems solved and unsolved. Contact Dermatitis 23: 217-220
16. Thomas P, Meurer M (1996) Immunopathien der Haut. In: Medizinische Immunologie (Hrsg Baenkler HW), Ecomed Verlag Landsberg, Kapitel III: 1-96
17. Thomas P, Thomas M, Summer B, Naumann T, Sander CA, Przybilla B. Intolerance of osteosynthesis material: evidence of dichromate contact allergy with concomitant oligoclonal T-cell infiltrate and Th1-type cytokine expression in the periimplantar tissue. Allergy 2000; 55: 969-972
18. Thomas P, Barnstorf S, Summer B, Willmann G, Przybilla B. Immuno-allergological properties of aluminium oxide (Al_2O_3) ceramics and nickel sulfate in humans. Biomaterials 2003; 24(6): 959-66
19. Goebeler M, Meinarddus-Hager G, Roth J, Goerdt S, Sorg C (1993) Nickel Chloride and Cobalt Chloride, two common contact sensitizers, directly induce expression of intercellular adhesion molecule-1 (ICAM-1), vascular cell adhesion molecule-1 (VCAM-1), and endothelial leukocyte adhesion molecule (ELAM-1) by endothelial cells. J Invest Dermatol 100(6): 759-765
20. Summer B, Ghoreschi K, Barnstorf S, Przybilla B, Thomas P (2003) Phenotype differences in monocyte derived dendritic cells from nickel allergic and non allergic donors upon nickel exposure. Int Arch All Clin Immunol (in press)

21. Sinigaglia F (1994) The molecular basis of metal recognition by T cells. J Invest Dermatol 102: 398-401
22. Willert HG, Brobäck LG, Buchhorn GH, Köster G, Lang I, Ochsner P, Schenk R (1996) Crevice corrosion of cemented titanium alloy stems in total hip replacements. Clin Orthop Rel Res 333: 51-75
23. Willmann G (2000) Bioceramics in orthopaedics: what did we learn in 25 years? Med Orth Tech 120: 10-16
24. Akatsu T, Takahashi N, Udagawa N, Imamura K, Yamaguchi A, Sato K, Nagata N, Suda T (1991) Role of prostaglandins in interleukin-1-induced bone resorption in mice in vitro. J Bone Miner Res 6: 183-190
25. Glant TT, Jacobs JJ, Molnar G, Shanbhag AS, Valyon M, Galante JO (1993) Bone resorption activity of particulate-stimulated macrophages. J Bone Miner Res 8: 1071-1079
26. Shanbhag AS, Jacobs JJ, Glant TT, Gilbert JL, Black J, Galante JO (1994) Composition and morphology of wear debris in failed uncemented total hip replacement arthroplasty. J Bone Joint Surg B 76: 60-67
27. Shanbhag AS, Jacobs JJ, Black J, Galante JO, Glant TT (1995) Cellular mediators secreted by interfacial membranes obtained at revision total hip arthroplasty. J Arthroplasty 10: 498-506
28. Yao J, Glant TT, Lark MW, Mikecz K, Jacobs JJ, Hutchinson NI, Hoerrner LA, Kuettner KE, Galante JO (1995) The potential role of fibroblasts in periprosthetic osteolysis. Fibroblast response to titanium particulates. J Bone Miner Res 10: 1417-1427
29. Scott P, Trinchieri G (1997) IL-12 as an adjuvant for cell mediated immunity. Semin Immunol 9: 285-291
30. Mitchison NA (1992) Specialisation, tolerance, memory, competition, latency, and strife among T-cells. Ann Rev Immunol 10: 1-12
31. Mozzanica N, Rizzolo L, Veneroni G, Diotti R, Hepeisen S, Finzi AF (1990) HLA-A, B, C and DR antigens in nickel contact sensitivity. Brit J Dermatol 122: 309-313
32. Summer B, Ghoreschi K, Barnstorf S, Roider G, Thomas P (2003) PBMC of nickel allergic and non allergic individuals display different apoptotic threshold upon exposure to nickel and metal ions released by coins. Arch Dermatol (in press)
33. Klaschka F, Ring J (1990) Systemically induced (hematogenous) contact eczema. Seminars in Dermatology 9: 210-215
34. Veien NK, Hattel T, Laurberg G (1994) Chromate allergic patients challenged orally with potassium dichromate. Contact Dermatitis 31: 137-139
35. Thomas P, Holz T, Messer G, Przybilla B (1999) Nickel allergic patients with or without reactions upon oral nickel challenge: lymphocyte reactivity and cytokine pattern. J Allergy Clin Immunol 103: 85 (A)
36. Cramers M, Lucht L (1977) Metal sensitivity in patients treated for tibial fractures with plates of stainless steel. Acta Orthop Scand 48: 245-249
37. Hildebrand HF, Veron C, Martin P (1988) In: Hildebrandt HF, Champy M (eds.) Biocompatibility of Co-Cr-Ni-alloys. Plenum press New York: 201-211
38. Mayor MB, Merritt K, Brown SA (1980) Metal allergy and the surgical patient. Am J Surg 139: 477-479
39. Waterman AH, Schrik JJ (1985) Allergy in hip arthroplasty. Contact Dermatitis 13: 294-301
40. Meyrick TRH, Rademaker M, Goddard NJ, Munro DD (1987) Severe eczema of the hands due to an orthopaedic plate made of Vitallium. Br Med J 294: 106-107
41. Rakoski J, von Mayenburg J, Düngemann H, Borelli S (1986) Metallallergien bei Patienten mit Metallimplantaten im Knochen. Allergologie 9: 160-163
42. Zemtsov A, Cameron GS, Montalvo-Lugo V (1997) Nickel-induced lymphocytoma cutis of the earlobe. Contact Dermatitis 36: 266

43. Summer B, Sander C, Przybilla B, Thomas P. Molecular analysis of T-cell clonality with concomitant specific T-cell proliferation in vitro in nickel-allergic individuals. Allergy 2001; 56: 767-770
44. Werfel T, Hentschel M, Kapp A, Renz H. Dichotomy of blood- and skin-derived IL-4-producing allergen specific T cells and restricted Vß repertoire in nickel mediated contact dermatitis. J Immunol 1997; 158: 2500-2505
45. Thomas P, Summer B, Sander C, Przybilla B. In vitro T cell reactivity in nickel allergy: comparison of T cell clonality, cytokine expression and mediator production. Int Arch Allergy and Immunol 2001; 124: 292-295
46. Fischer-Brandies E, Zeintl W, Schramel P, Benner KU (1992) Zum Nachweis von Titan im Organismus bei temporärer Alloplastik. Dtsch Zahnärztl Z 47: 526-528
47. Levenson T, Greenberger PA, Murphy R (1996) Peripheral blood eosinophilia, hyper-immunoglobulinemia A and fatigue: possible complications following rupture of silicone breast implants. Ann Allergy Asthma Immunol 77(2): 119-122
48. Pathak YV, Vanmeeteren R, Dwivedi C (1996) Aluminum polymeric implants: in vitro – in vivo evaluations. J Biomater Appl 11: 62-75

2.6 Allergic and Systemic Effects of Particles

R. M. Urban and J. J. Jacobs

Introduction

Total hip and knee replacement prostheses generate wear and corrosion products at their bearing surfaces, at modular junctions, and at interfaces with cement or bone. It is now well recognized that large numbers of these particles result in the formation of foreign-body granulation tissue, osteolysis and, in some cases, aseptic loosening requiring revision of an arthroplasty. Much less understood are potential immunologic phenomena and the possible systemic effects of widespread dissemination of metallic and polymeric degradation products [1, 6, 7, 8, 17]. The purpose of this paper is to summarize the histopathological and analytical findings from selected revision and postmortem retrieval studies and to communicate some of the emerging findings from our laboratory concerning the biocompatibility of conventional and alternative bearings.

Diosyncratic Reactions to Corrosion of Implants

Cobalt-chromium and titanium alloys are mainstays of modern joint replacement, providing high strength, resistance to corrosion, and the biocompatibility necessary for decades of in vivo service. Nonetheless, some concern persists regarding so-called "metal allergy" or specific immune hypersensitivity associated with metallic degradation products [3, 4].

Despite their excellent corrosion resistance, cobalt-chromium and titanium alloys do corrode in the biological milieu, as do all metallic biomaterials. Metallic ions released from the implant surface or from particles generated by wear and corrosion can form complexes with native proteins, resulting in organometallic species that may act as potential antigens. With regard to cobalt-based alloys in particular, the constituent elements of cobalt, chromium and nickel are known sensitizers with cross sensitivity reactions between nickel and cobalt thought to be frequent. Indeed, dermal hypersensitivity due to contact with metal or metallic corrosion products is a well-established phenomenon affecting an estimated 10 to 15% of the population. There are numerous case reports and cohort studies that temporally associate metal release from implants, primarily internal fixation devices, with an adverse immunologic response.

Documented hypersensitivity reactions to conventional metal-polyethylene total joint replacement prostheses are rare [3]. However, it is increasingly apparent that, in some individuals, unusual adverse tissue reactions can occur in settings of accelerated corrosion of metallic implants [9, 12, 15].

Lymphocytic Inflammation Associated with Contemporary Metal-Metal Bearings

There have been several reports of unusual lymphocytic aggregates in the periprosthetic tissues of contemporary metal-metal hip replacements. Willert [19, 20] and Davies [2] have described peri-vascular or diffuse lymphocytic infiltrates, including secondary lymphoid follicles, morphologically suggestive of hypersensitivity reactions. The lymphocytic infiltrate is believed to be a response to metallic degradation products generated by metal-metal bearings. In these studies, the findings of primarily lymphocytic inflammation in periprosthetic tissues from metal-metal bearings were contrasted to tissues surrounding metal-polyethylene or metal-ceramic bearings where inflammation was primarily histiocytic and lymphocytic infiltrates were rare. While initially described as possible delayed type hypersensitivity reactions, the optimal terminology to describe these unusual features has yet to be defined, and a working term of "aseptic lymphocytic vasculitis-associated lesions" has been suggested [14].

Particles of Chromium Phosphate Corrosion Products in Tissues Surrounding Metal-Metal Bearings

Our laboratory has examined the periprosthetic tissues from 5 metal-metal hip replacements revised for pain or aseptic loosening of the cemented femoral component after less than one year. The joint pseudocapsules were studied using standard hematoxylin and eosin stained sections and coordinated electron microprobe analysis with energy dispersive x-ray analysis. Histiocytes containing sub-micrometer size particles of CoCrMo alloy were present in all of the cases. Particles of $BaSO_4$ radiographic contrast material (0.3 to 0.7 micrometers in size) were detected in 4 of the cases. In each of these four cases, particles of chromium phosphate corrosion products (0.4 to 4 micrometers) were also present. The corrosion products were similar in composition to particles previously identified in association with corroded CoCrMo alloy modular head-neck junctions of hip replacement femoral stems [16]. The energy dispersive x-ray spectra of all but one of the chromium phosphate particles analyzed from the metal-metal bearings contained traces of barium (Figure 1).

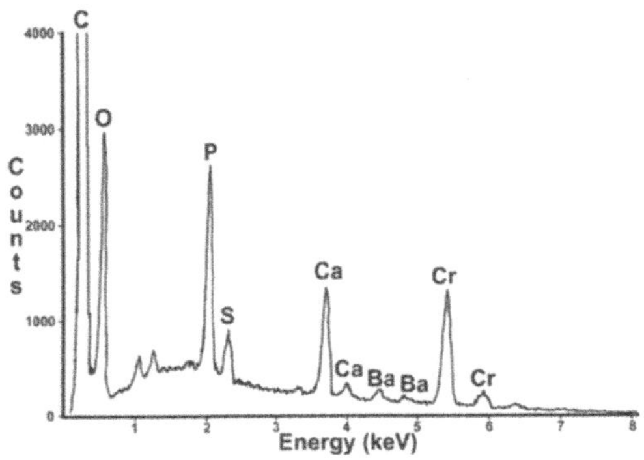

Figure 1:
Energy dispersive x-ray analysis spectrum of a 4-micrometer particle of chromium phosphate, a known corrosion product of CoCrMo alloys. This was one of many such particles detected in the joint pseudocapsule adjacent to a metal-metal bearing revised after less than 1 year for aseptic loosening of the cemented femoral component. The presence of trace levels of barium in these particles suggested the chromium phosphate had been abraded from the CoCrMo bearing surface by a three-body mechanism involving BaSO4 radiographic contrast material.

This finding was taken to suggest that chromium phosphate corrosion products had been abraded from the metal-metal bearing surface by a three-body process involving $BaSO_4$ particles. One of the cases with particles of chromium phosphate corrosion products in the periprosthetic tissues demonstrated extensive lymphocytic infiltrates similar to those reported by Willert for contemporary metal-metal bearings [19, 20].

Lymphocytic Inflammation, Late Dislocation and Corrosion of Head-Neck Junctions in Metal-Polyethylene Bearings

Histopathological features of lymphocytic inflammation, similar to those described for contemporary metal-metal bearings, have been observed in association with selected cases with severely corroded CoCrMo alloy modular head-neck junctions. All of the hips had been reconstructed using cementless titanium alloy components. Our laboratory has studied 5 such cases, all of which presented with late recurrent instability of the hip caused by the direct mechanical effect of a large intracapsular, granulomatous mass and/or gross destruction of the joint pseudocapsule and abductor mechanism. The initial dislocation occurred 14 to 54 months following primary hip replacement for osteoarthritis.

Four of the hips were revised after 16 to 60 months, and one was retrieved postmortem after 54 months in situ. Severe corrosion was evident at the CoCrMo alloy modular head-neck junction of all cases. Abundant black and green corrosion deposits surrounded the tapered junction on neck of the stem and the opening of the bore of the modular head. Evaluation of hematoxylin and eosin stained sections of the periprosthetic tissues showed widespread necrosis of the soft tissues as well as bone of the proximal femoral medulla. Only 2 of the cases had limited areas of viable tissue. The most characteristic histological features were extensive lymphocytic infiltration, both perivascular and in the form of follicles, high endothelial venules, and little foreign body reaction to particles (Figure 2). Large numbers of polyethylene wear particles were not seen. However, pale green particles identified as chromium phosphate corrosion products by energy dispersive x-ray analysis were scattered throughout the periprosthetic tissues. The widespread necrosis and lymphocytic inflammation in these cases were believed to be a reaction to soluble and insoluble metallic degradation products generated by corrosion at the modular head-neck coupling.

Fig. 2:
Light micrograph of an intra-articular soft tissue mass associated with severe corrosion at a modular junction between a CoCrMo head and a titanium alloy femoral stem. The hip prosthesis was revised for chronic instability 16 months following implantation for osteoarthritis. The mass was in large part necrotic, but limited areas of viable tissue seen here revealed extensive lymphocytic infiltrates forming follicles. There was a paucity of histiocytes, and particulate debris was rare with the exception of particles of chromium phosphate corrosion product from the corroded modular junction. Hematoxylin and eosin stain, X125

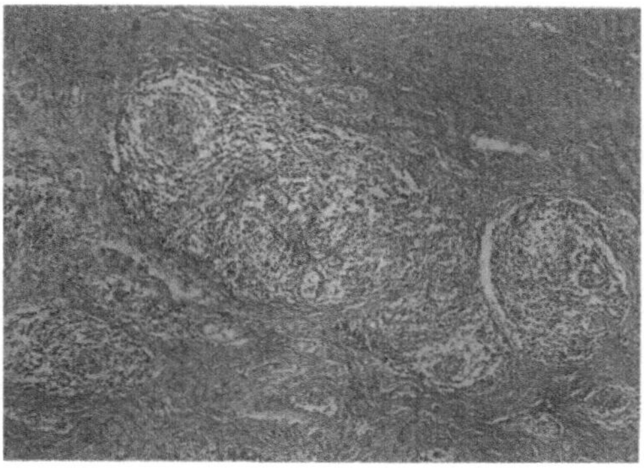

Discussion

In the vast majority of patients, permanent metallic orthopaedic implants are biocompatible and will continue to be crucial tools in the armamentarium of orthopaedic surgeons. When applied appropriately, these devices have had a history of success with few serious short and long-term sequelae. However, in certain situations and in particular individuals, adverse biological effects may occur which can compromise the clinical outcome. For this reason, it is important to continue to expand our knowledge of the host response to implant materials and to improve prosthetic materials and designs to minimize the generation of implant degradation products.

The pervasive use of modular connections and the reintroduction of metal-metal bearings have renewed concerns of corrosion and potential adverse responses to metallic degradation products. Both of these settings can introduce conditions that foster accelerated corrosion. Willert [18] reported that the preponderance of particles in the periprosthetic tissues of 19 patients with failed classic metal-metal total hip replacements were corrosion products, based on a reversal of the chromium/cobalt ratio in the tissues relative to the alloy. In this paper, we report the identification of particles of chromium phosphate in the joint pseudocapsules of 4 of 5 contemporary metal-metal bearings removed for aseptic loosening of the femoral prostheses. McKellop [13] described the chromium phosphate corrosion product as a "tenacious deposit formed on the bearing surface" during in vitro wear tests of CoCrMo metal-metal bearings. Our finding of particles of chromium phosphate in the capsular tissues confirms that this corrosion product does form in vivo in association with metal-metal bearings. The fact that the majority of particles had traces of barium suggests removal of the "tenacious deposit" by three-body wear involving particles of $BaSO_4$ radiographic contrast material.

The chromium (III) orthophosphate hydrate-rich corrosion product has been studied extensively with regard to corroded modular junctions [16]. The material forms adherent deposits surrounding sites of accelerated corrosion of chromium-containing alloys. The deposits fragment, forming particulates in the surrounding tissues. The corrosion product is amorphous by electron and x-ray diffraction, usually non-birefringent, translucent, and pale green to colorless in hematoxylin and eosin stained sections. Particles of chromium phosphate in the periprosthetic tissues range in size from several hundred micrometers down to nanometer size. These particles have been recovered from osteolytic lesions adjacent to corroded modular femoral stems [16] and have been shown to be capable of inducing the release of proinflammatory cytokines from macrophages in cell culture and bone resorption in organ culture [11]. Furthermore, similar debris generated from corrosion of modular stainless steel femoral intramedullary nails has been associated with diaphyseal osteolysis, in the absence of polyethylene wear debris, in the adjacent femur [10]. The elucidation of the role of solid corrosion products in the clinical performance of metal-metal bearings will require further study of implants and periprosthetic tissues retrieved postmortem and at revision surgery.

This paper has also reported an unusual tissue response to corrosion of modular head-neck couplings of metal-polyethylene hip replacements that is strikingly similar to the lymphocytic inflammation reported by Willert [19, 20] and Davies [2] in the tissues adjacent to contemporary metal-metal bearings. The features of lymphocytic infiltration, both perivascular and in the form of follicles, high endothelial venules, and little foreign body reaction was exactly the same as in sections from tissues adjacent to contemporary metal-metal bearings graciously provided by Professor Hans Willert for comparison. These findings support the notion that the unusual lymphocytic infiltrates are a response to corrosion of the metallic devices. A principal difference is that corrosion of the modular junctions resulted in such widespread necrosis of the capsular tissues and abductor mechanism as to cause chronic dislocation of the hip. To the best of our knowledge, dislocation of total hip replacements with metal-polyethylene bearings resulting directly from complications associated with corrosion of the prosthetic device has not been previously reported, nor has this complication as yet been reported in association with metal-metal bearings.

The prevalence of clinically significant local tissue reactions to metallic degradation products of joint replacement prostheses appears overall to be low. Unusual histopathological observations are not always reflective of the reason for revision. Clearly, additional well-documented and collected material from revisions as well as postmortem retrievals are essential to further our understanding of the undesirable findings described in this paper. In addition, further identification of the physical chemical form of degradation products is needed as an essential step prior to specific toxicological investigations in animal models and cell cultures to delineate the biological effects of corrosion of metallic implants.

Acknowledgements

This study was supported by NIH/NIAMS Grant AR39310, the Crown Family Chair of Orthopedic Surgery, and the Rush Arthritis and Orthopaedics Institute. We are also grateful for the cooperation in these studies of Davis W. Clark, MD; Melinda Harmon, MS; W. Andrew Hodge, MD; Jorge O. Galante, MD, Angel Peiro, MD; Aaron G. Rosenberg, MD; and Mitchell B. Sheinkop, MD.

References

1. Case CP, Langkamer VG, James C, Palmer MR, Kemp AJ, Heap PF, Solomon L (1994) Widespread dissemination of metal debris from implants. J Bone Joint Surg Br 76-B:701-712
2. Davies AP, Willert HG, Campbell PA, Case CP (2003) A histological comparison of periprosthetic tissues from metal-on-metal and metal-on-polyethylene total hip replacements. 70th Annual Meeting Proceedings, American Academy of Orthopaedic Surgeons 4:364
3. Hallab NJ, Merritt K, Jacobs JJ (2001) Metal sensitivity in patients with orthopaedic implants. J Bone Joint Surg Am 83-A:428-436
4. Jacobs JJ, Gilbert JL, Urban RM (1988) Corrosion of Orthopaedic Implants. J Bone Joint Surg Am 80-A:268-282
5. Jacobs JJ, Urban RM, Wall J, Black J, Reid JD and Veneman L (1995) Unusual foreign-body reaction to a failed total knee replacement: Simulation of a sarcoma clinically and a sarcoid histologically. A case report. J Bone Joint Surg Am 77-A:444-451
6 Jacobs JJ, Skipor AK, Doorn PF, Campbell P, Schmalzried TP, Black J, Amstutz HC (1996) Cobalt and chromium concentrations in patients with metal on metal total hip replacements. Clin Orthop 329S:256-263
7. Jacobs JJ, Skipor AK, Patterson LM, Hallab NJ, Paprosky WG, Black J, Galante JO (1998) Metal release in patients who have had a primary total hip arthroplasty. A prospective, controlled, longitudinal study. J Bone Joint Surg Am 80-A:1447-1458

8. Jacobs JJ, Silverton C, Hallab NJ, Skipor AK, Patterson LM, Black J, Galante JO (1999) Metal release and excretion from cementless titanium alloy total knee replacements. Clin Orthop 358:173-180
9. Jacobs JJ, Goodman SB, Sumner DR, Hallab NJ (2000) Biological response to orthopaedic implants. In: Buchwalter JA, Einhorn TA and Simon SR (eds) Orthopaedic basic science: biology and biomechanics of the musculoskeletal system, 2nd addition. American Academy of Orthopaedic Surgeons, Rosemont, IL, pp 401-426
10. Jones DM, Marsh JL, Nepola JV, Jacobs JJ, Skipor AK, Urban RM, Gilbert JL, Buckwalter A (2001) Focal osteolysis at the junctions of a modular stainless-steel femoral intramedullary nail. J Bone Joint Surg Am 83-A:537-548
11. Lee S-H, Brennen FR, Jacobs JJ, Urban RM, Ragasa DR, Glant TT (1997) Human Monocyte/macrophage response to cobalt-chromium corrosion products and titanium particles in patients with total joint replacements. J Orthop Res 15:40-49
12. Mathiesen EB, Lindgren JU, Blomgren GGA, and Reinholt FP (1991) Corrosion of modular hip prostheses. J Bone Joint Surg Br 73-B:569-575
13. McKellop H, Amstutz H, Lu B, Timmerman I, Carroll M (2001) A hip simulator study of the wear of large diameter, metal-on-metal hip surface replacements. Trans Soc for Biomaterials 24:339
14. Protocol of the Second Workshop on Immune Reaction to CoCr Implants, September 17, 2000, Zurich University, Zurich, Switzerland
15. Svensson O, Mathiesen EB, Reinholt FP, Blomgren G (1988) Formation of a fulminant soft-tissue pseudotumor after uncemented hip arthroplasty. J Bone Joint Surg Am 70-A:1238-1242
16. Urban RM, Jacobs JJ, Gilbert JL and Galante JO (1994) Migration of corrosion products from modular hip prostheses. Particle microanalysis and histopathological findings. J Bone Joint Surg Am 76-A:1345-1359
17. Urban RM, Jacobs JJ, Tomlinson MJ, Gavrilovic J, Black J, and Peoc'h M (2000) Dissemination of wear particles to the liver, spleen, and abdominal lymph nodes of patients with hip or knee replacement. J Bone Joint Surg Am 82-A:457-477
18. Willert HG, Buchhorn GHH, Gobel D, Koster G, Silvio S, Schenk R, Semlitsch M (1996) Wear behavior and histopathology of classic cemented metal on metal hip endoprostheses. Clin Orthop 329S:S160-S186.
19. Willert H-G, Buchhorn GH, Fayyazi A, and Lohmann CH (2000) Histopathologische veränderungen bei metall/metall-gelenken geben hinweise auf eine zellvermittelte überempfindlichkeit. Vorlaufige untersuchungsergebnisse von 14 fallen. Osteologie 2-16:1-3
20. Willert H-G, Buchhorn GH, Fayyazi A, Lohmann CH (2001) Signs of delayed hypersensitivity and histopathological changes around metal-metal hip joints. Trans Soc for Biomaterials 24:338

2.7 Loosening of Endoprosthesis caused by Staphylococcus epidermidis

D.P. König and J. Michael

Introduction

Several studies have implicated S. epidermidis as a causative agent for so called "aseptic loosened prosthesis" [2,4,9,26,27]. In 1969, CHARNLEY and EFTEKHAR [3] reported: "It is paradox that simple adherence to Listerian principles has abolished virulent postoperative infections, but infection by mildly pathogenic staphylococci appears to be increasingly common."
It is known that S. aureus shows a significantly greater preference for metals than polymers [8,10] while the opposite behaviour is seen in S. epidermidis [10,14]. The polysaccharide slime produced by the bacteria may cause the increased virulence of the bacteria in biomaterial-centered infections [4,10,25]. The polysaccharide slime is not responsible for the primary adherence but for the accumulation of the strain [12,24].
The frequency of pathological microorganisms in sepsis of totally replaced joints varies slightly [6,11]. Staphylococci including S.aureus and S.epidermidis comprise about half of the pathogenic agents [2]. Fitzgerald et al. [7] proved the accuracy of this statement showing that S.epidermidis was almost twice as common as S.aureus in 105 infected total joint arthroplasties treated during 1989-1992.
While infections with S.aureus cause significant clinical signs, infection with S. epidermidis is often difficult to recognize. Preoperative joint aspiration is often negative. Krimmer et al [17] have described detection of Staphylococci in clinical samples by 16S rRNA-Directed in situ hybridisation. This method is very sensitive but time consuming. There is increasing evidence that prosthetic hip loosening may be caused by a low grade infection with S.epidermidis [26,27]. S. epidermidis is known for its ability to adhere to various biomaterials, especially on polymer surfaces [10,22,23]. Barth et al. [1] showed that there were lower numbers of a poor exopolysaccharide producing strain of S.epidermidis (SP-2) on titanium-aluminium and polymethymethacrylate than of a good exopoly-saccharide producing strain (SE-360). In an in vitro study, the bacterial adherence of a slime-producing strain (RP 62 A) was compared with its isogenic slime-negative mutant (M7). Standardized biomaterial discs were incubated under growth conditions in tryptic soy broth containing either strain RP 62 A or M7. After 24h of incubation, the attached bacteria were removed by sonication and the colony-forming units were counted after plating of serial dilutions. We observed a significantly increased adherence and accumulation of the slime-producing strain (RP 62 A). In contrast to the slime negative mutant (M7) ($p=0.0001$). The highest colony counts were found for the slime-producing strain on polyethylene and polymethylmethacrylate. The slime-negative mutant lacked the ability of accumulation. Our in-vitro results show the relevance of slime production by S. epidermidis for in-vitro colonisation of biomaterials, with a preference for polyethylene and polymethylmethacrylate [13].

The effectiveness of bone cement containing antibiotics combined with systemic antibiotics in order to prevent implant infections in total hip replacement surgery, is well established [5,15,16]. Still, improvement of antibiotic loading of bone cements are under discussion. Tobramycin added to the bone cement reduced the number of adherent bacteria in contrast to pure bone cement [20]. An experimental study using an animal model indicated that the use of a tobramycin-impregnated polymethylmethacrylate pin sleeve can prevent the development of pin-tract infection [30].
It has to be kept in mind that the MBCs (minimum bactericidal concentrations) for biomaterial-adherent bacteria are higher than those obtained via clinical suspension techniques by as much as 2 to 250 fold [19,28]. Bacteria adherent to PMMA are commenly more resistant to antibiotics than organisms adherent to stainless steel [19]. Yaniv et al. [31] demonstrated a prolonged leaching time for peptide antibiotics (Vancomycin and polymyxin B nonapeptide) than that for gentamicin, novobiocin and erythromycin from acrylic bone cement. They suggested that peptide antibiotics alone or in combination with other antibiotics (polymyxin B nonapeptide and novobiocin) may provide longer periods of protection against a wide range of bacterial pathogens. This finding is supported by an in-vitro study (229) showing that vancomycin and ciprofloxacin were more active against 49 isolates recovered from orthopaedic implant infections than gentamicin. Case reports also show an effectiveness of vancomycin-impregnated polymethylmethacrylate beads in cases of methicillin-resistant Staphylococcus aureus (MRSA) implant infections [21]. Recommendations are to use 3.6 g of tobramycin and 1 g of vancomycin per 40g package of bone cement when antibiotic cement spacers are used in 2-stage exchange arthroplasty for infected total hip and knee arthroplasties[18].
As S. epidermidis shows a special affinity to polymers like polymethylmethacrylate (PMMA), uncemented joint replacements in revision surgery for previously infected joints should be preferred from the microbiological point of view. If bone cement is used, at least an antibiotic-loaded product should be chosen. The use of vancomycin/rifampicin as "slime buster" in combination with a cephalosporin should be considered as an i.v antibiotic regime in revision surgery for previously loosened and joints infected by S. epidermidis.
Taking into account that our in-vitro results have shown the least colonisation by S. epidermidis on stainless steal, this material could be considered as the first-choice implant material from a microbiological point of view. Future antimicrobially coated implants that can be used without bone cement may be a further step towards a reduction of implant-associated infections.

References

1. Barth E , Myrvik Q M, Wagner W, Gristina A G. In vitro and in vivo comparative colonization of Staphylococcus aureus and Staphylococcus epidermidis on orthopaedic implant materials. Biomaterials 10: 325-8 (1989).
2. Brause B D.: nfected orthopedic prothesis. In Bisno AL, Waldvogel FA: Infections associated with indwelling medical devices. American Society for Microbiology. Washington 111-127, (1989).
3. Charnley J. and N.Eftekhar: Postoperative infection in total prosthetic replacement arthroplasty of the hip-joint. Br.J.Surg. 56: 641-649 (1969).

4. Christensen G D, Baddour L M, Hasty D L, Lowrance J H, Simpson W A: Microbial and foreign body factors in the pathogenesis of medical devices infections. In: Bisno AL, Waldvogel FA: Infections associated with indwelling medical devices. American Society for Mikrobiology. Washington 27-60 (1989).
5. Espehaug B, Engesaeter LB, Vollset SE, Havelin LI, Langeland N: Antibiotic prophylaxis in total hip arthroplasty. Review of 10905 primary cemented total hip replacements reported to the Norwegian arthroplasty register, 1987 to 1995. J Bone Joint Surg Br 79: 590-595(1997).
6. Fitzgerald R H, Jones D R: Hip implant infection. Am J Med; 78 (Suppl. 6B): 225-8 (1985)
7. Fitzgerald R H, Randall K R, Brown W J, Nasser S. Treatment of the infected total hip arthroplasty. Curr Opin Orthop 5; I:26-30 (1994)
8. Gracia E, Fernandez A, Conchello P, Lacleriga A, Paniagua L, Seral F, Amorena B: Adherence of Staphylococcus aureus slime producing variants to biomaterials used in orthopaedic surgery. Int. Ortho. 21:46-51 (1997).
9. Gristina A G, Costerton J W: Bacterial adherence to biomaterials and tissue. J. Bone Joint Surg.[Am] 67-A: 264-273 (1985).
10. Gristina A G, Hobgood C D, Barth E: Biomaterial specifity, molecular mechanisms and clinical relevance of S.epidermidis and S.aureus infections in surgery. Zbl.Bakt.(Suppl.) 16: 143-157 (1987).
11. Inman J N,Gallegos K V, Brause B D, Redecha P B, Christian C L. Clinical and microbial features of prothetic joint infection. Am J Med 77: 47-53 (1984).
12. König D P, Perdreau-Remington F, Rütt J, Stoßberger P, Hilgers K.-D, Plum G: The increase of bacterial adherence and accumulation onto pure titanium due to slime production of Staphylococcus epidermidis. Acta Orthop Scand. 69(5): 523-6 (1998)
13. König D P, Perdreau-Remington F, Rütt J, Hilgers R.-D, Schierholz J.M: Adherence and accumulation of S.epidermidis onto different biomaterials due to extracellular slime production. Zent. bl. Bakteriol. 289: 355-364 (1999).
14. König D P, Schierholz J.M, Bertram C.: Decreased accumulation of S.epidermidis onto stainless steel in comparison to other biomaterials. J. Hosp. Inf. 44: 75-77 (2000).
15. König DP, Schierholz J M, Münnich U, Rütt .: Treatment of Staphylococcal Implant Infections with Rifampicin-Ciprofloxacin in Stable Implants. Arch Orthop Trauma Surg 121:297-299 (2001).
16. König D P, Schierholz J M, Hilgers R.-D, Bertram Ch, Perdreau-Remington F, Rütt J: In vitro adherence and accumulation of Staphylococcus epidermidis RP 62 A and Staphylococcus epidermidis M7 on four different bone cements. Langenbeck`s Arch Surg 386: 328-332 (2001).
17. Krimmer V, Merkert H, von Eiff c, Frosch M, Eulert J, Löhr J F, Hacker J, Ziebuhr W: Detection of Staphylococcus aureus and Staphylococcus epidermidis in clinical samples by 16S rRNA-Directed in situ hybridization. J Clin Microbiol 2667-2673 (1999).
18. Masri B A, Duncan C P, Beauchamp C P: Long-term elution of antibiotics from bone cement: an in vivo study using the prosthesis of antibiotic-loaded acrylic cement (PROSTALAC) system. J Arthroplasty 13: 331-338 (1998).
19. Naylor P T, Jennings R, Webb L X, Gristina A G: Antibiotic sensitivity of biomaterial-adherent Staphylococcus epidermidis. Orthop Trans 12: 524-525(1988).
20. Oga M, Arizono T, Sugioka Y: Inhibition of bacterial adhesion by tobramycin impregnated PMMA bone cement. Acta Orthop Scand 63: 301-304(1992).
21. Ozaki T, Yoshitaka T, Kunisada T, Dan' ura T, Naito N, Inoue H: Vancomycin-impregnated polymethylmethacrylate beads for methicillin-resistant Staphylococcus aureus (MRSA) infection: report of two cases. J Orthop Sci 3: 163-168 (1998).
22. Perdreau-Remington F, Stefanik D, Peters G, Ludwig C, Rütt J, Wenzel R, Pulverer,G. Microbial Ecology of Explanted Prosthetic Hips. A Four Year Prospective Study of 52 Patients with "Aseptic" Prosthetic Joint Loosening. Eur J Microbiol Inf Dis 15: 160-5(1996).

23. Peters G, Locci R, Pulverer G. Adherence and growth of coagulase-negative staphylococci on surfaces of intravenous catheters. J Inf Dis 146: 479-82(1982).
24. Peters G, Schumacher-Perdreau F, Jansen B, Bey M, Pulverer G: Biology of S.epidermidis extracellular slime. In Pathogenicity and Clinical Significance of Coagulase-negative Staphylococci (Pulverer G, Quie PG & Peters G Ed.) Fischer, Stuttgart 15-32(1987).
25. Peters G: New considerations in the pathogenesis of coagulase-negative staphylococcal foreign body infections. J Antimicrob. Chemother. 21(Suppl. C) 139-148 (1988).
26. Peters G, Schumacher-Perdreau F, Jansen B, Ludwig C , Rütt J: Aseptic prosthetic hip loosening - a chronic polymer-associated infection by coagulase-negative Staphylococci ? The Staphylococci, Zbl.Bakt. 21(Suppl.) 329-330(1991).
27. Rütt J, Ludwig C, Peters G, Schumacher-Perdreau F, G. Pulverer: Wird die schleichende aseptische TEP-Lockerung durch eine Infektion mit Staphylococcus epidermidis verursacht ? Orthop.Praxis 9 587-588(1990).
28. Schierholz J M, Beuth J, König D, Nürnberger A, Pulverer G Antimicrobial substances and effects on sessile bacteria. Zent bl Bakteriol 289:165-177(1998).
29. Tunney M M, Ramage G, Patrick S, Nixon J R, Murphy P G, Gorman SP: Antimicrobial susceptibility of bacteria isolated from orthopedic implants following revision surgery. Antimicrob Agents Chemother 42: 3002-3005(1998).
30. Voos K, Rosenberg B, Fagrhi M, Seligson D: Use of tobramycin-impregnated polymethylmethacrylate pin sleeve for the prevention of pin-tract infection in goats. J Orthop Trauma 13: 98-101(1999).
31. Yaniv M, Dabbi D, Amir H, Cohen S, Mozes M, Tsuberi H, Frietkin M, Dekel S, Ofek I: Prolonged leaching time of peptide antibiotics from acrylic bone cement. Clin Orthop 363: 232-239(1999).

2.8 Evidence-Based Infection Control Measures in THR

K. Weist and H. Rüden

State of the art infection control measures concerning reduction of surgical site infection risk are to be derived from recommendations which are categorized based on existing scientific data rather than on expert based opinions.

Objective

To highlight the most recent data on the epidemiology of surgical site infections (SSI) in total hip replacement (THR).
To describe important practices performed pre-, peri- and post-operatively to reduce the risk of SSI and unresolved issues in infection control.

Methods

The most important rationale is the Guideline for Prevention of Surgical Site Infection (1999) from the Hospital Infection Control Practices Committee (HICPAC) and the Centers for Disease Control and Prevention (CDC). The efficacy of these recommendations is categorized into four categories: strongly recommended for implementation and supported by well designed experimental, clinical or epidemiological studies (IA); or supported by some experimental, clinical, or epidemiological studies and strong theoretical rationale (IB); or suggested for implementation and supported by suggestive clinical or epidemiological studies or theoretical rationale for effective practices (II). One category exists with practices wherefore insufficient evidence or no consensus regarding efficacy is available.
Controlled studies concerning SSI prevention that have been published after 1999 have been taken into account as well.

Results

The National Nosocomial Infections Surveillance (NNIS) System with 176 participating US Hospitals shows pooled SSI rates (superficial, deep and organ spaced infections, all risk categories) for THR operations of 0.89 SSI per 100 operations. Several European surveillance systems are established. In 2002 the German surveillance system for nosocomial infections KISS (Krankenhaus-Infektions-Surveillance-System) includes 82 surgical departments with 33,580 THR. SSI infection rates are stratified in traumatology departments with 2.62 SSI per 100 operations and orthopedic departments with 1.41 SSI per 100 operations. The Dutch surveillance system (1996-2000) with 13,770 THR patients including a post-discharge surveillance module showed 2.4 SSI per 100 operations. The leading pathogens in the KISS-data causing SSI following THR were S. aureus (40%),

coagulase negative staphylococci (23%) and Enterococci (12%) respectively.
Pre-operatively, a recent randomized controlled trial with nasal application of mupirocin for patients colonized with S. aureus failed to reduce the SSI rate. The correct administration of perioperative antibiotic prophylaxis (PAP) is an indispensable practice (category IA). Nevertheless a recent German observational study in 627 surgical procedures including THR showed that only 45.3% of the PAP (397) were performed correctly. The performance of the surgical hand scrub with alcoholic solutions – widely accepted in European countries - is becoming a very important issue in US hospitals in regard to the HICPAC Guideline for Hand Hygiene in Health-Care Settings (2002).
Intra-operatively, the administration of supplemental oxygen (80%) proved to reduce SSI in elektive colorectal resections from 11.2% to 5.2% in a randomized controlled trial with 500 patients.
There are no studies supporting that differences in disinfecting surfaces or constructional formation of the operating room with respect to so called septic (dirty and infected) and aseptic operations (clean, clean-contaminated, contaminated) will lead to any improvement in reducing SSI. THR and total knee replacement are the only types of operation showing a significant SSI reduction using a laminar air flow system in one multi-center trial.
Post-operatively, a considerable number of SSI, between 12% and 84% are only diagnosed after discharge from the hospital.

Conclusion

Strict adherence to category IA practices (HICPAC-Guideline for prevention of surgical site infection) is mandatory. Surgical site infection rates in patients with THR are dependent on the patients' population (orthopedic surgery, traumatology). Performing surveillance of SSI is indispensable in order to obtain data for internal quality assurance. The optimal method to perform a post-discharge surveillance remains an unresolved issue especially in times of decreasing duration of patients' hospital stay.

SESSION 3

Future Ceramic Materials in Joint Arthroplasty

3.1 Enhancement of in vitro Bioactivity resulting from the Hydroxylation of Oxide Ceramic Surfaces

C. Niedhart, M. Sax, K. Geschwill, R. Telle and F.U. Niethard

Abstract

Oxide ceramics are excellent materials for implants and prostheses because of their biomechanical stability and low wear rate. However, oxide ceramics are bioinert, and after implantation failure rate is high. Aim of our study was to determine the influence of a surface modification via hydroxylation of oxide ceramics on the effects on human osteoblast like cells in vitro.

Alumina ceramic plates were sintered at 1600°C and the surface was polished to a mirror finish. The plates were then treated with 30 % sodium hydroxide solution for 24 or 96 hours (activation time) at 90°C or were left untreated (control). X-ray diffraction pattern of activated plates showed aluminium hydroxide at the surface. Bending strength was examined in a four point bending test. Weibull statistics showed no differences between treated and untreated ceramics.

Human osteoblast-like cells were prepared from bone obtained from knee surgery per explant technique and cultured in DMEM medium (10% CS, 1% penicillin/streptomycin). Cells were seeded with $4x10^4$ cells / probe. We examined cell attachment, survival and apoptosis rate after 24 hours and protein, alkaline phosphatase (AP) and osteocalcin (OC) secretion as well as mineralisation rate after 7 days. There was no sign of cytotoxicity or growth inhibition. Adhesion was significantly enhanced up to 136 % of control after 24 hours activation time ($p<0.01$), AP secretion was similar to control and OC secretion was enhanced to 229 % of control ($p<0.01$). Mineralisation was detectable at all probes.

Treating the surface of inert oxide ceramics with sodium hydroxide solution to produce biologically active OH-groups is a newly developed, simple and cheap technique. Bioactivity of alumina ceramics was clearly enhanced without cytotoxic effects or changes of material characteristics. In conclusion, this method "bioactivates" originally bioinert ceramics. In the future, it might be possible to design pure ceramic prostheses without the problem of early loosening.

Introduction

Ceramic components for endoprostheses have been successfully used for more than 25 years [29,31]. Their great advantage – in comparison with articulating metal-metal or metal-polyethylen combinations – is their low wear rate [4,5,7,11]. Wear debris can lead to osteolysis, resulting in aseptic loosening [19,30]. The problem of ceramic fractures has been solved, fracture rate of modern ceramic balls and cups has been reported between 0.004 and 0.02 % [32].

Oxide ceramics are bioinert and biocompatible, showing no cytotoxic effect in vitro and in vivo [3,12,15,22,23]. Additionally, they have no immunogenic

potential [28]. But one disadvantage of the oxide ceramics in joint replacement is their missing bioactivity. Experiments in the 1970´s with pure ceramic prostheses were not satisfactory. Due to their bioinertia, there was no osseous ongrowth, resulting in a fibrous interlayer without direct contact between ceramic and bone. This led to early loosening of the ceramic prostheses [3,9,16].
For the development of pure ceramic prostheses, for example small prostheses for finger or foot joints or resurfacing prostheses for the hip, a bioactive surface of the ceramic is necessary to enhance cell attachment and osseous ongrowth.
Some authors reported an enhanced bioactivity of oxide ceramics after surface modification, f. e. hydroxyapatite [14,27], multilayered apatite [33], glass ceramic [17] or ceramic [26] coating, but none of these implants came to clinical investigation.
The reason for the bioinertia is the high oxidation rate of oxide ceramics. There is under normal conditions no corrosion or ion release. If cells should attach to a surface, they need functional groups, like OH-groups or NH2-groups [6]. The surface of oxide ceramics shows no functional groups, resulting in a missing attachment of cells leading to a missing ongrowth of bone to pure ceramic implants.
In our laboratory, we developed a new, simple surface modification of oxide ceramics like alumina via hydroxylation with sodium hydroxide. This hydroxylation of the surface should enhance bioactivity because more active groups are representative at the surface, which can be detected by the target cells.
Aim of our study was to determine the influence of this surface modification of oxide ceramics on the stability and the bioactive effects on human osteoblast like cells in vitro.

Methods

Alumina HPA-0.5 w/MgO ceramic plates were sintered at 1600°C with a final diameter of 23 mm and the surface was polished to a mirror finish.
For the surface analysis and biomechanical testing, the plates were then treated with 30 % sodium hydroxide solution for 24 or 96 hours (activation time) at 90°C or were left untreated (control) [21].
Existence of alumina hydroxide (AlOH) groups at the surface was detected by X-ray diffraction pattern (Fa. Philips, CuKa, Ni filter, 30kV, 30 mA).
Ultimate strength values of activated and non-activated ceramics were examined in a four point bending test according to DIN EN 834-1 (Instron 1186). Test specimen had a size of 3x4x45 mm_. Span length was constant (20/10 mm), the press heads as well as the two support points were rounded to avoid shear load and cutting, the striker was driven at a constant rate (0.5 mm/min). Weibull statistics were evaluated according to DIN 51110.
For in vitro biocompatibility testing, round plates (23 mm diameter) were treated with 30 % sodium hydroxide solution for 24 hours (activation time) at 90°C or were left untreated (control). After activation, probes were washed intensely with distilled water.
Human osteoblast-like cells were prepared from bone obtained from knee surgery per explant technique [1] and cultured [25] in DMEM medium (10% calf serum, 1% penicillin/streptomycin). Cells of the second passage were seeded with 4x104 cells / probe. For the mineralisation assay, 5 mM b-glycerophosphate and 5 µg/ml ascorbic acid were added.

After 24 hours, cell attachment and cell vitality were determined by trypan blue and hematoxylin-eosin staining. Apoptosis rate was determined by TUNEL labelling (In situ cell death detection kit, Boehringer; Mannheim).
After seven days, determination of cell proliferation rate and cell vitality was repeated. Total protein content was measured with the BCA method (Pierce, Rockford), and alkaline phosphatase (AP) activity was assayed by determining the release of p-nitrophenol from p-nitrophenyl phosphate at 37.5°C, pH 10.5. Values were expressed as AP activity / total protein content. Determination of osteocalcin was performed with an enzyme immuno assay (NovoCalcin-Kit, Metro Biosystems , Osnabrück, Germany). Mineralisation was detected via von Kossa staining, AP staining was done with naphtol phosphate and fast blue (Sigma, Munich).
All experiments were done six times in duplicates. Mean and standard error of the mean were calculated, and mean values of untreated alumina were set as 100 %; values of activated probes were expressed in percent in relation to untreated alumina. Statistical analysis was done using the Wilcoxon nonparametric test. A confidence level of 95 % ($p<0.05$) was set as a measure of significance. Significant differences ($p<0.05$, $p<0.01$) were marked with * and **, respectively.

Results

X-ray diffraction pattern

After 24 hours activation time, aluminium hydroxide was clearly detectable by X-ray diffraction pattern (fig.1). This proves, that alumina is not completely chemically inert. Hydroxylation of the alumina surface is possible.

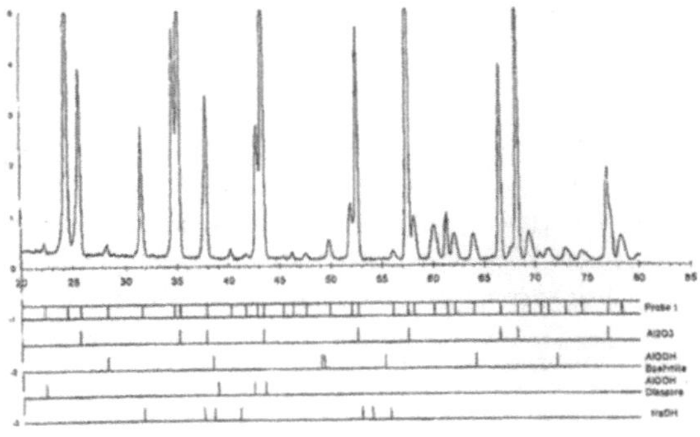

Figure 1:
X-ray diffraction pattern of sodium hydroxide treated alumina: Additionally to the alumina, aluminium hydroxide was detectable. Parts of sodium hydroxide were also seen.

Ultimate bending strength

The results of four different test specimen were compared: untreated alumina, alumina treated for 24 hours or 96 hours, and alumina treated for 24 hours and stored in calf serum for 96 hours (simulation of body fluid). As shown in figure 2, there were no differences in the curve characteristics of all four test specimen. So in conclusion, bending strength of alumina was not affected by hydroxylation treatment nor by simulating storage in body fluid.

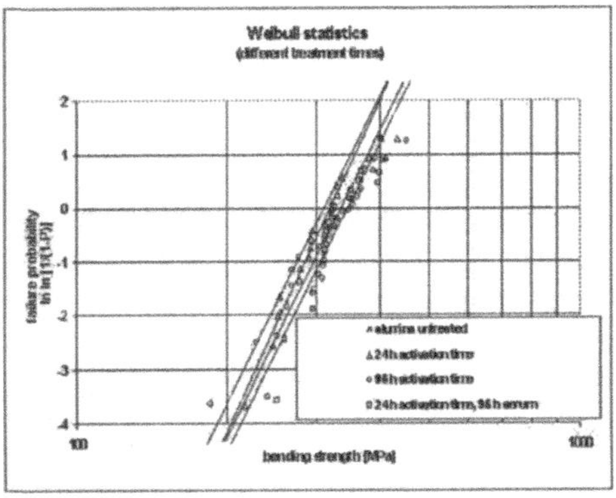

Figure 2:
Weibull statistics of untreated alumina, alumina after hydroxylation treatment for 24 hours and 96 hours, and alumina after hydroxylation treatment for 24 hours and storage in calf serum for 96 hours simulating body fluid.

In vitro bioactivity

Untreated alumina was compared with alumina after hydroxylation treatment for 24 hours. There was no sign of cytotoxicity or growth inhibition. The rate of attached cells (as a marker of cell attachment) on hydroxylated surfaces was significantly enhanced up to 136 % after 24 hours compared with untreated alumina ($p<0.01$). After seven days, cell count (as a marker for cell proliferation) was also enhanced up to 126 % compared with untreated alumina ($p<0.01$) (Fig. 3).

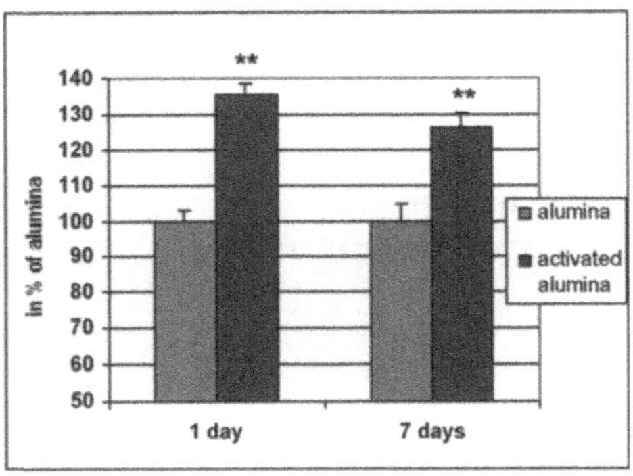

Figure 3:
Cell count after 1 and 7 days: Adhesion rate on hydroxylated alumina is enhanced to 136 % compared with untreated alumina after 24 hours; after 7 days, cell count is 26 % higher on hydroxylated ceramics.

Total protein content after seven days was increased to 130 % ($p<0.01$). Alkaline phosphatase secretion was not influenced by hydroxylation. Osteocalcin secretion as a marker of late osteoblast differentiation was more than doubled (229 %, $p<0.01$). Mineralisation was detectable at all probes. The rate of apoptotic cells was reduced from 0.32 +/- 0.19 % to 0.08 +/- 0.01 % ($p<0.05$) (Fig. 4).

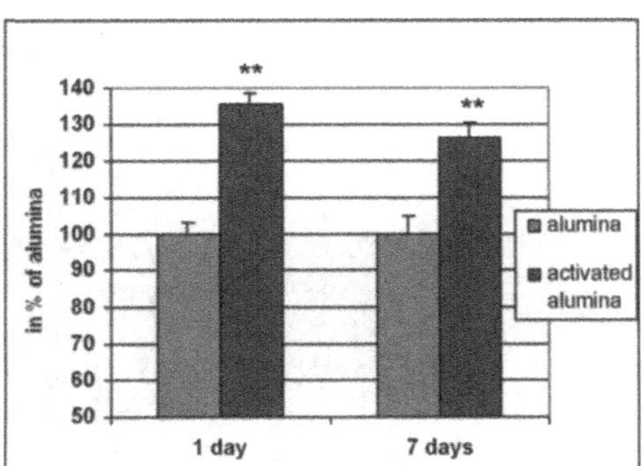

Figure 4:
Alkaline phosphatase (AP) and osteocalcin secretion of human osteoblastlike cells after seven days culture time: AP content was not influenced by hydroxylation, osteocalcin secretion was significantly enhanced to 229 %.

So in conclusion, all measured parameters, cell attachment, cell proliferation and cell differentiation were increased.

Discussion

Total joint replacement is one of the most successful operations in the last decades. Mobility and quality of life of millions of patients were improved. At the time, aseptic loosening of the prosthesis, induced by wear debris, is one of the most important problems in joint replacement [19,30] and is the reason for more than 75 % of all revision operations [18]. The use of ceramic-ceramic couples reduces wear debris [4,5,7] and should result in longer lifetime expectancy [10]. Usually ceramic components are used only as coupling partners, but not in contact to the surrounding bone. The reason is the bioinertia of oxide ceramics: If cells should attach to a surface, they need functional groups, like OH-groups or NH2-groups [6]. The surface of oxide ceramics shows no functional groups, resulting in a missing attachment of cells leading to a missing ongrowth of bone to pure ceramic implants. In clinical trials in the 70´s, pure ceramic implants showed a high rate of early aseptic loosening [3,9,168] because of the bioinertia of oxide ceramics. But pure ceramic prostheses are of high interest for the future: In small prostheses, for example finger or foot prostheses, it is difficult to combine different materials. Also bone saving resurfacing prostheses made of pure ceramic are of high interest. Pure ceramic prostheses need a "surface ceramic are of high interest. Pure ceramic prostheses need a "surface bioactivation" to avoid early loosening. One possibility is the coating of ceramics with bioactive materials, for example hydroxyapatite (HA) [14,27] as it is also known from metal implants. HA coating of metal implants has led to outweighing good results [8]. However, in explant series some of the hydroxyapatite coating was resorbed [2]. Data from the Norwegian arthroplasty register did not show a better performance of HA-coated cups [13]. In contrast to titanium- or cobalt-chrome alloys, alumina is bioinert. Resorption of HA coating will result in a loosening of alumina implants.

One alternative is the direct surface modification. Some authors allege, that alumina cannot be modified and shows no reaction with chemicals except hydrofluoric acid [24]. As we were able to show, treatment of alumina with sodium hydroxide over at least 24 hours at high temperatures leads to a surface reaction with the formation of alumina hydroxide groups at the surface of the ceramic. The creation of functional groups at the surface enhances the bioactivity of alumina ceramics, as we were able to show. Additionally, the covalent binding of bioactive peptides like BMP-2 or the RGD peptide sequence is possible, to further enhance the bioactivity [20].

So in conclusion, treating the surface of inert oxide ceramics with sodium hydroxide solution to produce biologically active OH-groups is a newly developed, simple and cheap technique. Bioactivity of alumina ceramics was clearly enhanced without cytotoxic effects or changes of material characteristics. In conclusion, this method "bioactivates" originally bioinert ceramics. In the future, it might be possible to design pure ceramic prostheses without the problem of early loosening.

Literature

1. Auf´m Kolk B, Hauschka PV, Schwartz ER (1985) Characterization of human bone cells in culture. Calcif Tissue Int 37:228-235
2. Bauer TW, Stulberg BN, Jiang M, Geesink RGT (1993) Uncemented acetabular components: Histologic analysis of retrieved components. J Arthroplasty 8:167-177
3. Böhler M, Knahr K, Plenk H Jr, Walter A, Salzer M, Schreiber V (1994) Long-term results of uncemented alumina acetabular cups. J Bone Joint Surg Br 76:53-59
4. Bos I, Willmann G (2001) Morphologic characteristics of periprosthetic tissues from hip prostheses with ceramic-ceramic couples. Acta Orthop Scand 72:335-342
5. Boutin P, Christel P, Dorlot JM, Meunier A, Roquancourt A, Blanquaert D, Herman S, Sedel L, Witvoet J (1988) The use of dense alumina-alumina ceramic combinatioon in total hip replacement. J Biomed Mater Res 22:1203-1232
6. Boyan BD, Hummert TW, Dean DD, Schwartz Z (1996) Role of material surfaces in regulating bone and cartilage cell response. Biomaterials 17:137-146
7. Dorlot JM, Christel P, Meunier A (1989) Wear analysis or retrieved alumina heads and sockets of hip prostheses. J Biomed Mater Res 23:299-310
8. Geesink RGT (2002) Osteoconductive coatings for total joint arthroplasty. Clin Orthop Rel Res 395:53-65
9. Griss P, Heimke G, Andrian-Werburg H, Krempien B, Reipa S, Lauterbach HJ, Hartung HJ (1975) Morphological and biochemical aspects of Al2O3 ceramic joint replacement. Experimental results and design considerations for human endoprostheses. J Biomed Mater Res 6:177-188
10. Griss P, Heimke G, Werner E, Bleicher J, Jentschura G (1978) Was bedeutet die Resorption des Calcar femuris nach der Totalendoprothesenoperation der Hüfte? Eine vergleichende Studie an Charnley-Müller und Oxidkeramikendoprothesen (Typ Lindenhof). Arch Orthop Trauma Surg 92:225-232
11. Hamadouche M, Boutin P, Daussange J, Bolander ME, Sedel L (2002) Alumina-on-alumina total hip arthroplasty: a minimum 18.5 year follow-up study. J Bone Joint Surg Am 84:69-77
12. Harms J, Mäusle E (1979) Tissue reaction to ceramic implant material. J Biomed Mater Res 13:67-87
13. Havelin LI, Espehaug B, Engesaeter LB (2002) The performance of two hydroxyapatite-coated acetabular cups compared with Charnley cups. J Bone Joint Surg Br 84B:839-845
14. Jiang G, Shi D (1998) Coating of hydroxyapatite on highly porous Al2O3 substrate for bone substitutes. J Biomed Mater Res B 43:77-81
15. Lerouge S, Huk O, Yahia LH, Sedel L (1996) Characterization of in vivo wear debris from ceramic-ceramic total hip arthroplasties. J Biomed Mater Res 32:627-633
16. Lerouge S, Huk O, Yahia LH, Witvoet J, Sedel L (1997) Ceramic-ceramic vs. metal-polyethylene total hip replacements: comparison of pseudomembranes after loosening. J Bone Joint Surg Br 79:135-139
17. Li Z, Kitsugi T, Yamamuro T, Chang YS, Senaha Y, Takagi H, Nakamura T, Oka M (1995) Bone-bonding behaviour under load-bearing conditions of an alumina ceramic implant incorporating beads coated with glass-ceramic containing apatite and wollastonite. J Biomed Mater Res 29:1081-1088
18. Malchau H, Herberts P, Eisler T, Garellick G, Södermann P (2002) The Swedish total hip replacement register. J Bone Joint Surg Am 84S2:2-20
19. Maloney WJ, Smith RL, Schmalzried TP, Chiba J, Huene D, Rubash H (1995) Isolation and characterization of wear particles generated in patients who have had failure of a hip arthroplasty without cement. J Bone Joint Surg Am 77:1301-1310

20. Niedhart C, Boeing R, Klee D, Niethard FU (2002) Short term bioactivity of titanium alloys is enhanced by covalent and adsorptive immobilisation of the RGD binding sequence. Acta Orthop Scand 73(S304):24
21. Niedhart C, Sax HM, Niethard FU, Telle R (2002) Bioactive implants and the method for the production thereof. European patent specification EP 1 140 237 B1
22. Pizzoferrato A, Cenni E, Ciapetti G (1992) In vitro cytocompatibility and tissue reaction to ceramics. In Raviglioli A, Krajewski A (eds): Bioceramics and the human body. Amsterdam, Elsevier 288-291
23. Plitz W, Griss P (1981) Clinical, histomorphological and material related observations on removed alumina-alumina hip joint components. In Weinstein, Gibbons, Brown (eds): Ruff implant retrieval: material and biological analysis. NBS special publication 601. New York, United States Department of Commerce 131-156
24. Sedel L (2000) Total hip arthroplasty using a ceramic prosthesis. Clin Orthop Rel Res 379:3-11
25. Siggelkow H, Niedhart C, Kurre W, Ihbe A, Atkinson MJ, Hüfner M (1998) In vitro differentiation potential of a new human osteosarcoma cell line (HOS 58). Differentiation 63:81-91
26. Takagi H, Yamamuro T, Hyakuna K, Nakamura T, Kotoura Y, Oka M (1989) Bone bonding behavior of bead-coated alumina ceramic under load-bearing conditions. J Biomed Mater Res Appl Biomater 23:161-181
26. Takaoka T, Okumura M, Ohgushi H, Inoue K, Takakura Y, Tamai S (1996) Histological and biomechanical evaluation of osteogenic response in porous hydroxyapatite coated alumina ceramics. Biomaterials 17:1499-1505
28. Thomas P, Barnstorf S, Summer B, Willmann G, Przybilla B (2003) Immuno-allergological properties of aluminium oxide (Al2O3) ceramics and nickel sulfate in humans. Biomaterials 24:959-966
29. Toni A, Sudanese A, Terzi S (1997) Ceramic in total hip arthroplasty. In: Puhl W: Performance of the wear couple biolox forte in hip arthroplasty. Enke Verlag, Stuttgart, 30-33
30. Willert HG (1977) Reaction of the articular capsule to wear products of artificial joint prostheses. J Biomed Mater Res 11:157-164
31. Willmann G (1996) Ceramics for total hip replacement. What a surgeon should know. Orthopaedics Int 21:1-5
32. Willmann G (2000) Ceramic femoral head retrieval data. Clin Orthop Rel Res 379:22-28
33. Yamashita K, Yonehara E, Ding X, Nagai M, Umegaki T, Matsuda M (1998) Electrophoretic coating of multilayered apatite composite on alumina ceramics. J Biomed Mater Res 43:46-53

3.2 Osseointegration of Ceramic Implants: Past, Present and Future

U. Schreiner and G. Scheller

Past

In the 1970ies cementless ceramic implants were introduced into total hip arthroplasty as monolithic ceramic screwed cups for the first time. Clinical and radiographical follow-ups revealed cup migration as a hint of instability of the implant and lack of osseointegration.
In 1974 Griss realised the first ceramic on ceramic coupling in THA in Germany. He introduced a cementless ceramic screwed cup in combination with a cemented stem and a modular ceramic ball head. The "Lindenhof" hip socket was a cylindrically shaped , monolithic screwed cup made of alumina ceramic with a smooth surface. The "Lindenhof" cup was evaluated in short- and mid-term follow-ups. Because of material related problems clinical use was stopped early. 1999 Griss presented longterm results of the "Lindenhof" cup [8]. 24 cups out of 67 well-known cases had to be revised due to loosening and migration. Amazingly the standing period of the revised cups varied between 1,5 and 21 years. 25 cups were still in situ at the presented follow-up, 21 of these were evaluated clinically and radiographically at an follow-up time of 22 years and 5 months. All cups were found migrated to a less or more extend.
An initial and early postoperative migration in 35% of the cases is reported by Gierse [7].
Mittelmeier introduced the "Autophor" cup in 1974 as well. This cup was a conically shaped, monolithic ceramic screwed cup (Fa. Feldmühle).
Follow-ups of this cup either showed high rates of implant loosening , i.e. 53% 12,3 years postoperatively [6]. (Fig. 1)

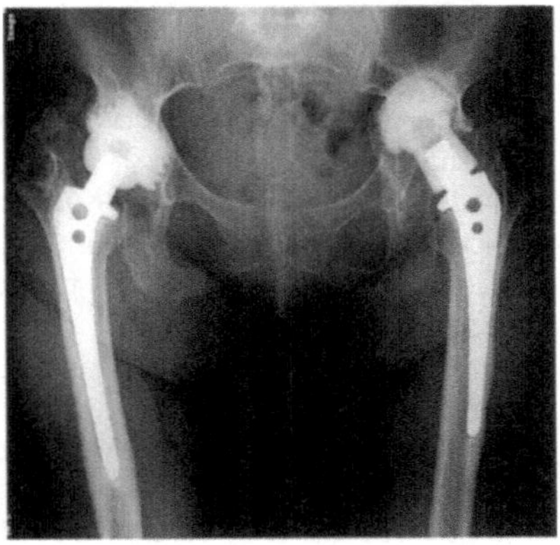

Figure 1:
Threaded ceramic cups implanted on both sides, cementless fixation. 15 years and 17 years after implantation. A layer of soft tissue can be observed. Right side: No migration, left side migration of the cup.

Even in the 70ies research was focussed on porous structured ceramic implants. Different working groups proved the osseointegration of ceramic implants with a rough or porous surface for dental implants [10,11,12]. This knowledge was not transferred to the field of orthopedic implantology.

Present

Nowadays a ceramic on ceramic coupling needs a metal shell as cementless acetabular component and a ceramic insert. This modular concept has disadvantages that could be avoided by a monolithic cup. Just to mention a certain minimum thickness of metal shell and insert together

- that restricts the realisation of small(er) cup sizes and
- restricts the realisation of larger head diameters .

Problems of insert fixation implied different technical solutions.

In the 1990ies the industry started to produce ceramics with porous or rough surface structures, supposedly with a better quality than twenty years before. Therefore the aim of an own experimental study was to screen different surface structures or surface treatments of bioinert alumina and zirconia ceramic cylinders for the ability to allow osseointegration. Test cylinders with different surfaces (smooth, macrostructured, rough and porous) were implanted "press-fit" in the femurs of Göttinger Minipigs. The standing period was 12 weeks. Macroradiographic and histological evaluation showed that the smooth and macrostructured cylinders were not osseointegrated. The cylinders with rough and porous surfaces were osseointegrated. Bone attachment varied between 20.5% to 52.8% of the implants' surface [13]. (Fig. 2)

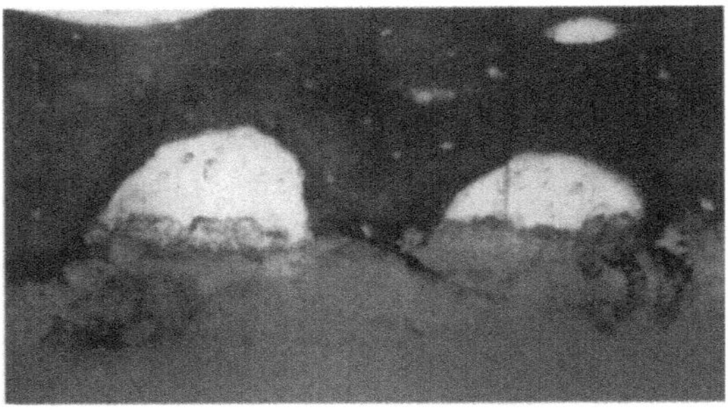

Figure 2:
Microscopical investigation of an alumina ceramic implant with rough surface. Direct contact can be observed at the interface with bone (upper figure: blue) and at the surface of the sample (figure below: beige)

Further experimental studies proved osseointegration of ceramic implants as well [1,5,11].

Weinstein et al. evaluated osseous tissue ingrowth into porous alumina cylinders implanted in canine femurs using a mechanical push-out-test. After a standing period of eight weeks they found a high interfacial shear strength due to osseointegration [14].

Coatings with bioactice materials are proved to enhance the osseointegration as well [9].

Summarizing the published studies it is evident that surface modifications like rough or porous structures enhance the osseointegration of ceramic implants as well as coatings with bioactive materials do.

As Cornell and Lane pointed out "osteoconduction is also observed in fabricated materials that have a porosity similar to that of bone structure". Even though growth factors, local cytokines and other proteins modulate the process, the three-dimansional structure of an implant or graft is the primary determinant of the speed and completeness of incorporation [3].

Polish working groups reported the clinical use of porous alumina ceramic implants. Forgon et al. observed the bone ingrowth into drill holes with a diameter of 500µm [4]. The study group intended the clinical use of a ceramic monoblock cup with a superficial, macroporous layer. Further results have unfortunately not been published.
Another polish working group tested porous alumina ceramic implants in an animal model and found bone ingrowth in outer and inner pores [2].

With regard to the development of cementless ceramic implants the reported results are encouraging. Nevertheless the mechanical data of the current alumina ceramic materials are still a problem concerning a "press-fit" implantation technique.

Future

A new generation of alumina matrix composites – Biolox delta®- with improved mechanical properties and promising tribological data enables the production of ceramic implants with a porous surface that are suitable for a "press-fit" implantation.
The osseointegration of implants made of Biolox delta® is going to be proved in experimental studies.
Therefore test cylinders with a porous surface have been implanted "press-fit" into the femurs of Göttinger Minipigs (Fig. 3 and 4). The test bodys are going to be tested by a push-out-test and by macroradiographical and histological evaluation. The study has not been finished yet.

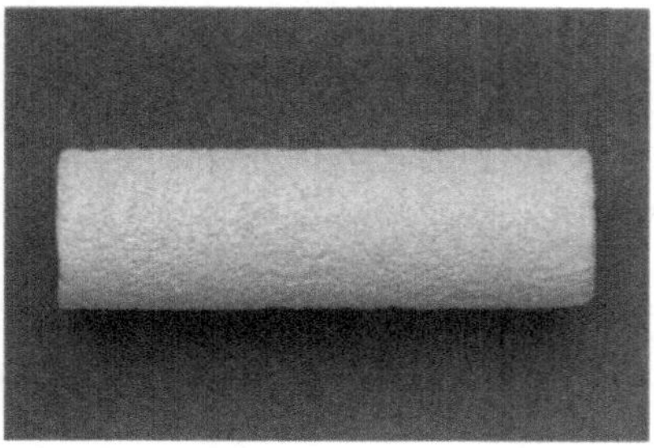

Figure 3:
Cylindrical sample made of Biolox delta®
with porous surface

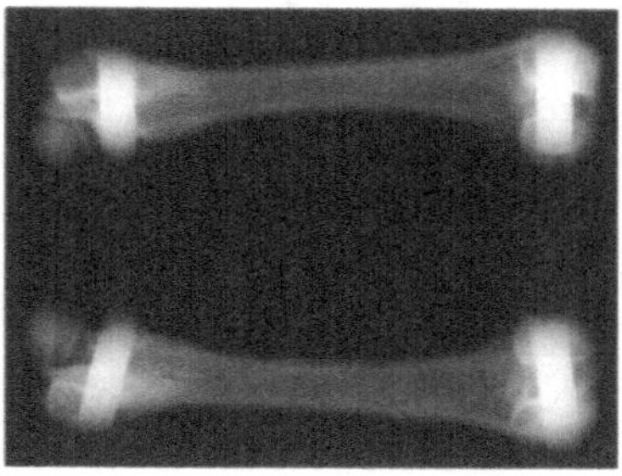

Figure 4:
X-ray of the femur of a pig with an
implanted Biolox delta® sample

Furthermore hemispheric, ceramic monoblock cups with a porous surface made of Biolox delta® have been implanted in sheep. The standing periods are 8 weeks and 1 year. The cups are going to be evaluated macroradiographically and histologically. This study has either not been finished yet.
Until now problems due to the material have not been observed in both studies.

Depending on the results of the mentioned studies a cementless monolithic ceramic cup is supposed to be developed for clinical use.
A renaissance of cementless ceramic monoblock cups seems possible.

References

1 Benum P, Lyng S, Bo O, Rafn I, Haffner JFW (1976). Porous ceramics as a bone substitute in the mediale condyle of the tibia. Acta Orthop Scand 47:158-166
2. Bienek J, Swiecki Z (1991). Porous and porous-compact ceramics in orthopedics. Clin Orthop 272:88-94
3. Cornell NC, Lane JM (1998). Current understanding of osteoconduction in bone regeneration. Clin Orthop 355S:S267-S273
4. Forgon M, Mammel E, Trombitas K, Kacsalova L, Draveczki I (1987). Morphological investigations of a porous aluminium oxide ceramic and the consequences for clinical application. Arch Orthop Trauma Surg 106:385-389
5. Furseth R, Pedersen KN (1978). Ultrastructure of tissue in intrabony and subperiostel porous ceramic implants. Int J Oral Surg 7:471-478
6. Garcia-Cimbrelo E, Martinez-Sayanes JM, Minuesa A, Munuera L (1996). Mittelmeier ceramic-ceramic prosthesis after 10 years. J Arthroplasty 11(7):773-781
7. Gierse H, Maaz B, Hofer C, Gruner S (1996). The ceramic cup type Lindenhof. Results 10-14 years after implantation. Arch Orthop Trauma Surg 115(3-4):167-170
8. Griss P, Claus A, Scheller G (1999). Analyse unserer Erfahrungen mit Keramik/Keramik-Hüftendoprothesen der ersten Generation. In: Sedel L, Willmann G (Hrsg): Reliability and Long-term Results of Ceramics in Orthopaedics. Thieme, Stuttgart, S 43-47
9. Kakutani Y, Yamamuro T, Nakamura T, Kotoura Y (1989). Strengthening of bone implant interface by the use of granule coatings on alumina ceramics. J Biomat Res 23:781-808
10. Pedersen KN, Haanaes HR, LyngS (1974). Tissue ingrowth into mandibular intrabony porous ceramic implants. Int J Oral Surg 3:158-165
11. Pedersen KN, Haanaes HR (1980). Further studies on tissue ingrowth into intrabony porous ceramic implants. Int J Oral Surg 9:140-143
12. Rhinelander FW, Rouweyha M, Milner JC (1971). Microvascular and histogenic responses to implantation of a porous ceramic into bone. J Biomed Mater Res 5(1):81-112
13. Schreiner U, Schroeder-Boersch H, Schwarz M, Scheller G (2002). Verbesserung der knöchernen Integraton bioinerter Keramiken durch Modifikation der Oberfläche – Ergebnisse eines Tierversuches. Biomed Technik 47:164-168
14. Weinstein AM, Klawitter JJ, Cleveland TW (1976). Electrical stimulationof bone growth into porous AL_2O_3. J Biomed Mater Res 10:231-47

Next Generation Ceramic Bearings

P. Merkert

Introduction

For the last 30 years Biolox® forte was the gold standard in ceramic materials for total hip arthroplasty. The new ceramic biocomposite Biolox® delta with its improved properties gives the designer the opportunity to create components, which were not previously possible, for example small-diameter ball heads, thin-walled cup inserts, knees and knee components and finger joints. Since the end of 2002 a stand-alone, validated production capability is available for ball heads.

Material properties

Biolox® delta, was developed by CeramTec AG. It is an alumina matrix composite consisting of an alumina matrix, zirconia grains within the matrix (approx. 25%) and strontium-platelets (Figure 1). Biological testing according to international standards has verified the material's biocompatibility [1].

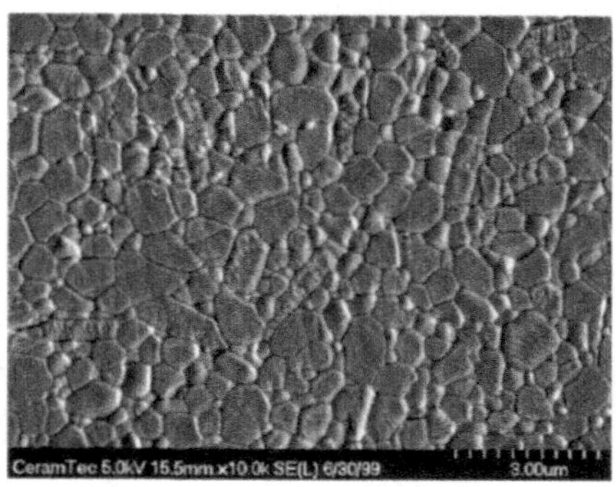

Figure 1:
Microstructure of Biolox® delta

The physical and mechanical properties are summarized in Table 1.

Table 1:
Typical values of some physical and mechanical properties of Biolox® delta

Property	Alumina Matrix Composite*
Density [g/cm³]	>4,36
Grain Size [µm]	≤ 1,5 (Alumina matrix)
4-pt-Strength [MPa]	>1000
K_{Ic} (SEVNB) [MPa√m]	5,7
Hardness [HV·}]	1975
Young´s Modulus [GPa]	350

Burst strength results showed that the material can achieve between 85 and 120 kN for a standard femoral ball head (which can be compared with the FDA requirement of > 46kN). The burst strength does not alter after multiple sterilization cycles in the autoclave even though the material consists of approx. 25 wt % zirconia (Figure 2 and 3). Zirconia, on the other hand, shows aging behavior [2].

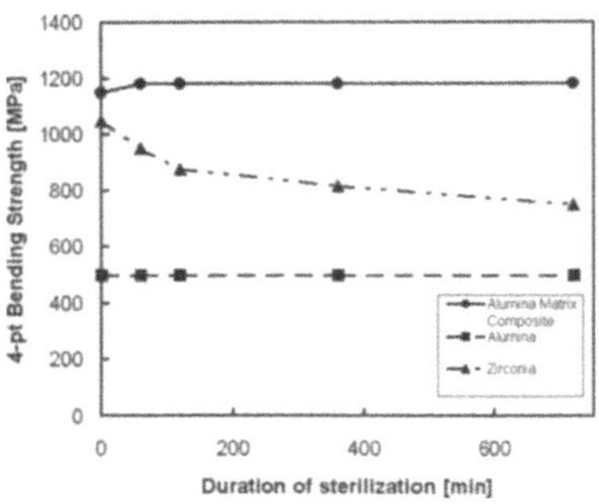

Figure 2:
Comparison of 4-pt bending strength of alumina, zirconia and Biolox® delta after autoclaving [2].

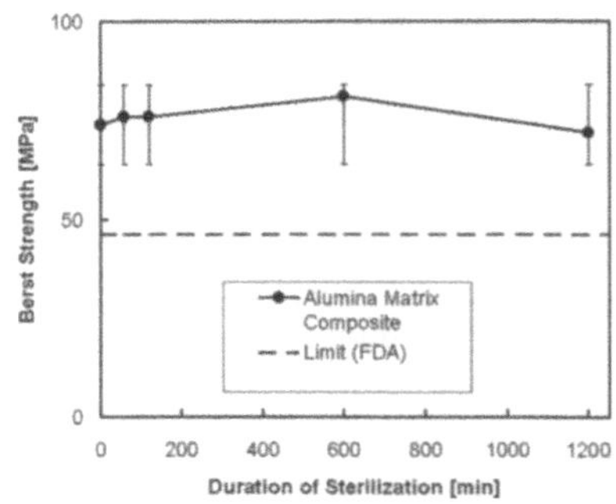

Figure 3:
Burst strength of standard ball heads after sterilization (autoclave) [2].

In hip simulator studies the wear of Biolox® delta-on-Biolox® delta is at least as low as that of alumina-on-alumina. Moreover the wear behaviour is not affected by gamma sterilization or by multiple sterilisation cycles in the autoclave (Figure 4).

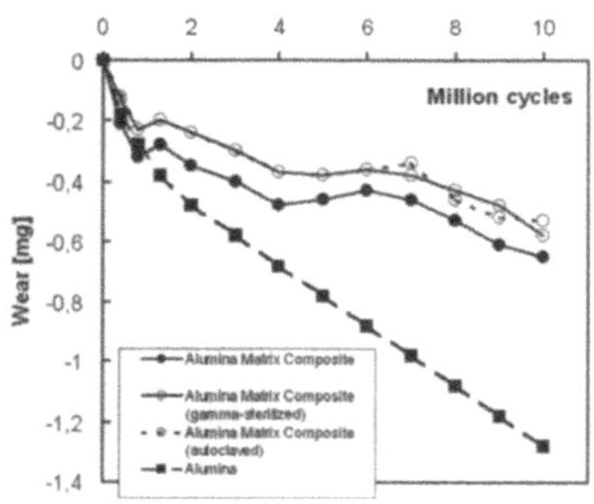

Figure 4:
Comparison of ceramic-on-ceramic hip simulator wear for Biolox® delta (non-sterile, gamma-sterilized and autoclaved) and alumina ball heads (Hip-simulator)

Developments during 2002

After several years of basic research and first part production in 2002, CeramTec developed a stand-alone production capability for Biolox® delta. To do this a team consisting of several engineers was dedicated to work on this task. Tasks for this team included establishing the sinter parameters, finding a sintering furnace having the necessary tight tolerances, working on hard machining and building up (and training) a production team. Approximately 2 million € was invested in machines, furnaces and first production batches. The resulting ball head production facility is only a small part of the entire production facility of the Medical Products Division and is only able to produce a small amount of ball heads at this time. For Biolox® delta two production methods are used. Small ball heads (diameter <28mm) are produced by solid ball head production. This involves the production of a solid ball which is turned, sintered, lapped and polished. Only then is the taper drilled. Large ball heads (diameter >28mm) are produced using the conventional ball head production method in which the ball heads are turned near net shape (including the taper) before sintering. All processes and machines used in the conventional production method are validated. The solid ball head production method will be validated within the next few months.

To further improve the acceptance of ceramic-on-ceramic bearings in arthroplasty CeramTec AG has decided to work with all of its customers in closer combined collaboration during the design development phase. In addition to following FDA design control requirements, CeramTec will define with its customers further test programs to be carried out as well as training activities intended to reduce as much as possible the risk of failure. This will benefit customers, surgeons and patients alike.

Conclusions

The new alumina matrix composite Biolox® delta is a high performance ceramic biocomposite material that combines the excellent material properties of alumina ceramics in terms of chemical stability, hydrothermal stability, biocompatibity and extremely low wear and of zirconia ceramics with its superior mechanical strength and fracture toughness.

Biolox, delta provides the opportunity to manufacture small and thin components, which will perform safely in patients even if they are young (have a long life expectancy) and active.

CeramTec AG is prepared to work with our customers on new developments in orthopaedics in Biolox® delta in order to realize the next generation of joint replacement implants.

References

1. Willmann, G., W. von Chamier, H.G. Pfaff. R. Rack, "Biocompatibility of a New Alumina Matrix Biocomposite AMC", Bioceramics 13, pp. 569 – 572, 2000.
2. Pfaff, H.-G., R. Rack, G. Willmann, "Long-term Performance of a Transformation Toughened Platelet Reinforced Alumina Matrix Composite", Bioceramics 14, pp. 541 – 542, 2001.
3. Burger, W., H.G. Richter, "High Strength and Toughness Alumina Matrix Composites by Transformation Toughened and 'In situ' Platelet Reinforcement (ZPTA) - The New Generation of Bioceramics", Bioceramics 13, pp. 545 – 548, 2000.

3.4 Hip-Spine Relations: Consequences for Acetabular Implantation New solutions with Delta Alumina Tripolar Implants

J.-Y. Lazennec

Dislocation remains one of the most common complications after total hip arthroplasty.

Some factors are related to prosthesis design and surgical implantation. Optimal adjustment of the acetabular cup is of the utmost importance. Precise 3D anatomical analysis shows the limits of pre- and per-operative planification and points out the interest of alternatives with tripolar system.

Anatomical study

Different morphological and functionnal parameters depend on the patient and are more or less controlled during surgical implantation:

- in the coronal plane: the Inclination of the acetabular cup
- in the sagittal plane: 2 angles easily evaluated on lateral X rays
  * the *Acetabular Tilt (AT)* which varies with the position of the pelvis
  * the *Sacro-acetabular Angle (SA)* (position of the acetabulum in relation to pelvic anatomy)
- in the transverse plane, *„functional or real anteversion"*, as anatomical anteversion varies with the position of the acetabular cup in the sagittal plane

Surgical consequences

1. The range of motion of a normal spine allows some adjustment as normal value for variation of Acetabular Tilt is about 30° between standing and sitting position. Those modifications of sagittal orientation are associated with less cup anteversion in standing position and more cup anteversion in sitting position.
2. Diseases affecting lumbosacral junction and prior surgical procedures (aging spine, lumbosacral fusion) reduce the adaptation of THA to sitting or standing position.

   In patients with limited spinal motion and, in many cases, permanent backward rotation of the pelvis, changes in anteversion between the sitting and standing position may be very small. This explains the possible catastrophic consequences of selecting an inappropriate anteversion angle during hip replacement.
3. Implantation of the acetabular cup may change the SA angle to a value outside the physiological range. Standardizing the position of the patient and the operative technique does not eliminate the risk of suboptimal acetabular cup positioning in patients with unusual anatomical characteristics.

   Regarding those morphological and functionnal parameters, *acetabular implantation is an arbitrary compromise.*

4. Bipolar arthroplasty has been proposed as a salvage treatment for recurrent instability, but the functional outcome was not very impressive. Surgical procedures *tripolar prosthesis* are increasing, mainly in Europe, where such devices have been commonly used since the 1980s for recurrent and, in some cases, primary THAs.
   Tripolar implants provide a greater stability than a conventional prosthesis.; several clinical studies support such hypothesis. Compared with bipolar prosthesis, tripolar cups have the advantage of a fixed acetabular component for pain relief. Nevertheless the future of the polyethylene component remains controversial for wear and loosening in those « classical implants ».
5. The use of *Delta Alumina tripolar THA* seems an interesting alternative to solve those difficult situations for adjustment and hip stability , as in some cases no ideal solution can be found for acetabular implantation. The additional outer-bearing surface motion, enlarges the « total dislocatable diameter »and increases range of motion and stability.
   The "self adaptation" of the intermediate cup can be demonstrated and explained geometrically and experimentally.

Conclusion

THA implantation remains a compromise for acetabular adjustment.
Delta alumina tripolar system offers new solutions in difficult cases .

3.5 Are Ceramics in Total Knee Replacement only a Vision to be seen through the pink glasses of Visionaries? – Collaborative Development of Ceramic Knee Components

S. Leyen

Ceramic for Total Knee Replacement

Manufacturing of "High-Tec" engineered Hip implant components from BIOLOX forte has proven to be very successful for Total Hip Replacement (THR). On the other hand, the number of safe advanced Ceramic products is still limited by several barriers like the high cost of development, the production of complex components and the problem to produce reliable high quality parts. The ability to penetrate significantly on the market is therefore more or less restricted to experienced companies. Hence, the existing of a manufacturing technique allowing to produce reliable high quality parts especially concerning complex components is a decisive step to produce knee components.

The prime goal is to develop and disseminate Ceramic Knee Components for Total Knee Replacement (TKR). For many visions which appeared rather plausible in the past (Stock et al. 1991), adequate ceramic materials had been missing. In their search for the optimum developers at CeramTec are entering the world of new "ceramic alloys" with BIOLOX delta (Burger and Richter 2000). A material allowing joint development projects on ceramic knee components together with partners from the orthopedic industry and surgeons. The improved values of the mechanical strength and reliability of the new BIOLOX delta ceramic as compared to the successfully used today's alumina ceramic justify the re-evaluation for the application of ceramics in TKR with the aim of a further reduction or complete avoidance of polyethylene particles and their contribution to implant loosening. Interdisciplinary teamwork of material supplier, implant manufacturer and surgeon allowing more easily product innovation and quicker response to market demands.

Objectives for ceramic in TKR are:

- BIOLOX delta components to reduce the wear debris,
- Reduction of PE back side wear, with no or lowest micro motion.,
- Production of components for metal sensitive patients,
- a safe methodology for product design and manufacture of custom made Ceramic implants,
- the use of BIOLOX delta to safeguard a higher degree of reliability and quality in TKR implants,
- and more depending on the knee design (e. g. Femur, Mobile Meniscal, Uni – MIS etc.).

State-of-the-Art and Degree of Innovation

Today knee components are made of CoCrMo alloy, which incorporate Nickel. Nickel is known to produce allergic reactions (Thomas 2001). A documentary search shows that in the eighties Japanese scientists investigated alumina femoral components (Oonishi and Hasegawa 1981). Furthermore their follow-up showed the reliability of ceramic femoral components; there were no cases of ceramic related fractures. The pioneers investigations started in 1972 by Prof. Langer at the Klinikum Jena have also shown positive results with advanced ceramic in the knee joint and structural reliability of the components (Langer 1992). Table 1 summarizes the material related expected improvements in comparison with the presently used material combinations for total or uni compartmental knee replacements.

Characterisation	**Concept**	**Observation an conclusion**
Ceramic femur on UHMW PE tibial articular insert	Al2O3/PE	• In vivo results are promising • Resistance to third-body rear • Reduced PE wear debris • Option for metal sensitive patients
	BIOLOX delta/PE	• Higher Body Mass Index (BMI) possible • Resistance to third-body rear • Reduced PE wear debris • Option for metal sensitive patients
Ceramic on Ceramic bearing in TKR	Al2O3 / Al2O3	• High resistance to third-body rear • No PE or metal wear debris • Option for a life time bearing • Solution for metal sensitive patients • Thick components
	AMC / AMC	• improved reliability • lowest bone loss • high BMI possible • thin wall components

Table1:
Future Trends for Ceramic TKR – What is next?

Today a CE-Mark has been granted to CeramTec AG for ceramic femoral components to be used on Polyethylene tibial components. Intensive lab-tests have shown that the new BIOLOX delta is suitable to take the body mass load of American and European patients. BIOLOX delta as a novel material has increased density and reduced structural flaws compared to many other industrial quality ceramics. The literature as well as the results of the ongoing feasibility study on ceramic knee components of CeramTec show clearly that there are positive effects of using ceramic in TKR. Is this a vision for ceramics in TKR only to be seen through the pink glasses of visionaries? No – a first published case study clearly shows the future potential (Garino 2002). Furthermore, in simulator studies a mobile bearing concept has proven that the wear could be decreased significantly. Fig. 1 shows the results in comparison to literature values.

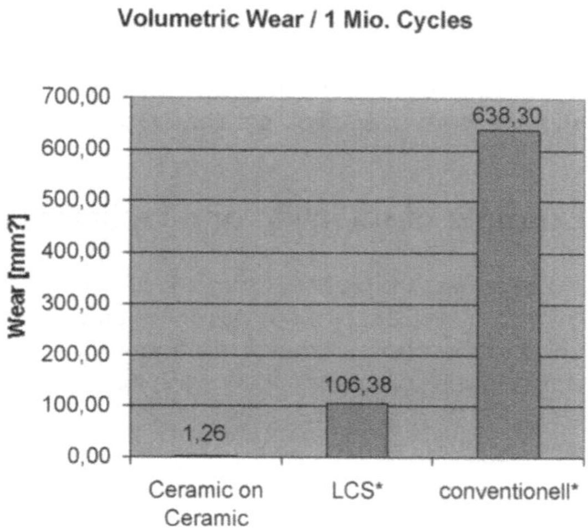

Figure 1:
Comparison of simulator wear performance of an experimental mobile bearing system,
(* Source: "DePuy 20 Jahre LCS Knie")

Components

High-end ceramic components can be produced by use modern compaction technology (Fig.2). Concerning relatively complex components this is a safe way of manufacturing. Alternatives are not so safe, for example:

- slip casting and paste extrusion, which are, due to their high water contents, less suitable and
- uniaxial pressing which is not adequate for large sized thick or three dimensional complex components.

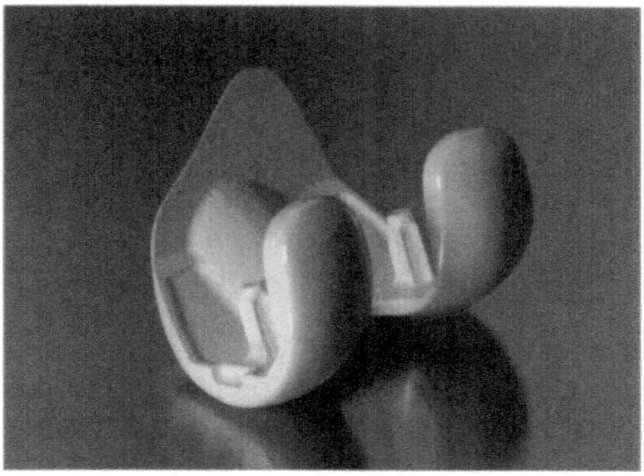

Figure 2:
Prototype femoral component manufactured in BIOLOX® delta

In subsequent green or white machining of pressed parts, even tight tolerances can be economically kept. In general, high quality materials must be used to avoid to introducing defects. These optimum materials are produced by CeramTec and are not comparable to others. The manufacturing capabilities are directly orientated to the needs of the implant manufacturer by optimizing the product to their component design and operating equipment as well as aiming at safe manufacturing process for high quality parts made of BIOLOX delta. The results for the implant manufacturers are expected to show substantial improvement over existing product ranges.

Example of scientific and technical collaboration

CeramTec´s project "Ceramic Knee Development" focuses on a new product and on an increase of the quality of produced bioceramic components. A flow chart of the chosen project methodology is given in Fig. 3. After the initial design data acquisition phase (Task 1) the partners will evaluate a given design for a

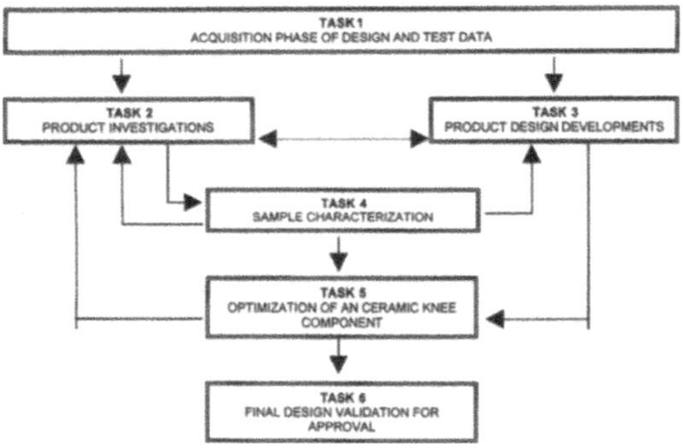

Figure 3:
Project Flow Chart for a typical joint development of a ceramic femur components

ceramic knee component. Detailed component testing (Task 2) will define the requirements for the future product. The component testing typically takes the following into consideration e.g.:

- Validating mechanical integrity of the product,
- Fatigue strength,
- Physiological load tests,
- Varus – Valgus stabilization test
- and, if useful, any combination of tests.

In the characterization phase (Task 4) the achieved results of the product investigations (Task 2) are discussed. They will form a further input for the design criteria of the product design (Task 3). The results of the product investigations will provide design optimization suggestions e.g. the necessary wall thickness and the desired bone fixation. This information is essential for the design of the targeted ceramic knee. By this knowledge the most promising concepts are integrated in an existing product range of knees in order to optimize it (Task 5). A subsequent design validation should deliver the inputs for the final approval (Task 6).

Discussion

The chosen project methodology reduces the product related safety risks to a minimum. All partners involved in projects like this already have gained considerable experience with knee designs. However, it can not be denied that some technical risk remains even with the chosen strategy. Future results are needed to show that the reduction of wear counteracts the more stringent load imposed on the knee in vivo. Furthermore it has to be proven that the new components result in a sufficient quality for young and active patients. This is why each step of the project is carefully adjusted to the others so that all steps shall be accessable. The differences caused by the variables showed to lie within the confidence interval of the chosen evaluation methods, so that significant results shall be achievable. The project milestones are to be chosen in a way, that allow a continuos verification of the achieved results. There shoud be a mid-term assessment so that the partners can decide weather the project is processing well. CeramTec hopes that the objectives of the project will be met with a high probability. All supporting development tasks are carried out in a collaborative development. The interdisciplinary partners are able to exploit the technical results in a far reaching possible way, except where information is commercially sensitive or covered by pending patents. The exisiting consortia intends to disseminate the results through the established channels of technical papers in scientific journals, and presentations at conferences in the near future.

Conclusion

The presently most wear resistant materials available for joint replacements are today's alumina ceramics as confirmed in hip surgery again and again. The much further improvements of the mechanical properties achieved with BIOLOX delta ceramics allow the production of appropriately sized components for TKR. For this reason CeramTec is hopeful that further improved long term success rates based on the complete elimination of polyethylene wear particles can be expected in TKR.

References

1. Burger W, Richter H (2000), High Strength and Toughness Alumina Matrix Composites by Transformation Toughening and `In Situ` Platelet Reinforcement (ZPTA) - The New Generation of Bioceramics Proceeding, Ceramic in Medicine, Bologna.
2. Garino J (2002)Ceramic Hemi-Unicondylar Arthroplasty: Case Study. In: Garino J P, Willmann G(Hrsg) Bioceramics in Joint Arthroplasty. Georg Thieme Verlag, Stuttgart, New York pp 121-124
3. Langer G (1972) Alloplastik am Kniegelenk mit Keramikprothesen, Paper presented at Fall Meeting of Medical and Scientific Society of Friedrich Schiller University Jena, Erfurt, 8th Dec.1992.
4. Oonishi H, Hasegawa T (1981), Cementless Alumina Ceramic total knee prostheses, Orthopedic Ceramic Implants, Vol. 1,.pp 157-160.
5. Stock D et al.(1991), United States Patent No. 5,064,437
6. Thomas P (2001), Allergologische Aspekte der Bioverträglichkeit von Titanbasisimplantaten, BIOmaterialien 2(1), pp 35-44

3.6 Ceramic Femoral Components in Total Knee Replacement

B. S. Bal and H. Oonishi

Introduction

Total knee arthroplasty is a surgical procedure with established success, and impressive survival rates at 15-20 years following the operation. Ultimately, total knee replacement components undergo aseptic loosening and failure. Progressive wear at the articulation of the artificial knee leads to the accumulation of microscopic wear particles in the periprosthetic tissues. The resulting inflammatory response can manifest as periprosthetic bone resorption that results in aseptic loosening of the implants, and late failure of the arthroplasty.

Alternative bearing surfaces have the potential of greatly reducing wear at the articulating surfaces of total hip and total knee replacements, thereby minimizing the possibility of periprosthetic osteolysis. While ceramic bearing surfaces have been used extensively in total hip replacement, the data for such biomaterials in total knees is relatively sparse. In this report, our experience with the use of ceramics in total knee replacements is summarized.

Design and Material Evolution

The impetus for a ceramic component in total knee replacement came from the encouraging wear data in total hip replacements with ceramic bearing surfaces. The senior author began using the KOM-1 (named after the Kokuritsu Osaka Minami Hospital) total knee system in 1982. The femoral component, tibia baseplate and the patella backing in the KOM-1 knee were made of alumina, with polyethylene inserts attached to the patella and tibia. These components were implanted without bone cement in 137 patients. At 15-18 years, in the 80% patients available for followup, a high incidence of failures was noted. Failures occurred because of inadequate fixation of the implants to bone, and not because of the use of ceramic.

The next evolutionary step was the second generation KOM-2 knee, developed in 1990. All components were now cemented to the underlying bone. A metal tibial tray was used to reduce component thickness. Articulating surfaces consisted of alumina-on-polyethylene. Of the 112 total knees implanted and available for followup at 4-10 years, none of the implants had failed. Periprosthetic radiolucent lines typically associated with total knee components were the only significant finding in this group.

The KOM-3 total knee was introduced in 1993. The principles of cement fixation were retained in this design, and the alumina femoral component now had beads to enhance cement fixation. Also, the patella was now all-polyethylene. In 111 patients that received a KOM-3 total knee, and that were available for followup at 2-7 years following the operation, occasional radiolucent lines around the implants were the only significant finding, with no clinical failures.

followup at 2-7 years following the operation, occasional radiolucent lines around the implants were the only significant finding, with no clinical failures.

More recently, in the year 2002, the senior author began using the Bisurface total knee, consisting of a zirconia femoral component, designed specially to enhance deep knee flexion. The knee is implanted with cement, and the posterior cruciate ligament is sacrificed. This design reflects the improvements and progress that began with the KOM-1 knee.

Separate from the above series, starting in 2001, thirty-five total knees were implanted in a clinical trial conducted in the United States, using a yttrium-stabilized zirconia femoral component. Cemented components from the Foundation Total Knee system (Encore Orthopaedics Inc, Austin, Texas, USA) were implanted. A deep-dish ultracongruent polyethylene insert substituted for the posterior cruciate ligament, which was sacrificed in each case. Early follow data demonstrate results that are identical to a control group, i.e., total knee replacements performed with the same components, except that the femoral component was made of cobalt-chrome instead.

Discussion

Knee simulator data have demonstrated at least a two-fold reduction in the generation of polyethylene wear with the zirconia femoral component. Comparable data have been reported for femoral components coated with oxidized zirconium. Ceramic femoral components have less surface roughness compared to those made of cobalt-chrome, and in vitro data have demonstrated that the depth of polyethylene wear is significantly less with a ceramic femoral component.

The theoretical concern of a ceramic component rupturing in service is not supported by the available clinical data. 223 total knees with the Bisurface ceramic femoral components were reported with a 2-9 year followup by Akagi et al. (JBJS 2000). Oonishi et al. reported on 360 total knees with an alumina ceramic femoral component at 3-18 years after implantation (Key Eng Mat 2001). Yasuda et al. reported on 32 total knees with a ceramic femoral component at 2-4 years after implantation (Bull Hosp Jt Dis 1993). Not a single instance of mechanical failure of the ceramic component was reported in any of these series.

Conclusions

Ceramics may have a role in extending the life of total knee replacements. Existing wear data, and the clinical information to date is encouraging. Clinical studies using ceramic femoral components in total knee systems with otherwise well proven designs and a long track record of clinical success will identify the precise role of this promising technology in total knee replacement surgery.

SESSION 4

Computer Assisted Knee Surgery: Development and Evaluation

4.1 Navigation in Knee Endoprosthetics: Merits and Disadvantages

K. Labs, G. Matziolis and C. Perka

Introduction

Among the factors that are decisive for the success of knee endoprosthesis are the patient group, the design of the prosthesis, the surgical technique used, alignment of the implant, soft-tissue balance, axial alignment and perioperative management.

Despite the availability of modern instruments enabling intramedullary and/or extramedullary alignment, considerable axial deviations can be observed postoperatively, which range between a varus malalignment of 20° and a valgus malalignment of 23° [2, 3, 5, 13, 20, 22, 23]. The correlation between axial malalignment and the occurrence of an increased rate of aseptic loosening of the prosthesis has been described in the relevant literature [5,7,8,21,29,31]. Axial malalignment also results in increased wear of the polyethylene components, which may require surgical revision.

Up to one third of all knee endoprostheses implanted by way of conventional surgical techniques exhibit malalignments of more than 3° in the frontal plane. Also, deviations in the sagittal plane will affect the rate of loosening [15]. The rates of aseptic loosening reported at a follow up of 8 years by Jeffery et al. [8] ranged at 3% for properly aligned and at 24% for improperly aligned prosthetic components.

It was shown by a publication of Rand und Coventry [21] that within a range of 0° to 4° of deviation from the mechanical axis, after 10 years a survival rate of 90% was observed, which was found to be reduced to 70% as soon as the axial deviation ranged beyond such limits. Hence, there is a direct correlation between the survival rate of knee endoprostheses and the accuracy of implantation.

The accuracy of conventional instruments for axis measurement is limited. For instance, the standard instruments generally available will not allow determination of the exact position of the femoral head or the ankle joint center. Apart from that, a standard bone geometry has been assumed in the design of such instruments, which will not be matched in every clinical case.

For this reason, the use of computer-aided surgery in the implantation of knee endoprostheses started in the mid-nineties. On the 21st of January 1997, the first computer-aided implantation of a prosthesis was performed by Saragaglia in Grenoble using the Orthopilot system (Aesculap AG, Tuttlingen, FRG). In the sequel, such technique was developed further and modified by a number of engineering companies. Currently, a number of nine different computer-aided navigation systems (ORTHOPILOT, Aesculap AG; SurgiGate, Medivision; Galileo, Endoplus; Navitrak, Centerpulse; Vector Vision, BrainLab; STRYKER-LEIBINGER, Stryker-Howmedica-Osteonics; MEDTRONIC and DISOS) and one robot-aided system (Robodoc, ISS) are used worldwide, the clinical application of which differs considerably as far as their functioning and operational characteristics are concerned. However, the aim shared by all of such systems is to optimise prosthesis alignment.

Computer-aided systems

Computer-aided systems basically integrate a number of three standardized components:

1 the therapeutical object
2 the virtual object
3 the anatomic environment

Basically, one distinguishes between passive systems such as for instance optoelectronic or electromagnetic navigation systems and active systems such as medical robots. Current R&D activities also concentrate on semiactive systems [12].
The above differentiation is due to the functional characteristics of such systems. Navigation systems work on the principle of passive elements, whereas robotics uses active components which perform autonomous operations. Latest system developments such as the Galileo system (Endoplus) integrate both system categories.
In addition, Picard et al. [18] distinguished between image and image-free navigation systems. While image systems require data acquisition using either preoperative CT or intraoperative fluoroscopy, the image-free systems enable intraoperative collection of necessary data using a kinematic model and an appropriate software without the need of any preoperative planning stage to enable exact positioning of the sawing gauge.

First results

1. The most comprehensive results of knee navigation have been obtained for the OrthoPilot system (Aesculap AG) from a multicenter study which was conducted by five orthopaedic and emergency surgery centers, and which included a total of 821 patients [1]. In the study, knee prostheses were implanted in 266 patients using conventional techniques, and in 555 patients using a navigation system. For this, an "image-free" navigation system was used. Radiological evaluation was performed for five axes (mechanical leg axis as well as frontal and sagittal orientation of both the femoral and the tibial prosthetic components).
The navigated group yielded a significantly higher accuracy of the mechanical axis, the femoral axis a/p, the tibial axis a/p and the sagittal plane. The cut-to-suture time varied between 56 and 165 (average 99.2 +/- 22.4) minutes in the conventional group, and between 70 and 193 (average 107.8 +/- 22.4) minutes in the navigated group, which means that the operating time was prolonged by 8.6 minutes at average. The rate of complications reported for the navigated group (6.1 %) was significantly lower than the one reported for the manual group (21.8 %).

The outcome of a comparative study which included 50 navigated (OrthoPilot, Aesculap AG) and 50 conventionally implanted prostheses was reported by Miehlke et al. [15]. The study yielded unacceptable results in 4 % of the navigated and in 8 % of the manual cases, the difference being statistically significant. Optimum results within a tolerance range of +/- 2° were achieved in 58 % of the navigated and in 44 % of the manual operations. Optimum results in

respect of a total of five radiological parameters were found to be much more frequent in the navigated group (n=22) than in the manual group (n=8). There wasn't any statistically significant difference in intraoperative blood loss, although such difference had been expected as a result of the necessity to open up the femoral medullary canal for manual instrumentation.
The operating time had been significantly longer in the first 30 cases reflecting the learning curve. From 40 cases onward, the operating times ranged between 60 and 75 minutes. Nowadays, the supplementary time required for navigation is approximately 12 to 15 minutes.

A number of 40 knee endoprostheses were implanted by Jenny and Boeri [9] using the OrthoPilot navigation system. A comparative number of the same prosthetic system (Search prosthesis, Aesculap AG) were implanted using conventional techniques. Proper alignment of the mechanical leg axis (≤3° varus/valgus error) was achieved in 85 % of the navigated cases and in 72 % of the manually implanted cases. Only 30 % of the conventionally implanted but 62 % of the computer-navigated cases complied a tolerance of ≤3° by all of the five axes.

2. The SurgiGate system (Medivision) also is a so called "image-free system" and is based on kinetic motion analysis. The system consists of an optoelectronic camera which registers the movements of the surgical instruments, and relates them to a coordinate system of the tibia and the femur. Referencing is performed subsequent to the establishment of basic dynamic reference data. The first 57 clinical applications were reported on by Strauss and Rüther [26]. There weren't any significant differences observed between navigated and conventional operations as far as the loss of blood, complications, Knee Society Score, ligament stability and the quality of alignment of the femoral component is concerned. The navigated operations allowed for significant improvements to be observed in respect of the mechanical leg axis, the position of the tibial plateau (a/p and slope) and the restoration of the articular line. The percentage of the prostheses which complied with a tolerance ≤3° for the mechanical leg axis was 93.3 % in the navigated group, and 77.8 % in the group of conventionally implanted prostheses. The mean deviation from the ideal axis in the frontal plane was 0.8° in the navigated and 1.4° in the conventional group. The mean cranial displacement of the articular line was 2.2 mm in the navigated and 5.9 mm in the conventional group. The use of navigation prolonged the operating time by 12 to 62 (average 19) minutes.

3. The Navitrak knee navigation system (Centerpulse, Winterthur) is a modular system working as well on an optoelectronic as on an electromagnetic principle. Electromagnetic navigation has been ousted to a very large extent by the benefits offered by optoelectronic coupling. Against the background of the CT-based application of the Navitrak system in spine surgery for positioning of pedicle screws, a CT-based application had been developed and used clinically in knee endoprosthetics [16]. Due to the costly and time-consuming preoperative phase an improved CT-free version, which is available since March 2002, has been developed on the basis of the gained clinical experiences [14]. The results obtained from initial clinical application of the CT-based version in a number of 31 operations were reported by MATTES and PUHL [14]. In the beginning, up to three hours were required for preoperative image reconstruction and planning. However, it was soon possible to reduce such time

to approximately 45 minutes. The average operating time has been 108 minutes (85–130 minutes). Further evaluation was performed based upon Knee Society recommendations using special alignment scores. In this evaluation system, perfectly aligned prostheses were assigned a maximum of 100 points. In this respect, an average alignment score of 80 (± 11.2) points was achieved. As far as the individual components were concerned, the worst score obtained for the femoral component (a/p) was 18 out of 25. There weren't any substantial complications reported. For reasons of the current data situation, it is not yet possible to make a final assessment of the CT-free application.

4. Knee-endoprosthetic navigation using the VectorVision system (BrainLAB) also offers the possibility of using either a CT-based or CT-free operating mode. So far, initial results have been available for CT- free navigation only. Perlick et al. [17] reported on their experience obtained from the navigated implantation of more than 16 TKAs, and compared such data to the data obtained for a number of 25 conventional implantations. Resulting from this was that in 86 % of the navigated group and in 52 % of the conventional group the mechanical leg axis was located in a varus/valgus range of +/-2°. When extending the tolerance to +/- 3° varus/valgus, 93 % of the navigated and 72 % of the conventionally instrumented prostheses were found to be in compliance. There is a tendency towards higher precision in the navigation-aided group. For reasons of small case figures, significance testing has not been performed.

5. The results obtained from knee navigation using the Stryker-Leibinger system (Stryker-Howmedica-Osteonics) in primary and revision implantations were reported by Sparmann and Wolke [25]. The system is an image-free system and works on the principle of kinematic analysis. Sparmann and Wolke compared the results obtained for two patient groups which included a number of 120 patients each. In one group, navigated instrumentation, and in the other group manual instrumentation had been used. The study yielded that in the navigated group the accuracy of implantation was improved to a highly significant degree.

6. A completely different navigation principle is offered by the Medtronic system. The image-generator-assisted navigation requires an intraoperative fluoroscopy of the hip, knee and ankle. On the basis of this fluoroscopic examination, the exact mechanical axis is calculated and represented threedimensionally. The time taken by such intraoperative examination for the purpose of evaluation by the image generator ranges at approx. 8 minutes, and for fluoroscopy is less than 1 minute, and hence can be considered to be of minor significance.
HAGENA et al. [6] reported on their experience obtained from the use of navigation in the implantation of 40 TKAs. For the purpose of evaluating the degree of accuracy offered by this navigation system, a prospective randomised study was initiated. Results are still unavailable. However, a high degree of accuracy of the intraoperatively obtained C-arm image for use in navigation has been reported [6].

7. The Disos system (Desktop Image Processing System for Orthopaedic Surgery) was developed by the German Helmholtz Institute of Aachen. The system provides the preoperative planning of the surgical procedure on the basis of obtained from CT data. The entire planning process is divided into the following

stages: analysis of individual biomechanical joint parameters, planning of implants and of the cutting planes, motion analysis and ligament balancing, as well as calculation of individual templates necessary for an intraoperative mechanical surface matching. Basically, data acquisition is possible not only on the basis of three dimensionally reconstructed CT scans but also on the basis of scout films (scout view, topogram) generated by a CT scanner. The two decisive benefits offered by the use of topograms consist in the reduction of radiation exposure and of cost in particular.
The planning results are being transferred to the patient by using individual templates. For this, the individual profile of the bone surface of a specific tibial or femoral area, reconstructed out of the CT data, is reproduced onto a separate polycarbonate block by way of computer-controlled milling after completion of the preoperative planning phase. Owing to the templates' exact adaptation to the bone structure, they can be used intraoperatively for the alignment of tools such as e.g. the above-mentioned cutting block for tibial or femoral osteotomy. Portheine et al. [19] reported on the results obtained from the first ten clinical applications of the system. Compared to other CAS systems, the template method used in knee endoprosthetics is superior especially by the fact that there aren't any supplementary technical aids required at the intraoperative stage, and that the surgical routine process is preserved to a large extent. Owing to the simple and exact alignment of the cutting block, which is enabled by the individual template, there no longer is any need to use intra- and extramedullary guide rods, which in the past proved to be time-consuming and inaccurate.

8. The Galileo system (Endoplus) consists of both a navigation and a robot part. Navigation is performed using an optoelectronic system which works in the infrared wavelength range. The system's minirobot can be autoclaved and is equipped with two linear shafts which are driven by servomotors. The robot's small dimensions enable its intraoperative use on the patient.
Registration of the skeleton geometry is performed by way of kinematic analysis. The center of the femoral head is determined kinematically without the use of any supplementary pin on the iliac crest. Relative movements of the pelvis are compensated for mathematically.
The system registers defined landmarks by way of scanning. For this, data relating to the mechanical axis, component size, femoral and tibial rotation and to the joint plane and the ankle joint are registered.
Computer-controlled positioning of the femur-cutting gauge is performed using the minirobot. The robot itself will not carry out any cutting or milling operations but positions the saw guide used for conventional oscillating bone saws. Currently, a surgical technique involving the measurement of ligament length and tension is being tested clinically.
First results obtained from a number of 41 clinical applications were reported by Ritschl et al. [24]. In these applications, the average deviation for the mechanical femoral axis in the frontal plane was 0.8° (0° – 2.3°) and 6 mm (0 – 14mm), respectively.

9. The Robodoc system (ISS) first was developed for use on the hip joint for milling prosthetic stems, and afterwards was developed further for use in knee endoprosthetics. The system allows for the optimum position of the implant components to be determined preoperatively on the basis of CT datasets, and enables calculation of the relevant milling paths. At the intraoperative stage, the

knee joint must be fixed firmly using two Schanz screws in order to avoid motion-induced artifacts. The first clinical applications of the system were reported on by Börner [12]. Evaluation of the results obtained from another study group which comprised a number of 52 robot-milled knee endoprostheses, and a number of 53 conventionally implanted prostheses yielded proper leg axes without any exceptions in the robot-milled group. In contrast to this, axial deviations of up to 7° were observed in 35% of the conventionally implanted prostheses [4].

Merits and disadvantages offered by navigation systems

In order to determine the merits or disadvantages offered by the aforementioned navigation and robotic systems, the system parameters listed below must be compared:

1. System admits the use of products of other manufacturers
2. Clearly structured and easy-to-use software
3. Modular structure of the navigation system
4. Uncomplicated data acquisition for alignment determination
5. CT-free data acquisition
6. Unrestricted rotational alignment of components
7. Detection of extra-articular deformities
8. Acceptable prolongation of operating times
9. Possibility of taking into account soft-tissue tension
10. Kinematic analysis including plausibility check
11. dentification and correction of registration errors
12. Possibility of changing over to conventional instrumentation without any difficulties
13. No supplementary pins required on the pelvis
14. Cost

	OrthoPilot	Surgigate	Navitrack	VectorVision	Stryker	Medtronic	Disos	Galileo	Robodoc
system admits products of other manufacturers	-	+	+	+	+	+	+	+	-
Software is cleary arranged and easy to use	+	+	+	+	+	+	-	+	+
modular structure of the navigation for determination of alignment	+	+	+	-	-	-	+	-	+
uncomplicated data acquisition for determination of alignment	+	+	+	+	+	+	-	+	-
CT-free data acquisition	+	+	both	both	+	+	-	+	-
unrestricted rotational alignment of components	-	-	-	-	-	-	-	-	-
detection and management of extra-articular deformities	-	-	+	+	-	+	+	-	+
acceptable prolongation of operating time	+	+	+	+	+	+	+	+	+
possibility of taking into account soft-tissue tension	-	+	-	-	-	-	-	-	-
kinematic analysis including plausibilit5y check	-	+	-	-	+	-	-	-	-
identification and correction of registration errors	-	-	-	-	-	-	-	-	-
possibility of changing over to conventional instrumentation without any difficulties	+	+	+	+	+	+	+	+	-
no supplementary pins required on the pelvis	-	-	+	+	-	+	-	+	+
high cost	+	+	+	+	+	-	-	+	+

Table 1:
Survey of available navigation and robot systems and their features

Up to now, it is not possible to establish a quality ranking by way of comparison of the systems. The only information which can be drawn from such comparison is a survey of the system requirements and of their application range.
It can be seen from the survey given in table 1 that currently there are six CT-free, two CT-aided and one fluoroscopy-aided systems available. The benefits offered by CT-free systems such as reduction of preoperative planning time, cut-down on cost and radiation exposure are relativized by the disadvantages existing in respect of kinematic data acquisition. Apart from that, intraoperative collection of data for the determination of axial conditions requires a lot of routine and is time-consuming. For the time being, CT-free systems will not enable the detection of extra-articular axial deviations. Moreover, the use of pivoting algorithms requires free-moving hip and ankle joints as a prerequisite. CT-free systems cannot be used in cases having a pathological hip center, e.g. serious cases of hip dysplasia or even congenital hip displacement. Apart from that, the results obtained when determining the femoral rotation using CT-free systems are still inaccurate and hardly reproducible. It is in this respect that the CT-aided systems offer distinct benefits. They also enable the detection of extra-articular deformities, and their integration into the planning process. Another benefit consists in representation of the epicondylar axis, which is essential for a correct determination of the femoral component rotation.
Currently, it is not yet possible to assess the more complex and more time-consuming and hence more expensive CT-based systems as far as improved accuracy of implant alignment is concerned. Relevant studies can only be conducted after completion of the software's planning and angle measuring module which currently is being tested and adapted [14]. In the case of extreme malalignment and acquired or congenital deformities of the lower extremity, the use of image-based navigation systems may offer better results. One aspect which is particularly valuable in respect of the surgical process and the operative result is the preoperative study of the patient's virtual 3D anatomy. It should be the objective of CT-based navigation to provide for exact determination of axial, torsional and rotational deficiencies or of bone defects as early as at the preoperative stage, and to enable exact planning and navigation of implant size and alignment. As far as standard implantations in the event of slightly changed anatomies are concerned, the benefit of three-dimensional planning seems to be of marginal significance to the outcome. In such cases, CT-free navigation will do.

Although it is true that the production of individual templates using the DISOS system which works on the basis of CT-aided planning is cost-efficient, it requires comprehensive technical equipment and is linked to the availability of a lab which offers the equipment needed. Compared to other systems, the principle on which this system works is not bound to classical navigation principles, and is based on CAD (Computer-Aided Design).

At present, intraoperative fluoroscopy can be considered to constitute a low-cost alternative to the use of CT-free or CT-aided systems. Regular adaptation and controls performed by the surgeon will have a positive effect on the surgical approach in TKA implantation. Owing to the three-dimensional reconstruction of the C-arm image, it is no longer necessary to perform expensive and time-consuming CT examinations and the calculations linked to them.

The disadvantage harboured by free-hand navigation systems generally lies in that the resection as such is performed using conventional bone saws although the resection cuts are determined by way of virtual control. This process neglects the saw blade's natural vibration also in respect of the quality of the bone involved. Possible deviations are detected to an insufficient extent only, and there haven't been any comprehensive plausibility checks developed so far. In contrast to this, the use of robots enables a much higher accuracy of milling paths.

The combination of navigation and robotics as used by the Galileo system seems to offer precious merits in respect of precise adjustment of the sawing cuts. Owing to such precise adjustment, the robot will work very accurately although it will not perform the bone milling operations as such. For the purpose of precisely balanced flexion and extension gaps, the system enables corrections in ventrodorsal and craniocaudal direction in increments of 0.5 mm. However, installation of the minirobot on the ventral distal corticalis of the femur seems to have an altering effect on the soft tissue.

Currently, ligament balancing and kinematic analysis of the surgical operations performed constitute the largest challenges to all of the systems. At present, symmetry and equity of the flexion and extension gaps are achieved using a distractor which allows for the tension of ligaments to be adjusted to the desired level. Current navigation systems indicate any remaining axial deviation in every plane. In the future, the quality of ligament balancing shall be improved by as a result of the introduction of more sophisticated measurement systems (pressure sensors).

The use of intraoperatively established kinematic analyses would be desirable for all of the systems, but currently is offered by some systems only. The kinematic graphs obtained from such analyses help to unmask medial and lateral instabilities. Measurements of this kind can be helpful in the analysis of malaligned implants for the purpose of revision surgery in order to determine the extent of malalignment.

Summary

Currently, the data available on computer-assisted surgery in knee endoprosthetics will not allow for any evaluation to be made as far as the superiority of individual systems is concerned. The consistent process of further development of modules and software applications offers an ever improving approach to the requirements of practical application.

There are first results available, which have been obtained from the use of individual systems, and which proved that partly significant improvements were achieved in implant alignment within the framework of comparative studies. The additional pre- and intraoperative time can be considered to be acceptable. Attention should be attached to the fact that complication figures did not increase.

So far, the systems used have not been in full compliance with the standards specified by the German Society for Orthopedics and Orthopedic Surgery as far as the admission of products of other manufacturers and kinematic analysis are concerned. Exact rotation alignment and controlled ligament balancing shall be the largest challenges in the future.

The studies which have been conducted so far, have reported on standard implants only, which were analyzed in respect of the accuracy of implantation on the basis of radiological geometry. These studies did not take into account special prosthetic designs such as fixed or mobile tibial inlay components or

implants for conservation or substitution of the posterior cruciate ligament. The alignment required especially in the sagittal tibial profile according to manufacturers' recommendations is substantially different.
The circumstance which must be criticized in all clinical studies which have been conducted to analyze the accuracy of systems is that three-dimensional problems were evaluated using two-dimensional radiological evaluation. The reproducibility of standard X-ray settings must be doubted to a very large extent, with individual measurement errors ranging at 1°. The extent of faulty assessment in the range of internal rotation of 20° and external rotation of 20° is estimated to range between 0° and 2° (SWANSON 2000). Hence, it is not possible to make any statement on the accuracy of femoral or tibial rotation using simple two-plane X-ray analysis.
The introduction of navigation systems offered potential merits in respect of higher precision for enabling the implantation of bicondylar knee endoprostheses without axial deficiencies. Surgeons are offered a valuable aid which after a certain learning process is likely to increase the precision of implantation. This becomes particularly clear when assessing the number of evaluated axes. While in conventional implantations it will probably be possible to implant a knee prosthesis properly in one or two axes only, the use of navigation systems allows for precise implantation in three or four axes at a time within a tolerance range of less than 2° which will be achieved at a much higher statistically significant probability rate [11].
The benefits offered by free-hand navigation systems consist in optimized alignment of the prosthetic components, and also in objectivation of the ligament conditions in the case of some systems. For the time being, it is not possible to completely eliminate sawing inaccuracies. The use of robots in the future could be very helpful in the optimization of sawing edges.
Critical intraoperative plausibility checks must be performed in order to detect possible malalignments and to remedy such mistakes. Preoperative radiography of the whole-leg in standing is necessary since it enables the detection of extra-articular femoral or tibial deviations. Any correction of such deformations by way of intra-articular intervention may cause irreversible instability of the collateral ligament since image free navigation systems base upon a normal anatomy of bones. In such cases and in the event of osseous defects, the use of image based modules is indicated since they offer the benefit of precise planning on the basis of image data records [17].

To enable the assessment of navigation or robot systems which are still at the stage of development, standardized evaluation criteria must be established. Apart from that, the benefits the patient gets out of the application of computer-assisted systems must be described and proved scientifically, which is a big challenge since especially the clinical results and the delayed results in particular are influenced by a number of additional factors [32].

References

1. Clemens U, Miehlke RK, Kohler S et al. (2003) Computerassistierte Navigation mit dem OrthoPilot-System und der Search-Evolution-Knieendoprothese. Ergebnisse einer Multicenter-Studie. In: Navigation und Robotic in der Gelenk- und Wirbelsäulenchirurgie. Hrsg. W. Konermann, R. Haaker, Springer-Verlag Berlin Heidelberg New York, pp 207-216
2. Coull R, Bankes MJK, Rossouw DJ (1999). Evaluation of tibial component angles in 79 consecutive total knee arthroplasty. Knee 5: 165-174
3. Feng EL, Stulberg SD, Wixson RL (1994). Progressive subluxation and polyethylene wear in total knee replacements with flat articular surfaces. Clin Orthop 299: 60-71
4. Gebhard F, Arand M, Fleiter T et al. (2001) Computer assistierte Chirurgie, Entwicklung und Perspektiven 2001. Unfallchirurg 104: 782-788
5. Goodfellow J.W., O'Connor J.J. (1986). Clinical results of the Oxford knee. Clin. Orthop 205: 21-24
6. Hagena FW, Kettrukat M, Christ R (2003) Fluoroskopieassistierte Navigation mit dem Medtronic-System. In: Navigation und Robotic in der Gelenk- und Wirbelsäulenchirurgie. Hrsg. W. Konermann, R. Haaker, Springer-Verlag Berlin Heidelberg New York, pp 256-261
7. Hsu HP, Garg A, Walker PS, Spector M, Ewald F.C. (1989). Effect of knee component alignment on tibial load distribution with clinical correlation. Clin Orthop. 1989: 135-44
8. Jeffery RS, Morris RW, Denham RA (1991) Coronal alignment after total knee replacement. J Bone Joint Surg 709-714
9. Jenny JY, Boeri C (2001) Computer-assisted implantation of total knee prostheses: a case control comparative study with classical instrumentation. Comput Aided Surg 6: 217-220
10. Insall JN, Binazzi R, Soudry M, Mestriner LA (1985) Total knee arthroplasty Clin Orthop 192: 13-22
11. Kiefer H (2003) Navigation in der Knieendoprothetik. In: Stand und Perspektiven der Computer-assistierten Chirurgie. Hrsg. K Labs, H Zippel, Uni-Med-Verlag Bremen London Boston, pp 105-108
12. Labs K (2002) Entwicklung und Perspektiven der computerassistierten Chirurgie. In: Stand und Perspektiven der Computer-assistierten Chirurgie. Hrsg. K Labs, H Zippel, Uni-Med-Verlag Bremen London Boston, pp 19-21
13. Laskin RS (1990) Total condylar knee replacement in patients who have rheumatoid arthritis. A ten year follow-up study. J. Bone Joint Surg 72A: 529-535
14. Mattes T, Puhl W (2003) Knieendoprothesennavigation mit dem Navitrack-System. In: Navigation und Robotic in der Gelenk- und Wirbelsäulenchirurgie. Hrsg. W. Konermann, R. Haaker, Springer-Verlag Berlin Heidelberg New York, pp 230-239
15. Miehlke RK (2002) Computerassistierte Instrumentation in der Knieend-oprothetik. In: Stand und Perspektiven der Computer-assistierten Chirurgie. Hrsg. K Labs, H Zippel, Uni-Med-Verlag Bremen London Boston, pp 98-100
16. Nizard R (2002) The navitrack system rationale and first experience. In: Stand und Perspektiven der Computer-assistierten Chirurgie. Hrsg. K Labs, H Zippel, Uni-Med-Verlag Bremen London Boston, pp 109-113
17. Perlick L, Bäthis H, Grifka J (2003) Knieendoprothesennavigation mit dem CT-freien Vector Vision System. In: Navigation und Robotic in der Gelenk- und Wirbelsäulenchirurgie. Hrsg. W. Konermann, R. Haaker, Springer-Verlag Berlin Heidelberg New York, pp 245-249
18. Picard F, Moody J, Jaramaz B, DiGioia AM, Nikou C, LaBaraca RS (2000) In: Proceedings 4th Annual North American Program on Computer Assisted Orthopaedic Surgery 89-90, Pittsburgh

19. Portheine F, Ohnsorge J, Schkommodau E, Radermacher K (2003) CT-basierte Planung und DISOS-Schablonennavigation in der Knieend-oprothetik. In: Navigation und Robotic in der Gelenk- und Wirbelsäulen-chirurgie. Hrsg. W. Konermann, R. Haaker, Springer-Verlag Berlin Heidelberg New York, pp 262-272
20. Ranawat CS, Flynn WF Jr, Saddler S, Hansraj KK, Maynard MJ (1993) Long-term results of the total condylar knee arthroplasty. A 15-year survivorship study. Clin Orthop 286: 94-102
21. Rand JA, Coventry MB (1988) Ten-year evaluation of geometric total knee arthroplasty. Clin Orthop 232: 168-173
22. Ritter MA, Herbst SA, Keating GM, Faris PM (1994) Radiolucency at the bone-cement interface in total knee replacement. J Bone Joint Surg 76A: 60-65
23. Ritter MA, Faris PM, Keating EM, Meding JB (1994) Postoperative alignment of total knee replacement. Its effect on survival. Clin Orthop 299: 153-6
24. Ritschl P, Machacek F, Fuiko R (2003) Das Galileo-System. Eine integrierte Lösung aus Navigation und Robotic zur Implantation von Knienedoprothesen. In: Navigation und Robotic in der Gelenk- und Wirbelsäulenchirurgie. Hrsg. W. Konermann, R. Haaker, Springer-Verlag Berlin Heidelberg New York, pp 225-229
25. Sparmann M, Wolke B (2003) Knieendoprothesennavigation mit dem Stryker-System. In: Navigation und Robotic in der Gelenk- und Wirbelsäulenchirurgie. Hrsg. W. Konermann, R. Haaker, Springer-Verlag Berlin Heidelberg New York, pp 250-256
26. Strauss JM, Rüther W (2003) Freihandnavigation mit dem SurgiGate-System unter Berücksichtigung der computerassistierten Weichteilbalance. In: Navigation und Robotic in der Gelenk- und Wirbelsäulenchirurgie. Hrsg. W. Konermann, R. Haaker, Springer-Verlag Berlin Heidelberg New York, pp 217-224
27. Stuhlberg D, Loan P, Sarin V (2002) Computer-assisted navigation in total knee replacement: results of an initial experience in thirty-five patients. J Bone and Joint Surg Am 84-A, Suppl 2: 90-98
28. Swanson KE, Stocks GW, Warren PD, Hazel MR, Janssen HF (2000) Does axial limb rotation affect the alignment measurements in deformed limbs? Clin Orthop 371: 246-252
29. Tew M, Waugh W (1985) Tibiofemoral alignment and the results of knee replacement. J Bone Joint Surg 67B: 551-6
30. Wiese M, Schmidt K (2003) Knieendoprothesennavigation mit dem CT-basierten Vector-Vision-System. In: Navigation und Robotic in der Gelenk- und Wirbelsäulenchirurgie. Hrsg. W. Konermann, R. Haaker, Springer-Verlag Berlin Heidelberg New York, pp 240-244
31. Windsor RE, Scuderi GR, Moran MC, Insall JN (1989). Mechanisms of failure of the femoral and tibial components in total knee arthroplasty. Clin Orthop. 248: 15-20
32. Zippel H (2003) Computerassistierte Chirurgie – Pro und Kontra. In: Stand und Perspektiven der Computer-assistierten Chirurgie. Hrsg. K Labs, H Zippel, Uni-Med-Verlag Bremen London Boston, pp 18-19

SESSION 5

Clinical Results in Hip Arthroplasty

5.1 Personal Indications of Alumina Against Alumina bearing surfaces in Total Hip Replacement

L. Kerboull

Introduction

For a long time user, exclusive and happy, of cemented implants with a couple of friction metal-polyethylene I learnt as one other which were the advantages and the inconveniences of this option. The acetabular loosening in the progress of osteolysis engendered by the wear debris of polyethylene having clearly been identified as the main cause of failure. Numerous researches were led to develop new techniques of manufacture and sterilization of which we can reasonably think that they will allow to improve the resistance in wear of this material in the years to come. Nevertheless, the physico-chemical structure of the polyethylene forbids to hope that it will be possible to obtain a perfect material, opening from then on a logical debate on the experiment of new materials in this application.
Among the various today proposed solutions, I held in a private capacity the couple alumina-alumina.
Can we replace in any event the couple metal-polyethylene by the couple alumina-alumina? The answer to this question is for me denial. Two main arguments oppose to it, the engendered additional cost and the conditions of mechanical contract of the use of alumina. From then on, it becomes thus indispensable to select the patients in functions of profits expected from alumina but also and especially from its use in the safest conditions , the main objective of this selection being to try to guarantee to the patient a result at least so durable as with one conventional couple of friction.
We shall not insist on the evident for all economic problem, which becomes regrettably fewer and fewer contournable in our daily practice.
I shall thus deal in this statement of the mechanical foundations of this choice as well as its current indications.

The historic reasons of the choice of alumina

The tribological qualities of alumina were demonstrated now for 30 years and stay today probably the best. Other unmistakable advantage of this material is the small quantity of the produced debris and especially their good tolerance avoiding osteolysis. It was blamed for a long time that the alumina fragility was responsible for a high risk of rupture. The improvement of the quality of the manufacture and the setting-up allowed to envisage the regular use of this type of implant with a reasonable risk of breakage. These various advantages made me retain alumina-alumina as the best alternative to metal polyethylene

Conditions of mechanical contract

The mechanical arguments seem important as far as they are sometimes maybe under estimated.
Three fundamental elements deserve to be known before using alumina.
The first one is the fragility of this material due to its hardness which is the inevitable corollary of its resistance in the wear. It thus exposes the patient to a risk of fracture unknown with modern prostheses metal polyethylene. Even if these risks appear to have been reduced by the improvement of the manufacture of alumina, they remain present and impose to the surgeon a big attentiveness both in the choice of the implant and in its setting-up. The choice of the prosthetic device is indeed fundamental because, as polyethylenes, the various available varieties of alumina are not equal. From then on, the education of the surgeon becomes important so that he can realize a enlightened choice. It is also up to the manufacturers to supply transparent information about the material and on its terms of service in the implant, as for instance the minimal thickness, the mode of fixation in the schell and design of the taper notably. If the use of a metal head does not impose particular technical precautions, besides the manipulation of the trunion, it does not also go away as regards the cup. It is now established that the position of the schell can have an incidence on the risk of fracture. So, the inclination of the cup must not be excessively vertical to avoid stresses concentrations and so favor the break of the acetabular implant.

The second element, which we have already approached is the indispensable modularity of these implants. If the relationships of the femoral trunion with the alumina head begin to be actually codified and reassured, it is not certain for those of the alumina insert with the metalback. The fixation of a massive alumina cup, cemented or not, was now abandoned because of the too big rigidity of the cup which subjected the cemented interface in stresses which it was impossible to it to assume in the long run. The improvement of the fixation of uncemented cup, largely due to the introduction of hydroxyapatite coating allows to hope to make reliable the setting-up of alumina cup. This good fixation is still subjected to certain conditions on which we are going to return. Being this the mechanical relationships of the alumina insert with its metal support can become conflicting if the drawing of both elements or the introduction of the alumina insert are deficient. So, the choice of the device remains difficult and only meticulous experiments and clinical experience will allow in the future to say what technological solution is the most reliable. For my part, I chose the Trident press-fit cup from Stryker, because the alumina insert of which is set in factory in a metal pit, it even fixed through a metal Morse taper system in the metal ring. This principle offers a bigger safety during the insertion of the alumina insert by eliminating the risks of bad positioning, sometimes very difficult to discover in the operating context. We could blame this system for increasing the global rigidity of the cup but that this is probably small compared with that inevitably imposed by the ceramic itself.

These considerations lead us naturally to evoke the last mechanical point of the conditions of contract represented by the relationships, immediate and future, of the bony tissue, with a stiff acetabular implant.
The first point to take into account is the shape of the acetabular cavity. The most appropriate mode of fixation of alumina metalback cup is up to day an uncimented fixation by impaction or screwing. This mode of fixation, essentially peripheral, obtains its primary stability of the expansion of the acetabulum walls and its secondary stability of the cup design and the osseous ingrowth in the contact of the porous coating. The first condition for success is thus that the bony acetabulum is continent and not deficient to assure a correct contact with the cup as well as a sufficient resistance in the deformation. As a consequence, when the osseous cavity is not spherical and insufficient any more in particular at the level of the anterior wall the fixation of such an impacted cup might be less good and more unpredictable. The addition of screws exposed to a risk of stress shielding. Some people recommend in this situation the increase of the diameter of reaming to achieve a spherical shape of the bony acetabulum. The problem is that this extensive reaming necessary to make spherical an oval cavity thins automatically the lateral walls making them weaker and impose to use a bigger cup thus stiffer. The higher setting-up of the cup also expose to the same problems while making more difficult the restoration of the center of rotation of the hip. So for us, the safe use of an uncemented press-fit cup imposes that the bony acetabulum still is anatomically respected.
The second parameter is the rigidity of the bony tissue determined by its mineralization. In the long run, the quality of the bone will determine the perpetuity of the fixation. Indeed, if the initial preparation or the osseous natural reshaping, by the ageing or by the drawing of the cup, lead to osteoporosis, the pressure gradient of rigidity between the bone and the cup and will increase and might expose this one to a risk of tilting or protrusion. It is for that reason that the quality of the bone, initial or future, is for us a fundamental criteria of selection, leading us to exclude the patients affected by osteoporosis or exposed to its arisen.

Selection of the patients

Considering the elements which have been discussed, we shall end by the selection of the patients. The first evident point is that alumina must be only proposed to the patients for whom there is an expected profit. So, the patients concerned are those having a big life expectation or a high level of activity exposing them to a rapid wear of the polyethylene. From then on, the young age and the male gender are mostly the reserved parameters. It does not seem to us reasonable not to include also the osseous criteria which we have just detailed because they will be probably determining in the future. It is the reason for which we propose alumina,, in our daily practice, only when the bony acetabulum is anatomically respected, formed by a dense tissue and when the patient is an active person but is exposed to a major risk of osteoporosis.

Conclusion

These criteria of selection will seem certainly excessive and too restrictive in some. In what concerns us, in the current state of the knowledge, and considering our experience with the metal-polyethylene couple, they seem to us corresponding to our concern to propose to our patients another solution only when the known conditions of its success, in short and long-term, seem most better.

5.2 American Experience with Alumina Ceramic-Ceramic Bearings in Total Hip Arthroplasty

S.B. Murphy, B. Bierbaum and R. W. Eberle

Introduction

Total hip arthroplasty (THA) is an effective surgical procedure for relief of pain and the restoration of diseased hip function. The most common method of THA in the United States currently consists of an uncemented titanium shell, an ultra-high molecular weight polyethylene (UHMWPE) liner, a modular cobalt-chrome femoral head, and either a cemented or non-cemented femoral component.

A consequence of the metal-polyethylene articulation is surface wear, liberating both polyethylene and metal wear debris. From this, resultant osteolysis secondary to wear debris has become the major cause of long-term failure of primary THA. Efforts have been made to improve the performance of the metal-polyethylene bearing by improving the wear resistance of the UHMWPE and by improving the design of the polyethylene-shell interface.

Attempts to improve the wear characteristics and slow the degradation of polyethylene include high dose gamma or electron beam irradiation at near melting-point, quenching free-radicals, and enhancing the cross-linking of the polymer chains. These various cross-linked polyethylenes have come into widespread use in the United States despite a lack of clinical studies supporting their use. These new processes may adversely affect the mechanical properties and fatigue characteristics of this material. While the wear resistance of crosslinked polyethylene in smooth counterface conditions are less than that of non-crosslinked polyethylene, in scratched counterface conditions the wear debris may be of less volume but are actually of a more adverse biologically active size (0.1μ – 0.5μ).[5] It has been shown that wear rates significantly accelerate in with increasing femoral head surface roughness and, subsequently, leads to the osteolysis cascade.[1] Moreover, Digas, et al, has recently reported in vivo radiostereometry (RSA) results of highly cross-linked polyethylene versus conventional polyethylene. Proximal penetration of the femoral head was statistically similar ($p>0.12$) for either polyethylene tested.[4]

Bearing materials that eliminate polyethylene debris and aim to reduce debris generation overall include both metal-metal and alumina ceramic-ceramic bearings. Each of these articulations has been reported to show significant differences in decreasing volumetric wear.[6] With the re-introduction of metal-metal articulating surfaces and the increased metal-ion release much work is currently being performed on the level and long-term effect of systemic metal-ion concentrations following metal-metal THA. However, the systemic affect of short, intermediate and long-term metal-ion release is not well understood and may result in adverse consequences not yet monitored and reported. Increased serum and urine metal concentrations in patients with metal-metal THA are considerably higher than in those patients that received traditional metal-polyethylene bearings. It has also been reported that there is a four-fold in crease in leukemia and lymphoma in patients with elevated serum and urine-metal levels.[9]

Alternatively, ceramic-on-ceramic bearings offer the opportunity to eliminate the metal-on-polyethylene bearing and polyethylene wear debris entirely. Ceramic material for implantation was reported thirty years earlier in the German patent literature.[13] In 1963, Lyman-Smith reported of the use and the body's tolerance of implanted ceramic materials. This was a porous ceramic (alumina – Al_2O_3) imbedded with epoxy resins.[3,14] However, the advantages of ceramic components for the articulation in primary THA include their relatively inert properties in body fluids, negligible amounts of toxic degradation products, and their resistance to scratching, third body debris and abrasive wear. In-vitro and retrieval studies continually report that ceramic-ceramic bearings produce the least amount of wear of any available bearing surface.[12]

The purpose of this article is to summarize the authors' clinical experience with alumina ceramic-ceramic bearings in THA.

Materials and Methods

Between June of 1997 and February of 2003, 363 THA's (363 hips in 325 patients) were performed using a ceramic-ceramic bearing surface. The acetabular component used in all cases was a press-fit, porous-coated titanium shell (Transcend™ Cup – Wright Medical Technology, Memphis, TN). An alumina ceramic acetabular bearing was inserted into the metal shell and locked with an 18° taper. The alumina acetabular bearing articulates with a modular alumina femoral head component (Figure 1). All acetabulae were under-reamed by 1 mm to ensure stability upon impaction. Screws to augment acetabular fixation were used in less than one percent of the cases performed. All patients were followed prospectively as part of an FDA/IDE monitored study and hospital IRB was received. The patients were evaluated clinically and radiographically pre-operatively, and post-operatively at 3, 6 and 12 months and annually thereafter. Outcome evaluation included Harris hips scores (HHS) on all patients.

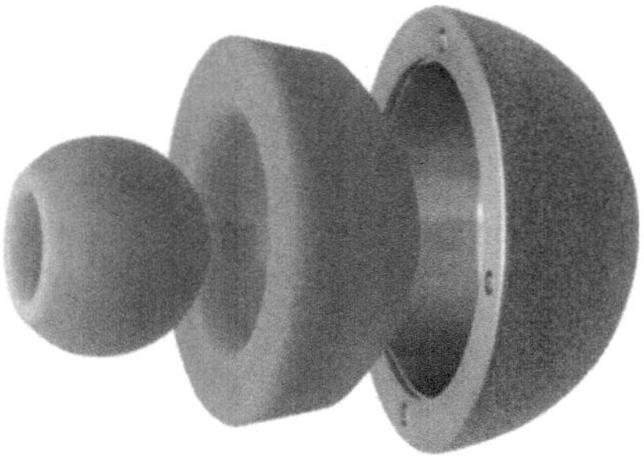

Figure 1:
Transcend™ Cup – Wright Medical Technology, Memphis, TN

There were 152 (47%) left hips, 136 (42%) right hips and 37 (11%) bilateral hips of which 128 (39%) were female and 197 (61%) were male. Mean patient age at surgery was 51 years (SD: 11 years, Range: 18 years – 78 years). By decade of age, the frequency of patients were as follows: less than 20 years old, 2 patients (< 1%); 20 to 29 years old, 7 patients (2%); 30 to 39 years old, 47 patients (14%); 40 to 49 years old, 102 patients (31%); 50 to 59 years old, 95 patients (29%); 60 to 69 years old, 53 patients (16%); 70 years and greater in 20 patients (6%). Pre-operative diagnoses included osteoarthritis 290 (80%), developmental dysplatic to 49 years old, 102 patients (31%); 50 to 59 years old, 95 patients (29%); 60 to 69 years old, 53 patients (16%); 70 years and greater in 20 patients (6%). Pre-operative diagnoses included osteoarthritis 290 (80%), developmental dysplatic hip 44 (12%), avascular necrosis 22 (6%), traumatic arthritis 6 (2%) and Legg-Calve-Perthes disease 1 (< 1%). A modified direct lateral approach was used in 199 hips (55%), posterior approach in 161 hips (44%) and a trans-trochanteric approach in 2 hips (1%). Mean ± SD follow-up time for all cases was 16 ± 14 months. Of those cases with a minimum of 2-years follow-up the average time to follow-up was 33 months (SD: 11 months, Range: 20 months – 61 months).

Results

To date, all components are well fixed. There have been no cases of ceramic head or liner fracture post-operatively and no signs of grossly visible wear. The acetabular component abduction angle averaged 42 degrees (Standard Deviation: 4 degrees, Range: 30 degrees – 55 degrees). Intraoperatively, one ceramic liner chipped when inserted eccentrically and was replaced at the time of surgery. One case involved a mismatch between head diameter and liner inside diameter. The ceramic femoral head was exchanged and the patient has had no further THA related problems. Postoperatively, one hip underwent irrigation and debridement three weeks postoperatively for increased pain and low-grade temperature and was culture negative. One liner was mal-seated and replaced on post-op day 3. There were three (1%) early dislocations and were in cases in which the posterior approach was used. There was one patient death from causes unrelated to the THA procedure.

The average pre-operative HHS was 51 ±13 (Range: 10 to 96) and, in those cases with 2-year minimal follow-up, improved to an average of 97 ±5 (Range: 78 to 100). Of a possible 44 points, the average pain component of the HSS preoperatively was 14 ±8 (Range: 0 to 44) and improved to 41 ±6 (Range: 10 to 44). The low HSS pain score was related to an aseptically loose femoral component with a stable, well functioning acetabular component. The average pre-operative range of motion was -3 degrees to 90 degrees and improved post-operatively to 0 degrees to 107 degrees with a maximum range of motion of 140 degrees.

Discussion

Early results from this study have demonstrated no major problems associated with ceramic-ceramic bearings in THA, such as bearing fracture or catastrophic wear. All preliminary series of ceramic-ceramic bearings have shown an incidence of liner chipping or mal-seating, especially early on. Nonetheless, ceramic liners are generally easier to insert than polyethylene liners but need to be properly seated by hand before impaction. In addition, to avoid the common technical errors in liner insertion, one-use ceramic liner seating / impaction devices have been developed to align the ceramic liner with the metal shell to avoid mal-seating and to avoid increased impaction forces. Unlike polyethylene, bearing thickness does not affect wear, thus ceramic-ceramic bearings are especially useful for dysplastic hips (Figure 2). These patients are typically young, with small socket components, where thin polyethylene typically leads to a high rate of polyethylene wear.

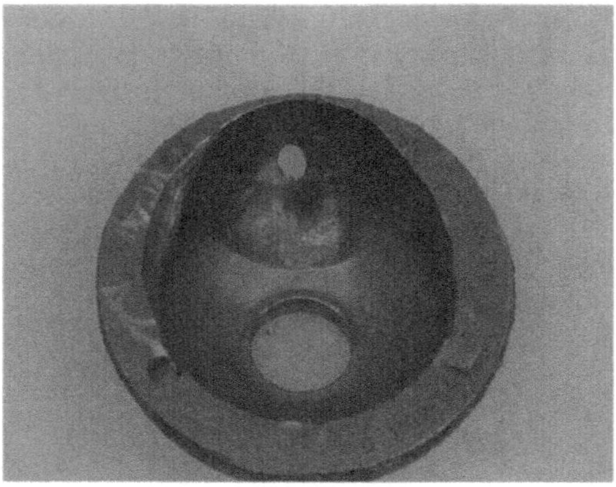

Figure 2:
Example of complete polyethylene wear-through and head penetration into the metal acetabular

In an FDA approved, multi-center, clinical trial of 333 THA's with the same ceramic-ceramic bearing (of which the author has participated and results are combined), Garino reported short-term results.[7] As with the current study, the preliminary results had no post-operative cases of ceramic bearing fracture or visible wear. There were 2 additional intraoperative liner "chip" fractures due to eccentric insertion treated by intraoperative exchange of the liner. The three dislocations we report is below the rate of combined reported results by Mallory being four percent in 11,000 hips.[11]

Similarly, Bizot, et al, reported 93.4% survivorship rate in 234 THA's with a non-cemented, metal-backed, ceramic-on-ceramic acetabular component, when revision was the end-point.[2] Of these cases, only one was ceramic related (fractured femoral head). There were three hips in which the acetabular component had a complete, non-progressive radiolucent line less than 1 mm thick. In each case, neither component migration nor osteolysis adjacent to the acetabular component was detected radiographically. Radiographically, we report no incidence of radiolucent lines or observed incidence of periprosthetic osteolysis in any cases. These intermediate reports of this ceramic-ceramic component show results equal to that of conventional THA with metal-on-polyethylene articulation.

Spontaneous ceramic component failure is a common argument for not using ceramic-ceramic bearings in THA. Interestingly, the incidence of polyethylene liner fracture or complete wear-through is a rarely discussed, but is somewhat a more common adverse event. Heck, et al, reported the results of the American Association of Hip and Knee Surgeons questionnaire sent to all members.[8] There were 77 hips (failure rate: 239/10,000), of all-polyethylene acetabular components that resulted in complete failure (polyethylene fracture or wear-through) and, in 172 hips (failure rate: 29 /10,000) involving metal backed acetabular components reported (Figure 2). Not reported were failures due to polyethylene wear-debris induced osteolysis and subsequent femoral / acetabular component revision. Comparatively, there were 11 ceramic femoral head failures (rate: 22/10,000) over the five-year study period reported. Likewise, Krikler, et al, reported 2 cases of ceramic femoral head fracture, five years following implantation, of 600 total cases and may have been related to the femoral neck Morse taper (14/16) which since has been changed to a 12/14 Morse taper.[10] This equates to a rate of 33:10,000 cases which is below the overall polyethylene failure rate as reported by Heck, et al, which does not include failure secondary to polyethylene wear debris. Moreover, the results from our reported study showed no failure due to ceramic component fracture in 363 hips. The decrease in wear-debris particles, in conjunction with the low rates of spontaneous component failure makes the benefit of ceramic-ceramic bearing a valid and proven option for THA.

Conclusion

The early results of the use of ceramic-ceramic bearings show promise in the elimination polyethylene debris and the reduction wear debris following THA. From this prospective study we report no cases of measurable wear, lysis, ceramic component fracture or postoperative chipping.

Current reports of wear rates involving ceramic-ceramic articulations are by far lower than any other materials currently available. The unknown affects of increased metal-ion release associated with metal-metal articulations, and the increase in particles per volume associated with crosslinked polyethylene may have introduced not only new adverse variables but also may have made the effects of polyethylene debris worse.

Therefore, because of the inert qualities of alumina ceramic materials, the significantly lower wear rates over other articular material combinations, and the durability associated with the new generation of ceramic materials, the use of alumina ceramic-ceramic bearing surfaces should be greatly considered as the alternative to the historic and traditional use of metal-polyethylene or metal-metal articulations in THA.

References

1. Barrack R, Castro FP, Jr, Szuszczewicz ES, Schmalzried TP: Analysis of retrieved uncemented porous-coated acetabular components in patients with and without pelvic osteolysis. Orthopaedics, 25(12): 2002.
2. Bizot P, Larrouy M, Witvoet J, Sedel L, Nizard R: Press-fit metal-backed alumina sockets: A minimum 5-year follow-up study. Clin Orthop, 379:134-142, 2000.
3. Boutin P: The classic: Total hip arthroplasty using a ceramic prosthesis. Clin Orthop, 379: 3-11, 2000.
4. Digas G, Kärrholm J, Thanner J, Malchau H, Herberts P: Highly Cross-Linked Polyethylene in Hip Arthroplasty. Randomized Study Using Radiostereometry (Preliminary Report). 31st Open Scientific Meeting & 9th Combined Open Meeting of the Hip Society & AAHKS, New Orleans, Louisiana, February 8, 2003.
5. Endo MM, Barbour PS, Barton DC, Fisher J, Tipper JL, Ingham E, Stone MH: Comparative wear and wear debris under three different counterfac conditions of crosslinked and non-crosslinked ultra high molecular weight polyethylene. Biomed Mater Eng, 11(1):23-35, 2001.
6. Fischer J, Besong AA, Firkins PJ, Barbour PSM, Nevelos JE, Tripper JL, Stone MH, Ingham E: Comarative wear and debris generation in UHMWPE on ceramic, metal on metal and ceramic on ceramic hip prostheses. 46th Annual Meeting of the Orthopaedic Research Society, Orlando, FL, March 12-15, 2002.
7. Garino JP: Modern ceramic-on-ceramic total hip systems in the United States: Early results. Clin Orthop, 379:41-47, 2000.

8. Heck DA, Partridge CM, Reuben JD, Lanzer WL, Lewis CG, Keating EM: Prosthetic component failures in hip arthroplasty surgery. J Arthroplasty, 10(5):575-580, 1995.
9. Jacobs J: Metal-metal: Metal ions – a cause for concern in metal-metal bearings. 31st Open Scientific Meeting & 9th Combined Open Meeting of the Hip Society & AAHKS, New Orleans, Louisiana, February 8, 2003.
10. Kirkler S, Schatzker J: Ceramic head failure. J Arthroplasty, 10(6):860-862, 1995.
11. Mallory TH, Lombardi AV, Jr, Fada RA, Herrington SM, Eberle RW: Dislocation after total hip arthroplasty using the anterolateral abductor split approach. Clin Orthop, 358:166-172, 1999.
12. Murphy SB: Ceramic-ceramic bearings in THA: The new gold standard – in the affirmative. Orthopaedics, 25(9):933-934, 2002.
13. Salzer M, Locke H, Plenk H, Punzet G, Stärk N, Zweymüller K: Experience with bioceramic endoprostheses of the hip joint. In: Advances in artificial hip and knee joint technology, Schaldach M, Hohmann D, eds. (Engineering in medicine series, vol. 2), Springer-Verlag, Berlin, p. 459, 1976.
14. Smith L: Ceramic-plastic material as a bone substitute. Arch Surg, 87:653, 1963.

5.3 All Alumina Articulation in the Stryker Howmedica-Osteonics THA A United States Experience 36-60 Months Follow-up

J. W. Mesko

Abstract

Five hundred fourteen total hip arthroplasties were performed in a prospective, randomized multicenter trial in the United States. All patients received a clinically proven hydroxyapatite (HA) coated, collarless, dual wedged titanium stem. While all acetabular shells had the same outside geometry, one third of the patients received a polyethylene liner mated with a Chrome Cobalt head and two thirds utilized a Ceramtec alumina acetabular bearing and femoral head. At the mean follow-up of 3.6 years, there were no statistical differences in the patient activity, satisfaction, or component performance. A 2.6% intraoperative insertional crack rate of the alumina liner resulted in an acetabular redesign with a second, non-randomized study of 209 additional hips. With a minimum of 24-month observation of this group, there have been no ceramic failures, and the clinical and radiographic results are not statistically different from the original control patients.

Introduction

The longevity of a total hip arthroplasty (THA) is dependent on many factors. Undeniably, the most important factor is precise surgical technique resulting in correctly oriented, well cemented, or well approximated cementless components to host bone in an aseptic environment. Other essential factors regarding the stem include metallurgy, geometry, proportionality, surface finish, femoral head material and polish, and manufacturing precision of femoral head articulation to the stem in modular components. The same factors are important on the cup side including the material property of the acetabular bearing surface and the design of its capture to the underlying metal shell in modular components. Much has been learned to optimize metallurgy and improve implant design and surface properties. Integrating this knowledge has resulted in greater predictability of 10-year successful outcomes in many THA systems [10, 5]. What appears to be impeding even greater longevity is the adverse interaction and secondary effects of the bearing couple. The degree of wear and the associated biological effects of the resulting debris can lead to host bone failure and late implant loosening. An all alumina ceramic bearing surface offers great promise to lessen wear and wear debris by virtue of its extreme hardness, biological inertness, and excellent tribiological properties [11, 9]. The first all ceramic bearing THA was introduced through an investigational study in the United States in the early 1980's with the Autophor by the Smith Nephews Richards corporation. This system showed high rates of early failure and revision and was consequently abandoned. The bearing failure was primarily attributed to poor design characteristics and not the ceramic couple. The hip ceramic-ceramic articulating couple is currently a class III investigational device regulated within a US investigational device exemption (IDE) study to demonstrate safety and efficacy prior to approval for general distribution. This study updates Bierbaum's [2] and D'Antonio's [4] reports on the results of a randomized study using a Stryker Howmedica-Osteonics (SHO) THA with a new generation alumina on alumina bearing compared to a metal on polyethylene couple.

Materials and Methods

Stryker Howmedica-Osteonics (SHO) sought a bearing couple that generated less wear debris than conventional metal on polyethylene surfaces. An alliance was forged with Ceramtec to produce a modular pressfit acetabular component. SHO modified the inside geometry and shell edge of their existing PSL acetabular component to accept an 18 degree tapered alumina ceramic insert (fig 1). The inserts were neutral in effacement and came in six sizes, fitting the range of 44 to 66 mm acetabular sizes.

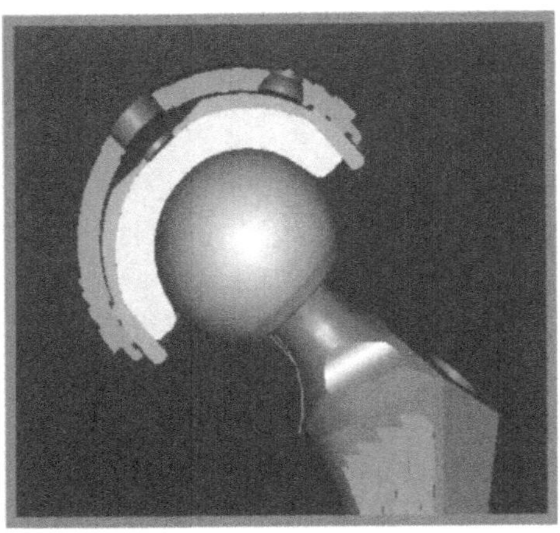

Figure 1:
ABC acetabular component cross section

Two liner sizes were manufactured for a 28-mm head in the 44-50 mm cups. Four liner sizes were manufactured for a 32-mm head in the remaining cup sizes. All cups were designed to recess the lateral edge of the ceramic liner below the margin of the metallic shell (fig 2). A picture of ABC assembled, like at end of bibliography. This prevents impingement of the prosthetic femoral neck on the ceramic shell at the extremes of motion, thus lessening the potential for impingement-related ceramic chipping and femoral neck notching that could lead to stem fracture at the trunion. Ceramtec Biolox forte alumina was used for all head and socket implants. The 28 and 32-mm alumina heads came in neutral and +5 lengths.

In October 1996 SHO initiated a prospective randomized US IDE study comparing alumina on alumina with a chrome cobalt on polyethylene total hip system with an established track record. Twenty-two surgeons from 16 centers who were familiar users of the SHO HA stem and PSL/HA cementless cup enrolled patients after gaining approval from their local hospital Institutional Review Board (IRB). Surgeons were mandated to adhere to inclusion and exclusion criteria.

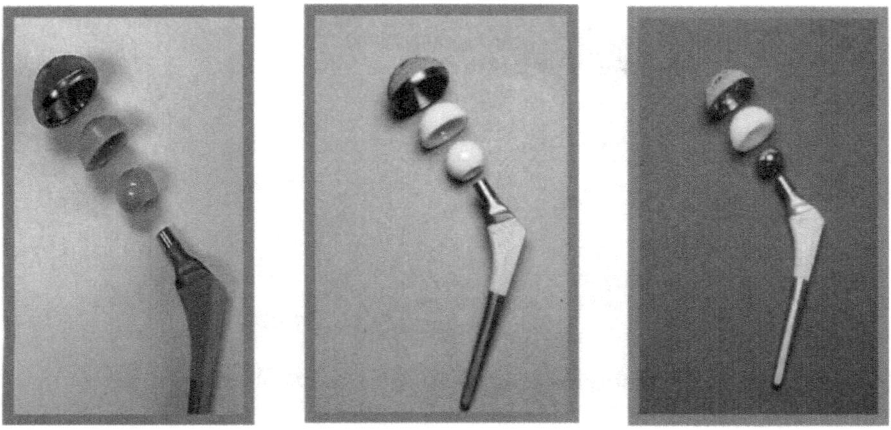

Figure 2: System I System II System III
Configurations for randomized ceramic study

Non-inflammatory etiologies of hip disease in patients who were greater than 20 years of age and not judged to be morbidly obese were some of these criteria. Each surgeon was given freedom to offer participation in this clinical trial to any eligible patient. Patients were given written informed consent, which became part of their permanent medical records. After consent was obtained SHO randomly assigned the patient the implants that were to be used.

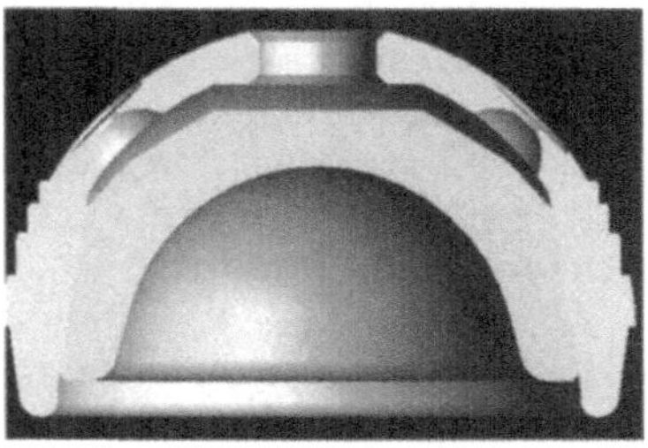

Figure 3:
Trident acetabular system cross section

Patients received one of three possible system configurations. Figure 3 shows all three configurations. The control system's (system 3) acetabular component was a PSL bead coated cup with screw holes and a neutral 28 or 32 mm ID. A UHMW polyethylene insert that was sterilized via ultraviolet radiation in an inert environment with subsequent vacuum packaging was also used. This was mated with a matched sized, highly polished nitrogen ion bombarded chrome cobalt alloyed femoral head. The other two study systems used a similarly modified PSL acetabular component as described above. Both cups had screw holes. This acetabular component was named the ABC (Alumina Bearing Couple) cup. Half of the ABC cups had the same bead coated surface as the control PSL shells (system 1). The other half had an arc-deposited titanium layer applied to the shell that was secondarily coated with HA (system 2). Both of these systems used the same ceramic liners and ceramic heads. The study was conducted between October 1996 and October 1998 (Appendix1). In all, 514 hips were enrolled. The following are the clinical results at a mean of 3.6 years postoperatively for these patients. As demonstrated in Table 1, the demographic distribution of these patients in regard to sex, age, height and weight were not statistically different.

Demographics	AL/AL (Study groups 1 and 2 combined)	CoCr/Poly (Study group 3)
Number of Cases	349	165
Number of Patients	318	161
Male/Female %	65%/35%	60%/40%
Mean Age (yrs.)	53	53
Mean Weight (lbs.)	189.8	188.5
Mean Height (ins.)	68.6	68.4
Mean Length of Follow-up	44.0 mo.	43.8 mo.
Diagnosis	78% OA, 4%PTA, 16%AVN, 2% other	76% OA, 5% PTA, 16% AVN, 3% other

Table 1

The introduction of the ceramic liner into the tapered titanium shell demands greater precision than conventional poly in metal shells. Failure to precisely seat the liner before final impaction can lead to insert cracks. This event occurred in 2.6% of the 349 ceramic liners in these experienced surgeons' hands. This condition led to a redesign of the alumina insert configuration. The new design was used in a fourth arm of the study begun in September 1999 at six of the original centers and expanded in 2001 to five additional centers. (Appendix 2). In this study arm, all patients received the same HA coated Omnifit stem as used in the initial group of patients as well as the modified acetabular system named the Trident® Acetabular system. (fig 4) Trident exploded cup like at end of bibliography. The Trident® shell's external geometry preserves the design as used in Secur-fit, PSL, and ABC cups. It has titanium arc deposition with HA coating as used in the series 2 ABC shell. The modified insert is a neutral alumina acetabular liner that is encased in a factory shrunk fit titanium sleeve. In the operating room, the tapered titanium sleeved ceramic insert is impacted into the taper of the shell. Extensive in vitro testing of this locking mechanism demonstrates greater push out force than most poly-metal locking mechanisms, with no fretting or corrosion at the interface.

Additionally the Trident® shell readily accepts polyethylene liners of various diameters and degrees of opening angles. This system permits the use of 36 mm alumina heads and alumina liners in all acetabular components 58 mm and larger. It also permits 36 mm chrome cobalt heads mated with 36mm ID cross-linked poly liners in shells 50 mm and larger

There are 209 hips in 194 patients enrolled in this study arm, with 188 hips (174 patients) having greater than 24 month follow-up. Although this group is more skewed toward male patients, the average age, weight and diagnosis is not statistically different than the previous groups (Table 2).

Demographics (as of12/30/02) 188 pts with > 24 month follow-up	Trident® Al/Al
Number of Cases	209
Number of Patients	194
Male/Female %	66%/34%
Mean Age (yrs.)	52.0
Mean Weight (lbs.)	189.7
Mean Height (ins.)	68.4
Length of Follow-up	24.1 mo.
Diagnosis	81% OA, 3% PTA, 11`% AVN, 4% SCFE, 0.5% other

Table 2

RESULTS

Clinical results are equally positive for both the ABC alumina group and the control group at a mean follow-up of 3.6 years (Table 3). Capello et al [3] reviewed the radiographic results of all hips with greater than 24 month (range 24-48 months) available follow-up. They found a statistically higher number of radiolucent lines in the Charnley-DeLee [6] zone 3 in both the alumina and control cups with porous coating as opposed to the arc-deposited HA coated cups (p=0.001). Ten control hips demonstrated scalloping in the Gruen [8] zone 8 region. This is in contrast to two in the system 1 alumina hips, and none in the system 2 (HA ABC cup) alumina hips. This observation is statistically significant (p = 0.001).

3-5 YR (MEAN 3.6 YRS)	Al/Al (n=271)	CoCr/Poly (n=128)
Pain none/slight	94%	94%
Limp none/mild	98%	95%
Mean Harris Score	96.7	96.4
Harris % G/E	96%	95%
Pt. Satisfaction (Are you satisfied with results?)	97%	96%

Table 3

Complications were seen in near equal proportion in both groups (Table 4). One system 1 hip had a stem revision due to a traumatic periprosthetic fracture and one hip revision arthroplasty was required for a deep sepsis five years post op. One system 2 hip had an early acetabular revision resulting from an anterior dislocation after an excessive cup anteversion. One system 2 stem was revised due to post-traumatic loosening 4.5 years post op, and 1 revision arthroplasty was performed as a result of infection at 11 months. There was also one system 2 revision arthroplasty for suspected, but not confirmed, sepsis. For the system 3

COMPLICATIONS	Al/Al	CoCr/Poly
Revision-Acetabular	1(0.3%)	3 (1.8%)
Revision-Femoral	2(0.6%)	2 (1.2%)
Revision-all	3 (0.9%)	0
Revision-Insert and/or head only	0	5 (3.0%)
Intra op Femoral Fx/Crack	13(3.7%)	7 (4.2%)
Post Op Femoral Fx.	6(1.7%)	2 (1.2%)
Dislocation	10(2.9%)	7 (4.2%)
Heterotopic Bone	12(3.4%)	10 (6.1%)
Intra Op Insert Chip	9(2.6%)	NA

Table 4

(control) hips, seven hips dislocated, with four needing revision surgery in which the head and insert were exchanged. One additional head and insert was revised due to polyethylene wear and osteolysis. Also in system 2, two stems were revised, one for painful leg length discrepancy, and one for loosening due to trauma. Finally, three cups were revised; two for loosening, and one for infection

Nine of the alumina couple hips had outside ceramic edge insert cracks due to eccentric insertion of the alumina into the ABC shell. In only one case was the liner and shell retained, with no adverse effects at 34 months. The remaining had liner, cup, or both exchanged at the index procedure and continue to do well at the time of this report. No alumina fractures have occurred in the remaining hips.

CLINICAL DATA: MINIMUM OF 24 MONTHS FOLLOW-UP

	Trident® (n=188)
Pain none/slight	**94%**
Limp none/mild	**99%**
Mean Harris Score	**97.0**
Harris % G/E	**97%**
Pt. Satisfaction (Are you satisfied with results?)	**99%**

Table 5

Enrollment continues in the Trident® group, with 625 implanted as of December 1, 2002 at all eleven investigational centers. Table 5 describes the results of the original 209 hips at the original 6 centers with implants in service greater than 24 months. The high satisfaction is not statistically different from the original ABC randomized patients. Radiographic analysis is of shorter duration, and does not suggest any adverse trends to date. Complications are as noted in Table 6 with this group. One stem was revised secondary to loosening following a periprosthetic fracture. Three acetabular components were revised or underwent liner exchanges; one as a result of loosening and two because of persistent hip instability. Of note, there are no ceramic fractures of any hip with this modified design.

COMPLICATIONS:

Revision-Acetabular**	1 (0.5%)
Revision-Femoral*	1(0.5%)
Revision-Both	0
Revision-Insert and/or head only	2 (1.0%)
Acetabular Component Loosening** (see rev acet)	1 (.0.5%)
Intra op Femoral Fx/Crack	4 (1.9%)
Post Op Femoral Fx.* (see rev fem)	1 (0.5%)
Dislocation	4 (1.9%)
Heterotopic Bone	8 (3.8%)
Intra Op Insert Chip	0

Table 6

Discussion

Both the ABC and Trident® alumina-alumina bearing utilize Ceramtec Biolox Forte alumina ceramic. This material is manufactured using hot isostatic pressing (HIP) which leads to decreased grain size and greater strength of any alumina to date. Other manufacturing improvements include proof testing, a strict quality controlled environment, and laser marking. These improvements have decreased the risk of implant fracture to an estimated 1/20,000 [12]. The ABC and Trident, systems have included a raised lateral margin of the shell in order to minimize the potential for late ceramic chipping as a result of femoral neck impingement [1]. This design allows an overall range of motion before impingement of 120 degrees in the 28mm liner, 128 degrees in the 32 mm liner, and 133 degrees in the 36 mm liner. Outside of the nine insertional cracks with the ABC design, there have been no additional ceramic fractures with a maximum of 6.25 years of observation. This correlates well to the international experience in which there are only two known acetabular liner fractures in greater than 7000 ABC cups inserted. These two fractures happened shortly after surgery in liners that were intentionally left in a canted, non-seated position [4]. The Trident, design improves this hip system in several ways. The factory shrink wrapping of the acetabular liner enhances its strength by 50%[7]. It does not demand a ceramic on metal alignment in the operating room, which led to marginal alumina fracture in a small percentage of such designs. Trident® gives an added advantage in that surgeons can easily remove the ceramic liner and revise to a polyethylene liner with various inside diameters, effacement angulations, and lip liners should the need arise. It also introduced a 36-mm head for larger acetabular components to allow enhanced range of motion.

The current clinical and radiographic information seen at a mean 3.6 years with the ABC prosthesis as well as the greater than 24 month with the Trident® prosthesis are very encouraging. No measurable wear, and fewer radiolucent lines in Gruen Zone 8 suggest that surrounding bone is less eroded by wear debris. Many of the complications seen in all groups were related to post operative trauma, or technical issues of insertion as noted in the outset of this paper. The future will reveal the degree of success an alumina-alumina bearing can achieve in decreasing osteolysis, and prolonging the life of a THA. Long-term results will also address other questions. How will the known routine distraction and subluxation of the bearing influence wear or bearing fracture? What will be the long-term complications of prosthetic impingement? Will there be a greater incidence of femoral prosthetic neck fracture or marginal ceramic liner fractures in designs that allow femoral prosthetic neck impingement on the rim of the ceramic liner? Will we see any adverse effects of the rigid metal-ceramic prosthesis composite in bone without the intervening "shock absorber" effect of polyethylene? Finally, will we see a higher incidence of instability resulting from surgeons that do not routinely use neutral liners?

As the US market awaits the FDA's approval for a more widespread release of this product, the health care payers have begun to weigh their willingness to provide the additional funding for this technology. The findings of this controlled group of patients begin to demonstrate the long-term cost savings alumina-alumina hip interfaces can provide in a young, active patient. This suggests that such a technology can provide a longer survivorship of the THA without the effects of bone loss and implant loosening resulting from poly wear debris.

References

1. Bader, R., Willman, G., Analysis of the range of motion of hip prosthesis based on design, position and type of acetabular cup. Bioceramics in Hip Joint Replacement, proceedings 5th International CeramTec Symposium, Feb 18/19, 2000, pg 66
2. Bierbaum, B.E., Barsoum, W.K., Puri, L., Headrick, j., Gomes, S., Alumina-Alumina Ceramic Bearings, Bioceramics in Joint Arthroplasty. Proceedings 6th international Biolox Symposium, March 23,24 2001, 22
3. Capello, W., D' Antonio, J., Bonutti, P., Manley, M., Comparison of Acetabular Surface Treatments in Alumina on Alumina Clinical Trial, Rochester, MN Presentation American Hip Society Meeting, Summer 2002
4. D'Antonio, J., Capello, W.N., Manley, M., Bierbaum, B., New Experience with Alumina-on-Alumina Ceramic Bearings for Total Hip Arthroplasty, J Arthroplasty 17:390, 2002
5. D'Antonio, J.A., Capello, W.N., Manley M.T., Geesink, R. Hydroxyapatite Femoral Stems for Total Hip Arthroplasty, 10-13 Year Follow up, CORR 393:101 2001
6. DeLee, J.G.; and Charnley, J.: Radiological demarcation of cemented sockets in total hip replacement. Clin. Orthop., 121: 20-32, 1976.
7. Epinette, J.A., Ceramic-ceramic Bearings:Why and for whom, Proceedings 6th International BIOLOX symposium, March 23/24, 2001, 27.
8. Gruen, T.A.; McNeice G.M.; and Amstutz, H.C.: "Modes of failure" of cemented stem-type femoral components: A radiographic analysis of loosening. Clin Orthop., 141: 17-27, 1979
9. Hamadouch, M., Boutin, P., Daussange, J., Bolander, M.E., Sedel, L., Alumina-on-Alumina Total Hip Arthroplasty, A Minimum 18.5 year Follow-up Study, JBJS, 84A:70, 2002.
10. Rasquinha, V.J., Dua, V., Rodriquez, J.A., Ranawat, C.S., Fifteen-Year Survivorship of the Omnifit Stem in Primary Hybrid Total Hip Arthroplasty. Scientific Presentation AAHKS 2002 meeting, Dallas, TX, 11/2002
11. Total Hip Replacement, NIH Consensus Statement 1994, 12-14:12(5): 1-31
12. Willman, G:, Ceramic ball retrieval Data. In: Proceedings of the 4th Symposium on Ceramic Wear Couple, Stuttgart, Germany, 1999

APPENDIX 1

Benjamin Bierbaum, M.D., Boston, MA
William Capello, M.D., Indianapolis, IN
Clifford Colwell, M.D., La Jolla, CA
Steven Copp, M.D., LaJolla, CA
James D'Antonio, M.D., Sewickley, PA
Paul DiCesare, M.D., New York, NY
Joseph Diamond III, M.D., Atlanta, GA
John Henry, M.D., Atlanta, GA
Edward Hellman, M.D., Indianapolis, IN
Jonathan Hottenstein, M.D., Sewickley, PA
William Hozack, M.D., Philadelphia. PA
William Jaffe, M.D., New York, NY
Ormonde Mahoney, M.D., Athens, GA
Kenneth Marks, M.D., Cleveland, OH
Patrick Meere, M.D., New York, NY
J. Wesley Mesko, M.D., Lansing, MI
Paul Pongor, M.D., Boston, MA
James Robertson, M.D., Atlanta, GA
Sean Scully, M.D., Durham, NC
Scott Siverhus, M.D., Toledo, OH
Richard Walker, M.D., La Jolla, CA
Robert Zann, M.D., Boca Raton, FL

APPENDIX 2

Benjamin Bierbaum, M.D., Boston, MA
Joseph McCarthy, M.D., Boston, MA
Arnold Scheller, M.D., Boston, MA
Donald Reilly, M.D., Boston, MA
William Capello, M.D., Indianapolis, IN
James D'Antonio, M.D., Sewickley, PA
Jonathan Hottenstein, M.D., Sewickley, PA
James Robertson, M.D., Atlanta, GA
Scott Siverhus, M.D., Toledo, OH
Robert Zann, M.D., Boca Raton, FL
William Hozak, M.D., Philadelphia, PA
William Jaffe, M.D., New York City, NY
Patrick Meere, M.D., New York City, NY
Ormond Mahoney, M.D., Athens, GA
Clifford Colwell, M.D., La Jolla, CA
Richard Walker, M.D., La Jolla, CA
Stephen Copp, M.D., La Jolla, CA
J. Wesley Mesko, M.D., Lansing, MI

5.4 Clinical Experience with the Hedrocel® Acetabular Cup

C. Perka, G. Möckel, K. Labs and G. Matziolis

Introduction

Cementless anchoring of orthopedic implants requires specific physical characteristics of the implant surface. While the primary implant stability is defined by the surface friction, the definite implant stability depends on the biological integration, which is correlated to the porosity of the implant. Different coating materials and techniques have been developed to improve both parameters, friction and porosity, e.g. sintered balls, fibre metals, plasma spray coatings and titanium blasting. Nevertheless, the achievable porosity and thickness of coatings have shown to underlie fundamental limitations.

In the past few years a new trabecular structured biomaterial, consisting of 98% tantal, the most corrosion resistant metal of all metals, and 2% vitreous carbon, was developed for use in acetabular cups (Hedrocel®) [1;2]. The cellular pores are dodecahedron in shape with a cellular pore diameter of about 550µm. The "portals" or "windows" connecting cellular structures are about 250-350 µm in diameter. The surface is 75 to 85% porous, e.g. 2-3-fold higher than traditional porous coatings [6]. Nevertheless, Hedrocel® is a bulk structural porous metal, not a coating. So the structural integrity does not dependent on "welds" between the rigid solid metal and the adjacent wires or beads. Additionally the stiffness of Hedrocel® is similar to bone, especially compared to the 25 to 100 times stiffness of traditional porous coated cups.

The Hedrocel® acetabular cup has an integral non-modular design, eliminating one source of polyethylen debris. The cross section shows 100% support of the direct compression molded polyethylene by metal backing without gaps or any possibility for motion and debris [5].

In this study we examined the postoperative results after implantation of 125 Hedrocel® acetabular cups in primary and revision total hip arthroplasty (THA).

Materials and Methods

Patients

105 primary and 20 revision THAs were performed in 125 patients using the cementless Hedroce® acetabular cup (Zimmer, Kiel, Germany) (Fig. 1). All patients having a minimum follow-up period of 24 months were included. The average follow-up period was 3.1 years (range 24 - 47 months). 3 patients (3.7%) died and 3 patients (3.7%) could not be traced, so that 64 hip endoprostheses (51 primary, 13 revision THAs) in 64 patients were finally evaluated.

The average age of the 27 men and 37 women at the time of surgery was 69.6 years (range 42 to 81 years). The average body mass index was 28 kg/m^2 (range 22-38 kg/m^2).

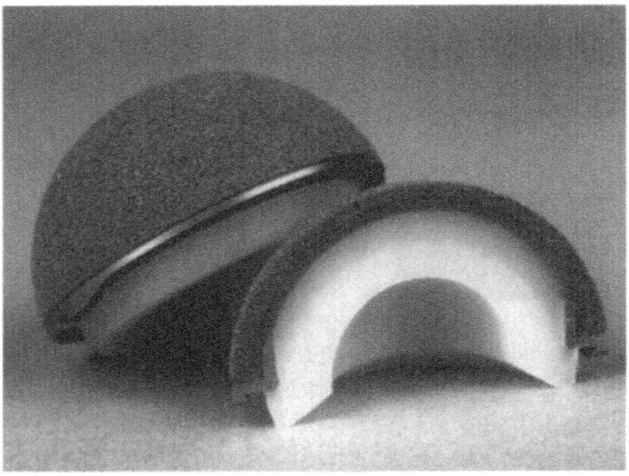

Figure 1:
Hedrocel® cup.

Medical treatment

40mg Enoxaparin was given once daily for thromboembolic prophylaxis in 63 cases. One patient had a thromboemboly in his history, so that unfractionated heparin was administered in individual, PTT controlled dosage.

Indomethacin (3 x 25mg for 21 days) was given for prevention of periarticular ossifications in all cases.

Surgical technique

The direct lateral approach was chosen in 62 cases and the anterolateral approach in 2 cases. All cups had direct molded UHMWPE with a diameter of 28mm.

The cup was reamed into the acetabulum until a firm anchorage of at least two third of the outer rim in autochthonous bone was achieved. In two cases having a hip dysplasia grade IV according to Crowe [8] an additional reconstruction of the deficient anterolateral acetabular margin had to be performed by structured bone grafting after a shortening derotating femur osteotomy. A cementless Zweymüller straight stem was implanted in all cases.

Follow-up examination

All complications were classified in accordance to their occurrence into intraoperative, early postoperative (within the first 3 post-operative months) and late ones.

The follow-up examination of all patients was performed by a single examiner (G.M.) using the Harris hip [14] and Merle d'Aubigné score [17] and also recording the functional leg length and the patient's subjective satisfaction.

2 examiners (C.P., G.M.) evaluated the pelvic and axial X-rays analyzing progressive and non-progressive radiolucent lines or osteolysis, as well as the presence of periarticular ossifications. They were classified according to Brooker [3], radiolucent lines surrounding the cup were evaluated according to the method of DeLee and Charnley [4;9]. Radiolucencies surrounding the stem were classified according to Gruen [12]. Signs of loosening or progressive component migration, signified by the presence of a continuous radiolucent line or component migration more than 2mm, were also evaluated.

Implant migration was assessed according to Nunn and Wetherell [19;21;22]. After correction of the magnification factor and pelvic rotation, horizontal and vertical cup migration and changes of inclination angle were determined.

Statistical analysis
With reference to an over all accuracy of 2mm, every migration greater than 2mm was defined as significant. The Kaplan-Meier product limit method was used to estimate the cumulative probabilities of loosening. Medians, mean values and ranges were specified where reasonable.

Results

Intraoperative complications
In none of the cases intraoperative complications occurred. Neither acetabular fractures nor nerve palsies were observed.

Early complications and revisions
5 specific early complications were observed: two dislocations (1.6%), two cases of non-revision-relevant haemorrhages (1.6%) and one case of deep infection (0.8%). One general complication (0.8%), a deep vein thrombosis, was recorded. Three revision operations had to be performed, two acetabular cup reorientations and close reductions due to dislocations and one implant removal because of a deep infection. The revised Hedrocel® cup showed a significant bony ingrowth only six weeks after implantation (Fig. 2).

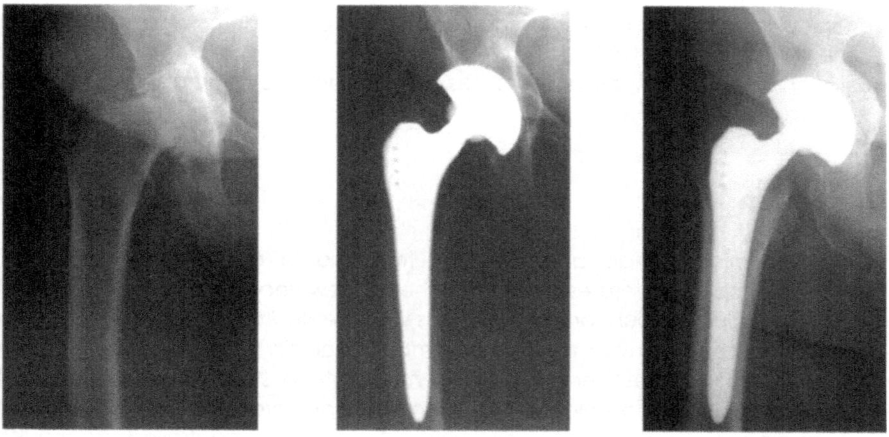

Figure 2:
(a) 73 year old woman having a coxarthrosis and an acetabular protrusion,
(b) 4 months after acetabular autologous bone grafting and implantation of a Hedrocel® cup, and
(c) follow-up examination 2 years postoperatively showing bone graft remodeling and a firmly incorporated cup.

Late complications
No additional aseptic or septic failures could be verified at the time of follow-up. Thus the implant survival curve according to Kaplan-Meier shows a 3.1 year overall survival rate of 100% with radiological loosening as the endpoint.

Clinical results

The average Harris hip score improved from 44.0 points (range 29-72 points, median 53 points) preoperatively to 87.1 points postoperatively (range 71-100 points, median 93 points). The Merle d'Aubigné score revealed a median improvement from 8.3 points preoperatively to 16.4 points after surgery. At the time of follow-up, the functional difference of leg length was less than 1cm in 62 cases (96.8%) and between 1 and 2,5cm in 2 cases (3.2%). No differences greater than 2cm were observed. Subjectively, the surgical outcome was described as excellent in 48 cases (75.0%), as good in 13 cases (20.3%) and as satisfactory in 3 cases (4.7%). None of the patients was dissatisfied.

Radiological evaluation

The images of 62 of the 64 cases (96.9%) could be evaluated for migration analysis at follow-up. Signs of loosening, reaming defect healing, radiolucent lines, osteolysis, bone resorption, sclerosis, osteointegration, bone remodelling (Fig. 2) and periarticular ossifications were determined for all 64 of the prostheses that were observed at follow-up.

Signs of loosening: Seam formation of the cup was verified in none of the patients. No continuous radiolucent lines, osteolysis or signs of loosening in the area of the cup were observed. Non-progressive incomplete radiolucent lines were found in six cases (9.4%). Sclerosis occurred in four cases (6.2%), exclusively in DeLee and Charnleys zones 1 and 2. Thus all cups were integrated stable into the acetabulum according to radiological criteria at follow-up.

Periarticular ossifications: Grade I ossifications were found in 6 cases (9.3%) and Grade II in one case (1.6%) according to Brooker.

Migration analysis: In none of the cases a significant migration of the cup could be revealed.

Discussion

Different biomaterials and surfaces for durable cementless fixation of orthopedic implants were established in the last few years.

Our study evaluated our early experiences with the Hedrocel® acetabular cup, a cup with improved physical properties, mainly porosity and friction, in primary and revision THA. These early results demonstrate a stable integration of all implants. No signs of loosening or migration could be revealed. 9.4% of the cases had incomplete radiolocent lines, which have to be controlled at regular intervals. They are known to appear in other implants, too, without being signs of implant loosening [7;11]. The introductorily described high surface friction of the Hedrocel® cup is detectable in the intraoperative handling of this implant [24]. In comparison to other implants significant higher forces have to be applied for cup impaction. Considerable complications, like fractures of the acetabulum, did not occur. Thus the high friction coefficient is a positive attribute of the Hedrocel® cup, giving it a great potential of simplifying hip revision surgery [5]. Furthermore a stable integration of soft tissue into the implant could be demonstrated [13].

The non-modular implant design has pros and cons. The UHMWPE is molded directly into the metal under high pressure and ultra-clean conditions with 100% support of the polyethylene by metal backing. On the one hand the complete avoidance of backside wear, which is being produced at the metal / inlay interface in modular acetabular cups and may potentially compromise the long term stability of the implant [23], is an advantage. On the other hand, due to their non-modularity, Hedrocel® cups are not suitable for resterilization, so that they have to be wasted if a stable anchorage is not achievable. Furthermore only 28mm heads can be used. This can cause an impingement between the neck of the stem and the outer rim of the cup in cases of XXL – heads being necessary [16], e.g. at cup revision, if a firmly incorporated stem should be left in situ. In addition an accessorily stabilization by screws is not possible. However this is not a disadvantage for an experienced surgeon in our experiences.

Because of the high friction and thus achievable primary stability we did not waste any Hedrocel® cup. Additionally we want to point out potential disadvantages of screw fixation of acetabular cups. The process of screwing in is, beside being a risk factor for cup dislocation, an additional step requiring time. Screws always affect the autochthone bone and may lacerate nerval and vascular structures [10;15]. Long term surveys have shown a high rate of progressive radiolucent lines and wear debris caused by acetabular cup screws [18;20]. In the case of screw breakage revision surgery becomes more difficult and screw removal is always associated with bone defects.

Our results document excellent clinical and radiological short-term results accompanied with a subjective complete satisfaction of the patients. For a definite evaluation of this implant's sufficiency further investigations, including more patients over longer periods of time, are necessary.

Reference List

1. Bobyn JD, Stackpool GJ, Hacking SA, Tanzer M, Krygier JJ (1999) Characteristics of bone ingrowth and interface mechanics of a new porous tantalum biomaterial. J.Bone Joint Surg.Br. 81:907-914
2. Bobyn JD, Toh KK, Hacking SA, Tanzer M, Krygier JJ (1999) Tissue response to porous tantalum acetabular cups: a canine model. J.Arthroplasty 14:347-354
3. Brooker AF, Bowerman JW, Robinson RA, Riley LH, Jr. (1973) Ectopic ossification following total hip replacement. Incidence and a method of classification. J Bone Joint Surg Am. 55:1629-1632
4. Charnley J, Feagin JA (1973) Low-friction arthroplasty in congenital subluxation of the hip. Clin Orthop 91:-1977
5. Christie MJ (2002) Clinical applications of Trabecular Metal. Am.J.Orthop. 31:219-220
6. Cohen R (2002) A porous tantalum trabecular metal: basic science. Am.J.Orthop. 31:216-217
7. Collis DK (1982) Long-term radiographic follow-up of total hip replacements. Hip.1-26
8. Crowe JF, Mani VJ, Ranawat CS (1979) Total hip replacement in congenital dislocation and dysplasia of the hip. J Bone Joint Surg Am. 61:15-23
9. DeLee JG, Charnley J (1976) Radiological demarcation of cemented sockets in total hip replacement. Clin Orthop20-32
10. Fruhwirth J, Koch G, Ivanic GM, Seibert FJ, Tesch NP (1997) [Vascular lesions in surgery of the hip joint]. Unfallchirurg 100:119-123
11. Green DL, Bahniuk E, Liebelt RA, Fender E, Mirkov P (1983) Biplane radiographic measurements of reversible displacement (including clinical loosening) and migration of total joint replacements. J.Bone Joint Surg.Am. 65:1134-1143
12. Gruen TA, McNeice GM, Amstutz HC (1979) "Modes of failure" of cemented stem-type femoral components: a radiographic analysis of loosening. Clin Orthop17-27

13. Hacking SA, Bobyn JD, Toh K, Tanzer M, Krygier JJ (2000) Fibrous tissue ingrowth and attachment to porous tantalum. J.Biomed.Mater.Res. 52:631-638
14. Harris WH (1969) Traumatic arthritis of the hip after dislocation and acetabular fractures: treatment by mold arthroplasty. An end-result study using a new method of result evaluation. J Bone Joint Surg Am. 51:737-755
15. Kirkpatrick JS, Callaghan JJ, Vandemark RM, Goldner RD (1990) The relationship of the intrapelvic vasculature to the acetabulum. Implications in screw-fixation acetabular components. Clin.Orthop.183-190
16. Krushell RJ, Burke DW, Harris WH (1991) Range of motion in contemporary total hip arthroplasty. The impact of modular head-neck components. J.Arthroplasty 6:97-101
17. Merle d´Aubigné R, Postel M (1954) Functional results of arthroplasty with acrylic prosthesis. J Bone Joint Surg Am. 36A:451-455
18. Morscher EW (1992) Current status of acetabular fixation in primary total hip arthroplasty. Clin.Orthop.172-193
19. Nunn D, Freeman MA, Hill PF, Evans SJ (1989) The measurement of migration of the acetabular component of hip prostheses. J Bone Joint Surg Br. 71:629-631
20. Puolakka TJ, Laine HJ, Moilanen TP, Koivisto AM, Pajamaki KJ (2001) Alarming wear of the first-generation polyethylene liner of the cementless porous-coated Biomet Universal cup: 107 hips followed for mean 6 years. Acta Orthop.Scand. 72:1-7
21. Wetherell RG, Amis AA, Heatley FW (1989) Measurement of acetabular erosion. The effect of pelvic rotation on common landmarks. J Bone Joint Surg Br. 71:447-451
22. Wetherell RG, Amis AA, Heatley FW (1989) Measurement of acetabular erosion. The effect of pelvic rotation on common landmarks. J Bone Joint Surg Br. 71:447-451
23. Williams VG, Whiteside LA, White SE, McCarthy DS (1997) Fixation of ultrahigh-molecular-weight polyethylene liners to metal- backed acetabular cups. J.Arthroplasty 12:25-31
24. Zardiackas LD, Parsell DE, Dillon LD, Mitchell DW, Nunnery LA, Poggie R (2001) Structure, metallurgy, and mechanical properties of a porous tantalum foam. J.Biomed.Mater.Res. 58:180-187

5.5 Wear Performance of 28 Millimeter Femoral Heads with the Harris Galante Cup: Comparison of Alumina and Cobalt Chrome

Ch. Hendrich, S. Goebel, Ch. Roller, S. Kirschner and J. M. Martell

Summary

Allthough hip simulator testing shows improved wear behavior for alumina ceramic femoral heads, this fact has not been supported by a clinical series.
The aim of this study was to compare the linear wear rates of 28 mm alumina (BIOLOX) vs. Cobalt-Chrome (CoCr) femoral heads in combination with the Harris-Galante-Porous-I and -II acetabular cup with conventional ultra high molecular weight polyethylene (UHMWPE) liners. A total of 209 implants were measured by using the computer assisted digital method of Martell. 109 implants received CoCr bearings (mean follow-up = 8 yr., range 2-13) while 100 received alumina bearings (mean follow-up = 5 yr., range 2-9).
While the linear wear rate of the metal bearings was at 0.14 ± 0.11 mm/yr, that of the alumina heads was observed to be 13 ± 0.08 mm/yr. This difference showed no significance (p= 0.46). Post-hoc power analysis indicated 80% power to detect a 0.038 mm/yr. (28%) difference in wear rates.
These results represent the first clinical data comparing wear rates for alumina ceramic vs. CoCr heads of 28 mm size. With an 80% power to detect a 28% wear reduction this series shows no advantage in wear performance for alumina ceramics on conventional UHMWPE in a modular cup design.

Introduction

Acetabular polyethylene wear with its associated pelvic and femoral osteolysis has been proven to limit the longevity of total hip arthroplasty. [4,8,22,23,25] Several prosthetic and patient factors have been shown to influence the amount of polyethylene wear. [1,6,9,16]
While the factors regarding the patient are hardly changeable, many prosthetic modifications have been discussed to reduce the wear rate for all patients. [1,19] To achieve lower wear, alumina ceramic femoral heads were introduced in the early seventies. Ceramic femoral heads have been shown to be harder than metal ones, which makes them more resistant to damage by third body wear particles. Additionally, ceramic bearing surfaces have increased wetability, which improves lubrication and decreases friction and wear. [5,7]
Hip simulator studies using water as a lubricant have proved the supposition of lower wear rates by using ceramic on polyethylene articulations. [14] However, it has not been confirmed whether this prevails clinically, since several studies have found higher wear rates for ceramic bearings in hip simulators using bovine serum as lubricant. [2,10] Elevations in temperature at the bearing interface, which is influenced by the concentration of the proteins in the lubricant, increases friction and therefore wear. [13]

Considering these facts, it is not known what the clinical performance of ceramic on polyethylene articulations will be. Unfortunately, the literature has few clinical studies investigating the wear performance of alumina on polyethylene. The few available studies are show both, reduction and an increase in wear. [3,21] New digital measuring methods for analyzing wear made it possible to evaluate a high number of hip prosthesis in a short time and with high accuracy. With the method of Martell a repeatability coefficient of 0.004 mm for the same and 0.006 mm for different observers. [11]

To our knowledge, no published series exist with adequate power (80%) to compare alumina and CoCr polyethylene wear rates in total hip arthroplasty. In this study the in vivo wear rates of alumina and CoCr femoral bearings in combination with the Harris-Galante Porous-I and -II acetabular components were evaluated using the method of Martell.

Patients, Materials and Methods

A retrospective series of patients with type I and II of Harris-Galante (Zimmer) with either 28 mm BIOLOX or CoCr femoral heads were analyzed for linear polyethylene wear using a computerized edge detection technique.[11] The UHMWE-liners were all sterilized by 3 Mrads of gamma irradiation in an air environment. Implants were packaged in air, however the average shelf life at both high volume centers was low. The two populations were analyzed independently at each site and the data combined for analysis by the senior author (JMM).

28 mm CoCr heads
The group with CoCr femoral heads consisted of 109 implants (mean follow-up = 8 yr. range 2-13) using the Harris-Galante-I and II cementless acetabular components with cementless femoral stems. These cases were performed at the Rush Presbyterian St. Lukes Medical Center in Chicago, Illinois, USA.

28 mm BIOLOX heads
The alumina group consisted of 100 implants with alumina (BIOLOX) femoral heads and identical Harris-Galante type I and II cementless acetabular components (mean follow-up = 5 yr. range 2-9). All of the alumina ceramic cases were performed at Würzburg University, Germany. Cementless and cemented femoral stems were used in this population.

Measuring method
Linear wear measurements were obtained using the method of Martell. [11] With this technique the distance between the center of the head and the center of the cup are compared over the course of time. Image analysis techniques provide superior reproducibility compared to conventional measuring systems. Head and cup edges are enhanced using custom edge operators. Those pixels making up the edge of the implant are used to determine best-fit circles around the head and the cup. In the case of poor picture quality, manual adjustment is possible. Once the cup center is located the magnitude and direction of head displacement relative to the cup center is calculated on serial radiographs. Linear wear is determined from the resultant vector for head displacement (Fig. 1).

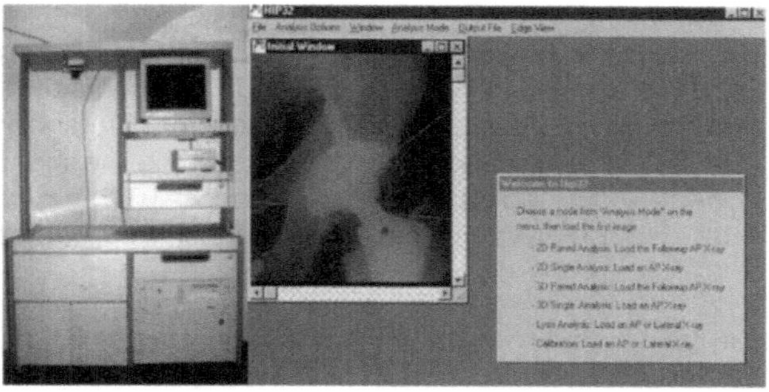

Figure 1:
12-bit CCD-Scanner and the method of Martell11 for clinical wear measurement.

Statistical analysis

The demographic characteristics of the two populations were tested for significant differences using the Chi-Square test. To test for significant correlations with the linear wear rates the demographic factors which differ between the two groups were evaluated using linear regression. The wear data were tested for normality and the appropriate transformation of the data was performed to achieve a normal distribution. The linear wear rates were adjusted for significant clinical covariates and tested at the 95% level using analysis of covariance. A post-hoc power analysis was then performed to assess the power of the study to detect differences in wear between the CoCr and alumina groups.

Results

Comparison of the two groups

Both groups showed significant demographic differences. The German cohort was significantly older ($p < 0.0001$), had an higher body-mass-index ($p = 0.001$), with larger cup size ($p < 0.0001$), and smaller inclination ($p = 0.001$). The two cohorts also differ significantly in regard to the diagnosis ($p < 0.001$). They showed no significant difference with respect to sex ($p = 0.61$) or radiographic anteversion ($p = 0.91$ – Fig 2) . While avascular necrosis and osteoarthritis are the most common diagnosis in both groups, avascular necrosis is less prevalent (16%vs. 28%) and osteoarthritis is more prevalent (72% vs. 60%) among the German patients. There was no difference in the wear rates whether the stems were implanted with or without cement ($p = 0.261$).

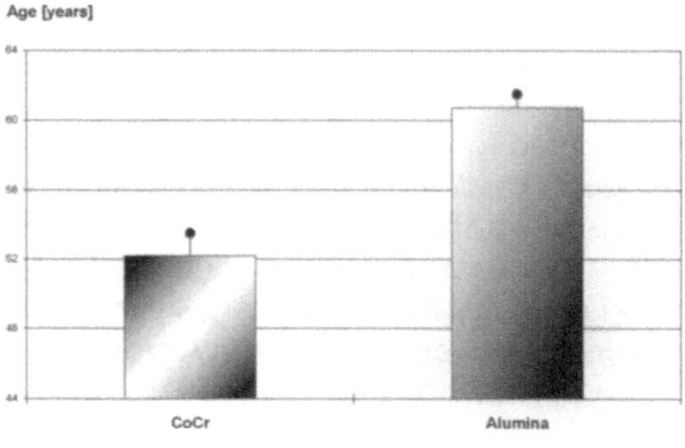

Figure 2:
The average age of the patients with CrCo and alumina (BIOLOX) heads. On the y-axis the age at implantation in [y], on the x-axis the type of the head is depicted. The difference between both group was significant (p<0.0001).

Linear rate of wear

The linear rate of wear among the CoCr metal bearings was 0.14 ± 0.11 mm per year. The alumina heads had an annual wear rate of 0.13 ± 0.08 mm (Fig. 3). The Mann-Whitney-U-test showed no significant difference between the two groups ($p = 0.46$). Post-hoc power analysis, using the mean standard deviation for both cohorts, indicated 80% power to detect a 0.038 mm/yr. (28%) difference in wear rates. No osteolysis was observed in either group at the last follow-up.

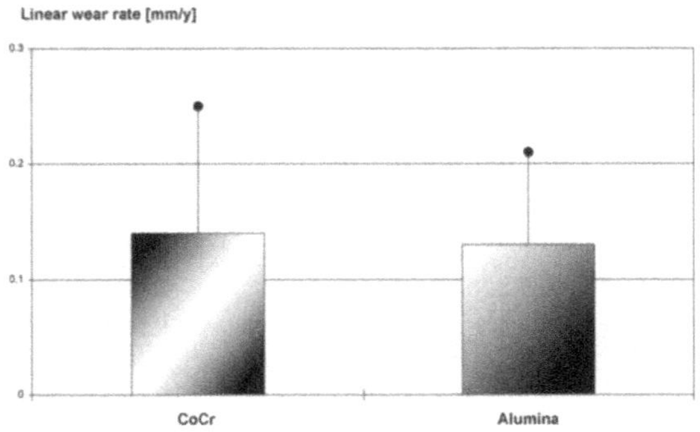

Figure 3:
Linear rate of wear of CrCo and alumina (BIOLOX) heads. On the y-axis the annual linear wear in [mm/y], on the x-axis the type of the head is shown.

Discussion

In this study the clinical wear rates of 28 mm CoCr and 28 mm BIOLOX femoral heads in combination with an uncemented modular spherical pressfit cup were compared. There was no significant difference in the linear polyethylene wear for both groups using the student t-test ($p = 0.73$) and after adjusting for covariates and using a non-parametric test (Mann-Whitney-U-test) ($p = 0.46$). Previous studies which showed no wear reduction with alumina bearings were under powered, and therefore one can not draw conclusions from the negative result. [3,18]

The linear wear rate we found for the CoCr heads agrees with previously published series [13,26], whereas the wear rate of the alumina heads was slightly higher than the ones reported in other studies. [15,17]

The retrospective nature of this study is one potential limitation. However the large size of both cohorts allows a high statistical power to detect differences in the wear rate of both types of heads. Another limitation is the larger follow up of the CoCr group compared to the alumina cohort (8 years vs. 5.2 years). However, both follow-up intervals are well beyond the 18-month bedding-in period and therefore reflect the true wear rates [3,12,20,24] The difference in follow-up was accounted for by reporting wear rates per year of service.

Although the two groups were significantly different with respect to prosthetic and demographic factors, only age was significantly correlated with the wear rate. This wear decreasing for each year of age by 0.0022 ± 0.0008 ($p= 0.004$). Using analysis of covariance to adjust for age continued to show no significant difference in wear between the two groups ($p=0.46$).

The results of our study showed no significantly better wear behavior of the BIOLOX alumina femoral head compared to a CoCr metal head. Despite the improved hardness of the ceramics relative to CoCr we could not show any evidence for a better performance of the alumina bearings. It is still unclear what benefit alumina bearings will provide in the face of third body wear mechanisms This was not the predominant mode of wear in this series, since all the implants studied were well fixed.

References

1. Bankston, A. B.; Faris, P. M.; Keating, E. M.; and Ritter, M. A.: Polyethylene wear in total hip arthroplasty in patient-matched groups. A comparison of stainless steel, cobalt chrome, and titanium-bearing surfaces. J Arthroplasty, 8(3): 315-22, 1993
2. Clarke, I. C.; Gustafson, A.; Jung, H.; and Fujisawa, A.: Hip-simulator ranking of polyethylene wear: comparisons between ceramic heads of different sizes. Acta Orthop Scand, 67(2): 128-32., 1996
3. Devane, P. A., and Horne, J. G.: Assessment of polyethylene wear in total hip replacement. Clin Orthop, (369): 59-72, 1999
4. Harris, W. H.: The problem is osteolysis. Clin Orthop, (311): 46-53, 1995
5. Izquierdo-Avino, R. J.; Siney, P. D.; and Wroblewski, B. M.: Polyethylene wear in the Charnley offset bore acetabular cup. A radiological analysis. J Bone Joint Surg Br, 78(1): 82-4, 1996
6. Jasty, M.; Goetz, D. D.; Bragdon, C. R.; Lee, K. R.; Hanson, A. E.; Elder, J. R.; and Harris, W. H.: Wear of polyethylene acetabular components in total hip arthroplasty. An analysis of one hundred and twenty-eight components retrieved at autopsy or revision operations [see comments]. J Bone Joint Surg Am, 79(3): 349-58, 1997
7. Jazrawi, L. M.; Kummer, F. J.; and DiCesare, P. E.: Alternative bearing surfaces for total joint arthroplasty. J Am Acad Orthop Surg, 6(4): 198-203, 1998
8. Joshi, A. B.; Markovic, L.; and Ilchmann, T.: Polyethylene wear and calcar osteolysis. Am J Orthop, 28(1): 45-8, 1999
9. Livermore, J.; Ilstrup, D.; and Morrey, B.: Effect of femoral head size on wear of the polyethylene acetabular component. J Bone Joint Surg [Am], 72(4): 518-28, 1990
10. Lu, Z., and McKellop, H.: Frictional heating of bearing materials tested in a hip joint wear simulator. Proc Inst Mech Eng [H], 211(1): 101-8, 1997
11. Martell, J. M., and Berdia, S.: Determination of polyethylene wear in total hip replacements with use of digital radiographs. J Bone Joint Surg Am, 79(11): 1635-41, 1997
12. Pedersen DR, Callaghan JJ, Johnston TL, Fetzer GB, Johnston RC. Comparison of femoral head penetration rates between cementless acetabular components with 22-mm and 28-mm heads. J Arthroplasty.,16:111-115, 2001
13. Phipatanakul, W. P.; Johnson, S. A.; Good, V.; and Clarke, I. C.: The fallacy of evaluating biomaterial wear-rates with water as lubricant: a hip simulator study of alumina-PTFE nd CoCr-PTFE combinations. J Biomed Mater Res, 39(2): 229-33., 1998
14. Saikko, V. O.; Paavolainen, P. O.; and Slatis, P.: Wear of the polyethylene acetabular cup. Metallic and ceramic heads compared in a hip simulator. Acta Orthop Scand, 64(4): 391-402., 1993
15. Saito M, Saito S, Ohzono K, Takaoka K, Ono K. Efficacy of alumina ceramic heads for cemented total hip arthroplasty. Clin Orthop.,171-177., 1992
16. Schmalzried, T. P. et al.: The John Charnley Award. Wear is a function of use, not time. Clin Orthop, (381): 36-46., 2000
17. Sugano N, Nishii T, Nakata K, Masuhara K, Takaoka K. Polyethylene sockets and alumina ceramic heads in cemented total hip arthroplasty. A ten-year study. J Bone Joint Surg Br.,77:548-556., 1995

18. Sychterz, C. J.; Engh, C. A., Jr.; Young, A. M.; Hopper, R. H., Jr.; and Engh, C. A.: Comparison of in vivo wear between polyethylene liners articulating with ceramic and cobalt-chrome femoral heads. J Bone Joint Surg Br, 82(7): 948-51., 2000
19. Sychterz, C. J.; Shah, N.; and Engh, C. A.: Examination of wear in Duraloc acetabular components: two- to five-year evaluation of Hylamer and Enduron liners. J Arthroplasty, 13(5): 508-14., 1998
20. Sychterz, C. J.; Engh, C. A., Jr.; Yang, A.; and Engh, C. A.: Analysis of temporal wear patterns of porous-coated acetabular components: distinguishing between true wear and so-called bedding-in. J Bone Joint Surg Am, 81(6): 821-30, 1999
21. Urban, J. A.; Garvin, K. L.; Boese, C. K.; Bryson, L.; Pedersen, D. R.; Callaghan, J. J.; and Miller, R. K.: Ceramic-on-polyethylene bearing surfaces in total hip arthroplasty. Seventeen to twenty-one-year results. J Bone Joint Surg Am, 83-A(11): 1688-94., 2001
22. Wan, Z., and Dorr, L. D.: Natural history of femoral focal osteolysis with proximal ingrowth smooth stem implant. J Arthroplasty, 11(6): 718-25, 1996
23. Willert, H. G.; Bertram, H.; and Buchhorn, G. H.: Osteolysis in alloarthroplasty of the hip. The role of ultra-high molecular weight polyethylene wear particles. Clin Orthop, (258): 95-107, 1990
24. Wroblewski BM, Siney PD, Dowson D, Collins SN. Prospective clinical and joint simulator studies of a new total hip arthroplasty using alumina ceramic heads and cross-linked polyethylene cups. J Bone Joint Surg Br.,78:280-285,1996
25. Zicat, B.; Engh, C. A.; and Gokcen, E.: Patterns of osteolysis around total hip components inserted with and without cement. J Bone Joint Surg Am, 77(3): 432-9, 1995
26. Zichner, L. P., and Willert, H. G.: Comparison of alumina-polyethylene and metal-polyethylene in clinical trials. Clin Orthop, (282): 86-94, 1992

5.6 Alumina-on-Alumina Coupling with 36 mm Heads

R. Giacometti-Ceroni and L. Zagra

Abstract

According to Charnley, the rationale to have a 22mm head is in reducing the friction torque and the volumetric wear.
This fact is absolutely true for metal-poly coupling and partially true also for ceramic-poly, but if we employ a ceramic-ceramic coupling, a diameter of heads of 36mm doesn't increase the volumetric wear nor the friction torque, compared with a 22 mm metal-poly coupling.
On the other hand, a bigger diameter leads to more stable artificial joints and to a wider range of motion.
In the last two years we have developed and used an acetabular component, with a 36 mm liner-head alumina-alumina coupling.
We performed a perspective study to investigate the rate of dislocation of the prostheses in the first two month after operation.
We analysed two groups: the first one (225 cases, from March 2001 to December 2002, mean age 64 years and 9 months) in which 36 mm heads were implanted, and the second (151 cases, from January 2001 to December 2002, mean age 66 years and 9 months) in which the surgical technique was the same, but heads of 28 mm were used.
We compared the number of dislocations, 2 (0,88%) in the first group and 7 (4,63%) in the second, and the data confirmed that there is a statistically significant (p=0,020) decrease in dislocations in the group of 36 mm heads.

5.7 Uncemented Alumina on Alumina THR: a retrospective study

A. Berizzi, G. Castiello and L. Colognese

Alumina on Alumina bearing surfaces were introduced in the early 70s as an alternative to metal on polyethylene articulation, as part of an effort to reduce the complications related to polyethylene wear debris.

In this paper we present a consecutive series of patients who received a cementless Alumina on Alumina total hip replacement, with a minimum follow-up of 54 months.

Materials and method

Between January 1997 and June 1998 we performed 110 consecutive Total Hip Replacement (THR) in 110 patients, 60 women and 50 men.

The mean age at the time of intervention was 62,5 years (43 – 77). The initial diagnosis was primary osteoarthritis in 87; congenital hip dysplasia in 10; avascular necrosis of the hip (AVN) in 4; revision for aseptic loosening in 3; rheumatoid arthritis in 2; coxa profunda in 2 and arthrodesis in 2.

The implantation was performed utilizing a lateral approach (Watson-Jones) without osteotomy of the greater trochanter in all the patients.

The same uncemented hip prosthesis was implanted in all the patients. The stem (C2 type, LIMA-LTO spa, San Daniele del Friuli – Italy) is straight, collarless, with antero-posterior and latero-medial conicity, rectangular cross-section and sharp edges. The stem is made of a Ti_6Al_4V Titanium alloy and has a rough sandblasted finish.

The acetabular cup (SPH Peg, LIMA-LTO spa, San Daniele del Friuli, Italy) is hemispherical and made of a Ti6Al4V Titanium alloy. The bone interphase surface with five small pegs is coated with Hydroxyapatite. The design also incorporates three screw holes for additional screw fixation if needed.

The femoral head is made of high-purity aluminium oxide ceramic (BIOLOX®forte, CeramTec AG, Germany), with a diameter of 28 mm and is attached to the stem by means of a Morse taper 12/14.

The acetabular insert uses a sandwich system (Al_2O_3+UHMWPE, made by LIMA-LTO spa, San Daniele del Fruli, Italy). The ceramic insert and UHMWPE liner lock by means of a taper system. This sandwich (PolyLock® CeramTec AG, Germany) then interlocks with the outer titanium shell.

All the patients were subjected to the same rehabilitation program: passive motion from the first post-operative day and partial (30 Kg) weight bearing starting on the second or third post-operative day. Full weight bearing, with crutches, was allowed four weeks after the operation and complete unassited walking was allowed six to seven weeks after operation. Light muscular reinforcement was encouraged four weeks after the operation (bicycle, swimming).

All of the patients have been evaluated preoperatively. The surviving patients were asked to answer a detailed questionnaire and to return for a clinical and radiological evaluation. All evaluations were performed by the same observer. Hip functional results were rated according to the Harris Hip Score (HHS) system. The X-ray evaluation included both pelvic and femoral side. The inclination of the socket relative to the horizontal line and the presence of radiolucent lines in the zones described by Charnley were studied on the pelvic side. The alignment of the stem with respect to the axis of the femur, the presence of radiolucent lines in the zones described by Gruen, subsidence of the stem and resorption of the calcar were studied on the femoral side.

Results

At the time of follow up, we were able to contact and to evaluate 85 patients. Of the initial 110 patients ten died of causes unrelated to the THR, and 15 were untraceable. None of the contacted patients refused the evaluation.

The mean preoperative HHS, in the primary osteoarthritis, was 54,1 (24 – 82), at the follow-up the HHS in the same group was 85,5 (37 – 100). In the dysplastic group the preoperative HHS was 48 (12 – 68) and the last HHS was 84 (58 – 100). In the group of the AVN the preoperative HHS was 33 (16 – 49) and 85 (61 – 100) at the follow-up.

We have had two early dislocations, easily reduced under anesthesia, and without impairment of the late results.

We have had 3 deep vein thrombosis, without pulmonary embolism.

We have had only one infection of the soft tissues around the prosthesis, treated with surgical debridement and systemic antimicrobial therapy; at the follow-up the patient was in good health, without any signs of infection or loosening.

There have been three revisions due to aseptic loosening, two acetabular cups and one stem.

A full analysis of the X-ray controls is still underway.

Squeaking in a Ceramic on Ceramic Total Hip

T. H. Eickmann, I. C. Clarke and G. A. Gustafson

Introduction

Three causes of squeaking have been described in the literature. In one case squeaking was thought to be due to a mismatch material wear couple, zirconia on alumina [1]. Another case involved a Biolox ceramic head which had worn through a 3 millimeter (mm) ultra high molecular weight polyethylene (UHMWPE) liner [2]. Three squeaking cases were reported in a retrieval study of "AML Plus" stems and "ACS" polyethylene liners. The metal heads were found to be articulating with the acetabular metal backings [3]. Garino has observed squeaking in a case where a 28 mm ceramic head was paired with a 32 mm inner diameter ceramic liner (J. Garino, personal communication 2002). Heros reported squeaking in two cases where a 32 mm ceramic head was paired with a 28 mm inner diameter ceramic liner (R. Heros, personal communication, 2002). The common finding in all cases was two hard surfaces coming into contact. We were unable to find a case in the literature implicating polyethylene as a source of squeaking.

We encountered squeaking in a patient with an alumina ceramic on ceramic hip arthroplasty. The squeaking was audible from across the room and caused her to seek treatment. In this report we present indications for revision surgery, findings at surgery, and discuss ways to minimize impingement and squeaking.

Case Report

A 54 year old female with rheumatoid arthritis underwent primary cementless total hip arthroplasty in March 1999. The stem and 50 mm O.D. cup were made of Ti-6A1-4V (Encore, Austin, Texas). The head and liner were alumina Biolox forte (Ceramtec Inc). The alumina head diameter was 28 mm with a -3.5 mm neck length.

Painless squeaking was noted six months postoperatively with normal ambulation. Two years after primary surgery radiographs demonstrated a notch on the posterior aspect of the neck of the femoral component (Fig. 1). This finding coupled with persistent squeaking were the indications for revision in April 2002.

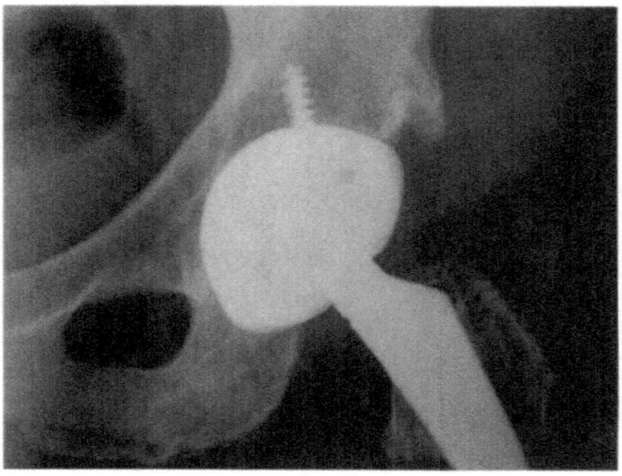

Figure 1:
Preoperative radiographs showing notching of the femoral neck.

At revision surgery, metal staining was noted in the surrounding soft tissues. The femoral neck had two distinct notches about 1 mm wide and deep, extending 10 mm and 14 mm transversely around the femoral neck (Fig. 2). The elevated posterior-rim of the metal-backed cup had also been partially destroyed by impingement and abrasion with the femoral neck. The cup and stem appeared to be in acceptable position and were well fixed. The metal shell and stem were retained and a CoCr head with a longer neck and UHMWPE liner were placed.

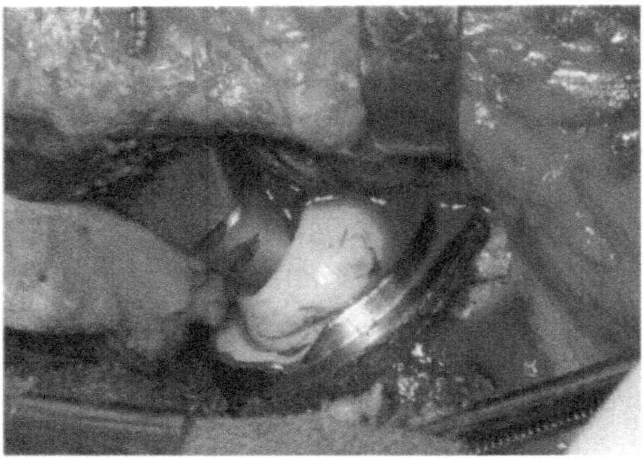

Figure 2:
Posterior aspect of titanium femoral neck with two notches. Titanium acetabular shell with a portion of the elevated metal rim worn away.

To avoid continued impingement, the elevated metal "protective" rim was removed along 30 percent of the circumference of the metal shell with a high-speed burr. The hip was stable without impingement after the modifications to the metal-backing and postoperatively the squeaking had resolved.

Six weeks postoperatively the patient dislocated her hip while stretching in bed. She underwent closed reduction and was given a hip abduction brace. One week later she again dislocated her hip, this time while climbing into the bathtub without her brace. Computerized tomography was obtained for component positioning, the inclination of the cup was 55 degrees, the planar anteversion was 30 degrees, and the femoral anteversion was 16 degrees (Fig. 3, Table 1). Open reduction of her anterior hip dislocation was performed and the components were again judged to be in acceptable position. The patient was taken through a full range of motion without impingement or dislocation and then placed in a cast postoperatively.

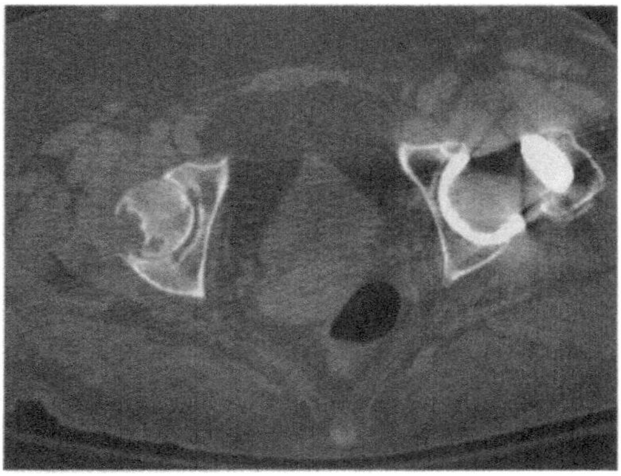

Figure 3:
Computerized tomography showing cup anteversion

	Left THA Side (Degrees)	Right Side (Degrees)
Cup Inclination	55	47
Cup Anteversion	35	28
Planar Anteversion	30	21
Femoral Anteversion	16	2

Table 1:
Comparison of Component Positioning to Patient Anatomy

Discussion

Squeaking has been reported in a case of mismatch wear couple, with zirconia on alumina [1]. Squeaking was also reported by Bono in three metal on polyethylene hips. The femoral head had penetrated the polyethylene liner and was articulating with the metal shell [3]. Simon reports squeaking in a ceramic on poly hip which was found to have articulation of the ceramic head on the metal backing [2]. The last two scenarios result in a low contact area. Pitto says that squeaking is a joint tolerance issue [4]. Garino and Heros cases of squeaking, in which the ceramic head and liner were incorrectly paired, support Pitto's statement. In this case neck-socket impingement found at revision was an obvious explanation for the squeaking. Another possibility is metal acting as a third body in ceramic articulations may cause squeaking by the same mechanism as the ceramic head that wore through the liner and articulated with the metal shell. In this mechanism impingement which creates metal wear debris is still the problem. Willmann reports the bearing surfaces were not responsible in the cases of squeaking he has encountered. Squeaking has not been seen in the Peterson Tribology Lab in ceramic articulations. Squeaking was due to cup design, positioning, or a combination of both (G. Willmann, personal communication 2002).

In this cup design an elevated metal rim was incorporated on the metal backing to "protect" the ceramic [5]. With this cup design, size of the cup (50 mm) and neck length (-3.5 mm) determine whether the neck impinges with the liner or metal backing (Table 2).

Cup Size	Range of Motion Prior to Component Impingement			
	-3.5 mm neck		+3.5 mm neck	
	Impingement on Cup	Impingement on Liner	Impingement on Cup	Impingement on Liner
48 to 50 mm	116	122	118	118
52 to 54 mm	120	124	126	122
56 to 58 mm	124	124	125	119
60 to 62 mm	127	123	129	119

Table 2:
The effect of cup size and neck length on range of motion prior to component impingement.

The metal rim decreases the range of motion 6 degrees in this case. The elevated rim on the metal-backing of cups puts the neck at risk in cases of neck-socket impingement [6, 7]. The metal rim also creates a fulcrum for subluxation and dislocation in our case (Fig. 4).

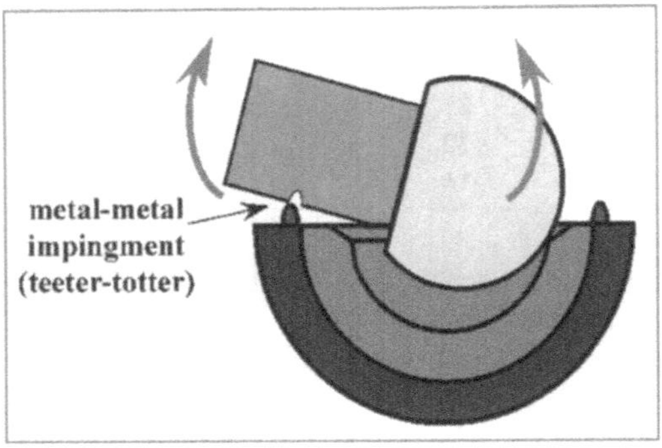

Figure 4:
Impingement teeter-tooter creates notching of the neck with subluxation

Concerns have been raised about chipping of the ceramic liner in cup designs where the metal backing does not fully cover the ceramic liner [5, 8, 9]. The clinical relevance of chipping is uncertain. Sedel reports it has not been a problem in 3,500 ceramic hip arthroplasties (L. Sedel, personal communication, 2002). Hamadouche reports no liner fractures in 18.5 years follow up using designs like the Ceraver in which the femoral neck comes in contact with the ceramic liner in cases of component impingement [10].

Rigid on rigid bearings eliminated the soft polyethylene "bumper" between the stem and cup (Fig. 5). Impingement with notching of the femoral neck has been reported with metal on metal articulations [11, 12]. In this case neck-socket

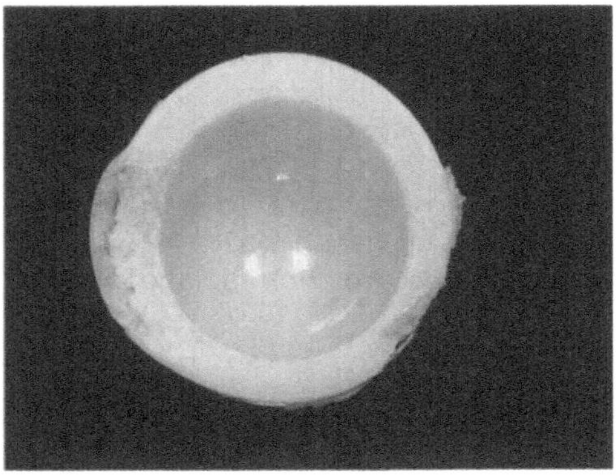

Figure 5:
Polyethylene liner acting as a bumper in cases of component impingement

impingement resulted in notching of the femoral neck, abrasion of the "protective" metal rim, and metal contamination of the ceramic bearing surfaces. At revision, the porous stem was well fixed and was left in situ. The notches on the neck pose a risk for fatigue fracture of the neck. The cup was not revised because intraoperatively the cup appeared to be in good position and the hip was stable.

Many optimal orientations have been described for cup placement [13, 14, 15, 16]. Garino suggests that more horizontal cup positioning (< 45 degrees) may be ideal and additional anteversion (20-30 degrees) may be needed in ceramic on ceramic articulations [17, 18,19]. Bader recommends 45 degrees inclination and 15 degrees of anteversion [20]. If the cup is too vertical the risk of ceramic fracture and dislocation increases [21]. The cup position by CT scan was 55 degrees of inclination and 30 degrees of planar anteversion. The cup in this case is positioned out of the "safe zone" for dislocation of 30 to 50 degrees inclination and 5 to 25 degrees of planar anteversion described by Lewinnek [16]. Experienced surgeons placed the cup out of the "safe zone" in 78 percent of the cases when positioning was determined by a navigational system [22]. This suggests that a surgeon cannot be expected to consistently place the cup in an ideal position.

In this case both the cup and stem were more anteverted then the unoperated side, which put her at risk for component impingement [23, 24]. Without the protective bumper effect of a polyethylene liner, positioning of rigid on rigid bearings may be less forgiving [7, 19]. Patients with activities and hobbies requiring the extremes of range of motion may not be good candidates for hard on hard bearing systems. These patients increase there odds of impingement especially if component positioning is suboptimal. In cases of hard on hard bearings would the need for precise positioning offset the $ 250,000 cost of a navigational system?

Conclusion

Squeaking occurred as a result of neck-socket impingement. Impingement can be minimized by component design and positioning. Omitting the elevated metal rim on the metal backing in this cup design would allow greater range of motion prior to component impingement. Rigid on rigid bearings are less forgiving then metal on polyethylene. Optimal component positioning is crucial when hard on hard bearings are used.

References

1 Morlock M, Nassutt R, Janssen R, et al: Mismatched Wear Couple Zirconium Oxide and Aluminum Oxide in Total Hip Arthroplasty. J Arthroplasty 16: 1071, 2001

2 Simon J, Dayan A, Ergas E, et al: Catastrophic Failure of the Acetabular Component in a Ceramic-Polyethylene Bearing Total Hip Arthroplasty. J Arthroplasty 13: 108, 1998

3 Bono J, Sanford L, Toussaint J: Severe Polyethylene Wear in Total Hip Arthroplasty. J Arthroplasty 9: 119, 1994

4 Pitto R: Contemporary Concepts of Ceramic Cups. Proceedings of the Masters Series in Ceramic Hip Arthroplasty, Costa Mesa, California, 2002

5 Siverhus S: Design Considerations and Preliminary Results with the Osteonics Acetabular Cup System. Bioceramics in Orthopaedics-New Applications. Proceedings of the third International Symposium on Ceramic Wear Couple, 1998

6 D'Antonio J, Capell W, Manley M, et al: New Experience with Alumina-on-Alumina Ceramic Bearings for Total Hip Arthroplasty. J Arthroplasty 17: 390, 2002

7 Clarke I: Role of Ceramic Implants. Design and Clinical Success with Total Hip Prosthetic Ceramic-to-Ceramic Bearings. Clin Orthop 282: 19, 1992

8 Rueda D, A'lvarez M, Barahoona F, et al: Ceramic Inserts in Metal Cups. A Five-year Experience. Performance of the Wear Couple BIOLOX forte in Hip Arthroplasty. Enke Verlag, Stuttgart 97

9 Willmann G: Design of Ceramic Acetabular Components: A Retrospective. Key Engineering Materials 192-195: 525, 2001
10 Hamadouche M, Boutin P, Daussange J, et al: Alumina-on-Alumina Total Hip Arthroplasty. J Bone Joint Surg. 84-A: 69, 2002
11 Iida H, Kaneda E, Takada H, et al: Metallosis Due to Impingement Between the Socket and the Femoral Neck in a Metal-on-Metal Bearing Total Hip Prosthesis. J Bone Joint Surg 81-A: 400, 1999
12 Schmalzried T, Peters P, Maurer B, et al: Long-duration Metal-on-metal Total Hip Arthroplasties With Low Wear of the Articulating Surfaces. J Arthroplasty 11: 322, 1996
13 Harris W: Advances in Surgical Technique for Total Hip Replacement. Clin Orthop 146: 195, 1980
14 Kummer F, Shah S, Iyer S, et al: The effect of Acetabular Cup Orientations on Limiting Hip Rotation. J Arthroplasty 14: 509, 1999
15 McCollum D, Gray W: Dislocation after Total Hip Arthroplasty. Clin Orthop 261: 159, 1990
16 Lewinnek G, Lewis J, Tarr R, et al: Dislocations after total hip replacement arthroplasties. J Bone Joint Surg Am 60: 217, 1978
17 Garino J: Modern Ceramic-on-Ceramic Total Hip Systems in the United States. Clin Orthop 379: 41, 2000
18 Garino J: Design Considerations and Preliminary Results with the Wright Medical „Transcend" Acetabular Cup System. Bioceramics in Orthopaedics-New Applications. Proceedings of the third International Symposium on Ceramic Wear Couple, 1998
19 Garino J: Ceramic-Ceramic Total Hip Replacement: Intraoperative Considerations. Bioceramics in Joint Arthroplasty. Proceedings Sixth International Biolox Symposium, 2001
20 Bader R, Steinhauser E, Gradinger R, et al: Computer-based motion simulation of total hip prostheses with ceramic-on-ceramic wear couple. Analysis of implant design and orientation as influence parameters. Z Orthop Ihre Grenzgeb 140(3): 310, 2002
21 Bader R, Willmann G: Ceramic Cups for hip endoprostheses. 6: Cup design, inclination and antetorsion angle modify range of motion and impingement. Biomed Tech 44:212, 1999
22 DiGioia III A, Jaramaz B, Plakseychuk A, et al: Comparison of a Mechanical Acetabular Alignment Guide With Computer Placement of the Socket. J Arthroplasty 17: 359, 2002
23 Pitto R, Schmidt S, Meller S, et al: The effect of the Orientation of the Acetabular and Femoral Component on the Range of Motion and Impingement in Total Hip Arthroplasty. Bioceramics in Joint Arthroplasty. Proceedings Sixth International Biolox Symposium, 2001
24 Seki M, Yuasa N, Ohkuni K: Analysis of Optimal Range of Socket Orientations in Total Hip Arthroplasty with Use of Computer-Aided Design Simulation. J Ortho Res 16: 513, 1998

5.9 Fiction and Facts Concerning the Reliability of Ceramics in THR

G. Willmann

Ceramics for THR

The use of bioceramics in total hip replacement (THR) dates back to the early 1970s. There are two wear couples that proved to work successfully: ceramic femoral heads articulating against a polyethylene acetabular component (ceramic-on-polyethylene) and ceramic femoral heads articulating against ceramic acetabular inserts (ceramic-on-ceramic). In these applications BIOLOX® forte is the most widely used ceramic.

Ceramic-on-polyethylene and ceramic-on-ceramic wear couples are now accepted state-of-the-art, since they enable the wear rate to be reduced and the problem of particle-induced osteolysis to be solved. Clinical studies show that the in vivo wear rate of ceramic-on-polyethylene is below 0.1mm per year and that for ceramic-on-ceramic is 0.005mm per year. In comparison the typical wear rate for metal-on-polyethylene more than 0.2mm per year. Based on these results it is fair to state that ceramics reduce wear debris and offer the solution to solve the problem of particle induced osteolysis in THR. Acceptance of these benefits is almost universal.

Historical Fracture Rate

Ceramics exhibit a range of excellent properties. They are extremely hard, stiff, synoviaphilic and wear resistant. They produce no metal ion release, and no allergic reactions. On the other hand they are brittle materials, which means that there will always be a small risk of ceramic fracture [3,7,8].

In 1998 and Heros et al [3] reviewed the literature and found 35 different articles in which the fracture rate was reported. They found that in some studies the fracture rate was as low as 0 while in others it was as high as 13%. In attempting to explain the high rates reported in their review, they pointed out the importance of sample size, product design, product manufacture, surgical and clinical factors, etc. For example, in some studies the sample size was only 50 units, in others the product design was old-fashioned, in others the products were made by companies which are no longer in existence and in yet others clinical factors were important.

Results based on large units have been performed in France, Japan, and with BIOLOX®. Sedel at al [5] reported for the French ceramics that the in vivo fracture rate was 0.03%. In Japan Oonishi et al [4] reported similar values. Heros et al [3] reported for 1st and 2nd generation BIOLOX® 0.026% and 0.014%, respectively. The prerequisite for these low failure rates are good product design, good manufacturing, a good quality assurance for ceramics, and well trained surgeons. The results verify that provided these prerequisites are respected, a very low fracture rate could be obtained.

Today's fracture rate

As reported by Heros et al [3] there have been further improvements of ceramic properties, e.g. by introducing clean room processing, hot isostatic pressing, laser marking, and proof-testing. We present here data obtained for today's BIOLOX® forte (3rd generation ceramics).

We present data for ball heads and inserts of today's ceramics manufactured by CeramTec AG between 1995 and December 2002. The number of fractures was determined using information reported to CeramTec. It includes all causes of fracture including trauma, metal taper damage, combination with not-approved taper, incorrect surgical or clinical use, etc. The number of components implanted was based on CeramTec sales figures. Some results of the analysis are shown in Table 1. It can be seen that the rates are very low. Much lower than the rates for other complications.

Revision due to fracture of	*Complication rate*
BIOLOX® forte head 28mm	0.01%
BIOLOX® forte head 32mm	0.004%
CeraLock® inserts (direct fixation)	0.01%
PolyLock® inserts (sandwich)	0,01% and higher
Revision due to	
Aseptic loosening	Far more than 1 %
Inflammation	Approx. 1 %

Table 1: Complication rates

The update presented is of status Dec 2002. The components discussed are 28mm and 32mm standard femoral heads. Between 1995 and 2002 1.3 million BIOLOX® forte heads have been implanted. In the 1970s and 1980s the femoral heads used were 32mm heads, today the mostly used head is the 28mm femoral head. 70% of the standard heads used are 28mm heads.

The failure rate of ceramic inserts (= inlay, liner) was analyzed, too. The inserts that are fixed in the metal shell of the acetabular component by taper fixation are called CeraLock® inserts, the ones with polyethylene between the metal shell and the ceramic insert are called PolyLock, (sandwich concept). Up to 2002 approx. 350.000 ceramic inserts have been sold. The majority of the inserts had been of CeraLock® type.

The large number of ceramic components implanted worldwide is an excellent basis for statistics.

In our analysis we include all reasons of fracture, e.g. trauma, damaged metal taper, combination with not-approved taper, mal-handling by hospital staff and surgeons etc.

The results (see table 1) are based on the cases reported to CeramTec.

The average value of the in vivo fracture rate of all 28mm BIOLOX® forte femoral heads is 0.01% (1:10.000), the one of 32mm BIOLOX® forte heads is smaller. It is 0.004% (=4:100.000). The 28mm and 32mm heads have been used worldwide in combination with various THR stems of different manufactures.

The ceramic heads never fractured because specifications or standards were not met, e.g. specifications of material properties or specifications of the ceramic taper .

The average value of the in vivo fracture rate of all CeraLock® inserts manufactured between 1995 and 2002 is 0.01% (=1:10.000) for all types and for all sizes. Again the ceramic inserts never fractured because specifications or standards were not met. These excellent results can only be achieved if the optimum combination of technical and surgical demands can be achieved, i.e. if the design of the metal shell, the ceramic inserts, all interface properties, and all surgical aspects are in optimum solutions. Example for typical problems that can initiate ceramic fracture are mal-handling [2,6], impingement [1], patient's behavior [9], and cup position not according to recommendations [1].

There are some reports on fracture during surgery. One problem is tilting of insert [2]. Tilting causes stress concentration in the ceramics and may cause fracture. The problems depends very much on the design of the cup and the angle of tilting. Quite often the ceramic fracture is caused by mal-handling [4], e.g. damage of the taper of the acetabular shell may cause stress concentration in the ceramic insert and enhances the risk of failure. Mal-handling can easily be eliminated by training the surgeons (Learning curve).

Repeated impingement between the rim of the insert and the stem of the neck may be initiated by mal-positioning of the acetabular cup [1] or by not-recommended patient's activities [9] or combination of both.

Clinical experience with ceramic inserts proves that the correct position of cups with ceramic CeraLock® and PolyLock® inserts is essential. Even with an good cup design it is important to minimize the risk of impingement between the neck of the stem and the rim of the ceramic insert. Orthopedic companies recommend angles of cup position in their manuals on surgical technique. As a rule of thumb the inclination angle should be approx. 45° and the anteversion angle between 12° and 15° [1].

The in vivo fracture rate of PolyLock® inserts varies. It depends very much on the design of the acetabular components and the insert-polyethylene interface. There are acetabular systems that experience a fracture rate as low as the one of CeraLock®, but there are some that have a higher failure rate. If so: Corrective actions that had been initiated are re-designing the whole system. When the re-designed system passed all laboratory tests for approval follow up studies have to be performed. The follow up studies are still ongoing.

Since the number of PolyLock® inserts is much smaller than the one of CeraLock® inserts there is not a sufficiently good basis for publishing numbers and statistics.

Summary

1. The average value of the in vivo fracture rate of the mostly used BIOLOX® forte 28mm heads is 0.01%, the one for 32mm heads is 0.004%.
2. The average value of the in vivo fracture rate of CeraLock® insert is 0.01%.
3. These excellent results can only be achieved if all demands are in optimum solutions, i.e. technical and surgical ones.
4. Some acetabular components with PolyLock® inserts experience higher fracture rates due to design issues. Corrective actions have been initiated. The follow up studies are ongoing.
5. Evaluating the complication rate of ceramic components it may be fair to state that the risk of ceramic fracture is very low when comparing to clinical complications, e.g. revision due to aseptic loosening, early and late inflammation etc. All these complications are in the order of 1% and more.

References

1. Bader R, Steinhauser E, Willmann G, Gradinger R (2001) The Effects of Implant Design, Position and Wear on the Range of Motion after Total Hip Arthroplasty. Hip Int. 11: 80-90
2. Beaver R J, Cormick C, Kop A (2002) Fractures in Misaligned Ceramic Acetabular Liners: A Laboratory Study. In: J. Garino, G. Willmann (eds.) Bioceramics in Joint Replacement. Georg Thieme Verlag, Stuttgart, New York, p 65-71
3. Heros RJ, Willmann G (1998) Ceramics in Total Hip Arthroplasty: History, Mechanical Properties, Clinical Results, and Current Manufacturing State of the Art. Seminars of Arthroplasty 9: 114-122
4. Oonishi H, Amino H, Ueno M, Yunoki H (1999) Concepts and Designs with Ceramics for Total Hip and Knee Replacement. In: Sedel L, Willmann G (eds.) Reliability and Long-term Results of Ceramics in Orthopaedics, Georg Thieme Verlag Stuttgart 1999, p 7-28
5. Sedel L, Nizard R, Bizot P, Meunier A (1998) Perspective on a 20-Year Experience with Ceramic-on-ceramic Articulation in Total Hip Repacement. Seminars of Arthroplasty 9:123 – 134
6. Steinhauser E, Willmann G, Bader R, Gradinger R (2002) Keramische Einsätze für Hüftgelenkpfannen: Vermeidbare, handhabungsbedingte Brüche [Ceramic inserts for acetabular cups: Avoidable fractures caused by handling]. Z f Orthop 140: S15
7. Toni A., Sudanese A, Terzi S, Tabaaroni M, Calista F, Giunti A (1995) Ceramics in Total Hip Arthroplasty. In: Wise D L et al. (eds.) Encyclopedic Handbook of Biomaterials and Bio-engeneering. Marcel Dekker, Inc. New York, Basel, Hong Kong, Part A, Vol. 2, p1501 – 1544
8. Willmann G (2000) Ceramic Femoral Head Retrieval Data. Clin. Orthop. Rel. Res. 379: 22-28
9. Willmann G (2002) Hüftgelenkspfannen mit Keramik: Patientenverhalten verursacht Impingement und Subluxation [Ceramic acetabular cups: Patient's bevaviour initiates impingement and subluxation]. Z f Orthop 140:165

SESSION 6

Complications in THR using Ceramics

Panel Discussion:	J.-Y. Lazennec (France) C. Perka (Germany) L. Sedel (France) A. Toni (Italy)
Case Reports:	Fractured Ceramic Ball Head How to solve the Problem Impingement How to solve the Problem Not favourable in cup positions How to solve the problem

SESSION 7

Quality and Regulatory Issues

7.1 Ceramics and Joint Replacement – Post Market Surveillance and Best Practice

J. H. Shaw

Ceramic femoral heads made from aluminium oxide (alumina) or zirconium oxide (zirconia) are used as an alternative to heads manufactured from various metal alloys in total hip replacements. Alumina femoral heads can be used in conjunction with alumina or polyethylene acetabular cups; zirconia femoral heads are usually used in conjunction with polyethylene. Hip replacements using ceramic femoral heads have been reported in some studies to show better wear properties compared to metallic femoral heads, and are generally associated with satisfactory clinical performance.

However, the UK Medical Devices Agency (MDA), the Agency of the UK Government's Department of Health responsible for medical device safety, receives periodic reports of fracture of ceramic femoral heads. Although often it is impossible to identify the reasons for the failure in individual cases, clinical practice can affect the performance of ceramic femoral heads.

This paper describes steps that can be taken in terms of post market monitoring and best practice to monitor and improve the performance of these devices.

Post Market Surveillance

Ceramic femoral heads are a component in a hip joint replacement implant, and are therefore moderate to high-risk devices that are intended for long term use and offer significant benefit to a patient's quality of life. Premature failure of these implants has considerable clinical implications for patients who may need to undergo revision surgery, a procedure that has significant associated risks.

Annex I of the Medical Devices Directive [1], which regulates hip implants in the European Union, sets out the essential requirements covering aspects of safety and performance for all medical devices. For joint replacement implants, clinical data will, as a general rule, be required to demonstrate compliance with the relevant essential requirements. Before placing on to the market a joint replacement implant that has new design features, uses new materials or comprises a new product range, the manufacturer should demonstrate that such clinical data are already available from pre-market clinical investigations run within the framework of the Regulations and/or from reviews of the relevant scientific literature. The requirements are set out in Annex X of the Medical Devices Directive [1]. Details of any proposed pre-market clinical investigations of a medical device must be submitted to the relevant Competent Authorities within the European Union prior to commencement.

Based on the clinical data obtained in the pre-market phase, a manufacturer may place the CE marking on a joint replacement implant before the medium and long term clinical performance of that implant is known.

However, the Medical Devices Directive requires manufacturers to

institute and keep up to date a systematic procedure to review experience gained from devices in the post production phase and to implement appropriate means to apply any corrective action.

It is therefore primarily for the manufacturer, in conjunction with the Notified Body that audits the manufacturer, to establish appropriate post market surveillance (PMS) mechanisms. As pointed out in the Medical Devices Agency guidance document on post market surveillance for orthopaedic implants [2], for any joint replacement implant these mechanisms should include properly structured post-market clinical studies designed to confirm the medium and long-term performance of the implant. The studies should also be designed to ensure that the manufacturer's claims on performance are justified. This applies equally to implants that are the subject of pre-market clinical investigations prior to CE marking and to those that are introduced to the market on the basis of pre-existing clinical data.

Post-market clinical studies should

- *be carried out in accordance with a defined written protocol;*
- *define specific objectives and the end points that will demonstrate these objectives;*
- *consist of a sample large enough to produce statistically valid data to demonstrate achievement of the specified end points for each implant using a recognised technique (e.g. Kaplan Meier method of calculating survivorship data).*

Three key elements which form a basis of good PMS have been identified [2] as implant registries, structured clinical follow up of a statistically relevant subset of patients, and adverse incident reporting. The latter of these three steps, adverse incident reporting, is also a requirement of the Medical Devices Directive under the Vigilance reporting mechanism to Competent Authorities in Europe.

Best Practice

Modern ceramic femoral heads are individually tested to a load equivalent to around twenty-five times body weight before they are released for sale in order to minimise the risk of head fracture once they are implanted. However, between 1996 and January 2002, MDA received eleven reports through post market surveillance of fractured ceramic femoral heads. This is in a context of an estimated 40,000 hip replacement implant operations annually in the NHS in England, of which MDA estimates that around 5 per cent may have used ceramic femoral heads.

In general, it has been difficult to establish the exact cause for the failure. Taper damage, which can occur during revision, may lead to an increased risk of ceramic head failure. MDA is aware of one clinical failure of a ceramic femoral head which was associated with the use of a femoral head/stem adaptor sleeve supplied by the stem manufacturer for use with another manufacturer's ceramic femoral head.

However, in the majority of cases reported to MDA, the nature of the failure was such that it was not possible to determine the exact reason for the device fracture. Nevertheless, MDA considered that it would be helpful to reinforce best practice for these devices, to reduce the risk of future failures. For this reason, in February 2002, MDA consulted with all suppliers of hip replacements to the UK health service, and with manufacturers of ceramic femoral heads, to prepare and issue a Safety Notice [3] to the UK health service addressing best practice for these products.

The main messages fell into four categories as follows: Mix and match of design/manufacturer, surgical technique, revision technique and sterilization. The overriding message was that surgeons should follow manufacturers' instructions when using alumina or zirconia ceramic femoral heads in hip replacement implants.

The specific advice in the four categories broke down as follows:

Mix and match of design/manufacturer

1. Do not use a ceramic femoral head supplied by one manufacturer with a femoral stem supplied by another manufacturer;
2. Only use ceramic femoral heads in combination with stems or cups specifically recommended by the manufacturer;
3. Do not use femoral stem taper adaptor sleeves at the head/neck interface unless they are part of a head-sleeve-neck system provided by one manufacturer;

Surgical Technique

4. Do not use excessive force (particularly impact) during attachment of a ceramic femoral head to a stem; do not allow a metal hammer/mallet or other hard item to come into contact with the ceramic head during impaction;
5. Do not implant used, dropped or damaged ceramic femoral heads;
6. Ensure that femoral stem and ceramic femoral head tapers are clean and dry prior to implantation;

Revision

7. Do not implant a ceramic femoral head during hip replacement revision if the stem is not being revised, unless the head is specifically designed by the manufacturer for use in revision surgery;

Sterilization

8. Do not resterilize zirconia femoral heads using steam. MDA had previously advised users [4] not to resterilize zirconia ceramic femoral heads using steam sterilization because this process may cause roughening of the articulating surface.

Summary

The design loop for all medical devices is an ongoing one, and requires the feedback of information from the field through post market surveillance. It is important that this post market surveillance is monitored and analysed, and if appropriate fed back in turn to the field in the form of corrective guidance. This will hopefully lead to risk reduction, improved awareness, and a better clinical result for patients in the future.

References

1. Council Directive 93/42/EEC concerning medical devices, OJ L169 of 12 July 1993.
2. Post-market surveillance of CE marked joint replacement implants including guidance to manufacturers on post market clinical studies – Medical Devices Agency, September 2000.
3. Medical Devices Agency Safety Notice SN2002(05) – February 2002 Best practice in use of ceramic femoral heads in hip replacement
4. Medical Devices Agency Safety Notice SN9617 - June 1996 - Zirconia Ceramic Heads for Modular Total Hip Femoral Components: Advice to Users on Resterilization.

7.2 Quality Improvement Resulting from Legal and Regulatory Developments

H. S. Dobbs

Introduction

The last thirty years have seen the development of a large quantity of ever-more demanding legal and voluntary requirements. The orthopaedic industry has worked hard to meet these requirements. In this respect CeramTec has been a leader. In fact, it has actively participated in the development of standards and has created state-of-the-art research, product development and quality assurance programs. All of this work has been done for a single purpose only, namely to ensure that its products and processes comfortably exceed both current requirements and customer expectations.

Legal and Regulatory Requirements

Thirty years ago, the medical device industry was largely unregulated. In the USA, for instance, there were no medical device regulations until the introduction of the Medical Device Amendment of 1976. In Europe each country had its own national laws, but it was not until the publication of the Medical Devices Directive in 1993 that these were harmonized into pan-European legislation. To meet these requirements manufacturers must produce and in most cases submit to the appropriate authorities documentation verifying the suitability of their products. Today most CeramTec products have the CE mark, which is the European mark of regulatory approval, and are cleared or approved for sale in the USA and in most important markets worldwide.

Table 1: Legal and regulatory requirements

1976:	Medical Device Amendment (USA)
1990:	Safe Medical Device Act (USA)
1993:	EC Medical devices Directive (93/42/EEC)
1997:	Food and Drug Administration (FDA) Modernization Act (USA)

High Purity Alumina: Material Properties

The first recognised requirements for alumina in orthopaedics were published by the German Standards' Institute (DIN) in 1979 as DIN 58835. This standard was adopted two years later by the International Standards Organization (ISO) as ISO 6474 and two years later still by the American Society for Testing and Materials (ASTM) as ASTM F603. Subsequently the DIN standard was replaced, but both the ISO and the ASTM standard are still in existence (see Table 2). The ISO standard was revised in 1994 and this revision resulted in the requirements for bulk density, grain size and biaxial flexural strength being made tougher (see Table 3). These standards also list a number of additional requirements that must be satisfied including purity, allowed constituents, compression strength, wear resistance and fatigue strength. CeramTec components are able to comfortably exceed all these requirements.

Table 2: Standards for high purity alumina for orthopaedic implant use

1979:	DIN 58835, Aluminiumoxidkeramik (Chirurgische Implantate)
1981:	ISO 6474, Ceramic materials based on alumina (Implants for surgery)
1983:	ASTM F603, High-Purity Dense Aluminum Oxide for Surgical Implant application
1994:	ISO 6474 Revision 2, Ceramic materials based on high purity alumina
2000:	ASTM F603 Revision, High-Purity Dense Aluminum Oxide for Medical application
2003:	ISO 6474 Revision 3, Ceramic materials based on high purity alumina

Table 3: Evolution of material property requirements and BIOLOX forte values

	Units	**ISO 6474 1981**	**ISO 6474 1994**	**CeramTec BIOLOX forte**
Bulk Density	g/m^3	>3.90	>3.94	>3.96
Grain Size	µm	<7.0	<4.5	<2.0
Flexural Strength	MPa	NA	>250	250*

*>400 MPa is normally obtained in practice.

Quality Assurance

The first European country to publish a quality system standard was the UK with the publication of British Standard, BS 5750 in 1979. This was adopted by ISO in 1987, when it became the now-famous ISO 9000. ISO 9000 was revised in 1994 and was substantially revised in 2000, when requirements for continuous improvement and customer satisfaction were added. Quality system requirements for medical devices were introduced by the UK Department of Health with the publication of their notorious guides (Blue, Green, Gold, etc) and these formed the basis of the resulting European standard, EN 46001, which was published in 1993 and internationalized in 1996 as ISO 13485. In the USA quality system requirements for medical devices were introduced in 1978 with the publication by the FDA of its Good Manufacturing Practice Regulation (21 CFR Part 820). This was revised in 1996 with the publication of the FDA's Quality System Regulation, which included for the first time design control requirements, and was further systematized in 1998 with the publication of the Quality System Instructional Technique Handbook (see Table 4).

From the early days of manufacture of ceramic components for the medical device industry (this was in the 1970s) CeramTec, formerly Feldmuehle and Cerasiv, has been committed to quality. It was one of the first companies to implement a quality system and to obtain third party certification. Faced with the above-mentioned array of quality requirements the company has made many improvement to its quality assurance system. Proof of the success of these improvements has been the fact that within the last three months the company has undergone and passed quality system audits from the FDA, from its European notified body and from at least four of its most important customers.

Table 4: Quality assurance requirements and standards

1978:	FDA Good Manufacturing Practice Regulation (21 CFR Part 820)
1979:	BS 5750, Quality systems. Pt 1: Specification for design, manufacture and installation.
1987:	ISO 9000, Quality systems - Model for quality assurance in ...
1993:	EN 46000, Quality systems - Medical devices
1994:	ISO 9000 Revised, Quality systems - Model for quality assurance in ...
1996:	ISO 13485, Quality systems - Medical devices
1996:	FDA Quality Systems Regulation (QSR) (21 CFR Part 820)
1998:	FDA Quality System Instructional Technique
2000:	ISO 9000 Revised, Quality management systems - Requirements

Process and Software Validation

Although ISO 9000 mentions validation, it was the FDA that put process validation on the quality map with the publication of its Guideline on General Principle of Process Validation in 1987. Later it incorporated process and software validation requirements in its QSR. This was followed by a guidance document on software validation and a rule on electronic records and signatures (see Table 5). Following these requirements CeramTec undertook a multi-million Euro validation program to ensure that its processes are in full compliance and will remain so in the future.

Table 5: Validation milestones

1987:	FDA Guidelines on General Principle of Process validation
1996:	FDA Quality System Regulation (21 CFR Part 820)
1997:	FDA General Principles of Software Validation Guidance Document
1997:	FDA Final Rule on Electronic Records and Signatures (21 CFR Part 11)
1998:	Global Harmonization Task Force Validation Guidance Document

Biological Safety

Work on the biological safety of medical devices was undertaken by ISO in the late 1980s and its seminal standard for Evaluation and Testing was published in 1990, ISO 10993-1. This standard indicates which tests are likely to be required in order to verify the acceptability of any given material or device for implant use. Since then ISO has published 18 standards in this series, all of which specify test methods and requirements. Such tests are less important for well established materials with proven clinical performance such as BIOLOX forte, but are essential when a new material is introduced such as CeramTec's new BIOLOX delta. Table 6 list some of the tests recently performed on Biolox delta in order to demonstrate its acceptable biological response.

Table 6: Some biological safety tests performed on BIOLOX delta

Test Type	Applicable ISO Standard
Carcinogenicity	10993: 3
Genotoxicity	10993: 3
Cytoxicity	10993: 5
Implantation	10993: 6
Sensitization	10993: 10
Chronic Toxicity	10993: 11

Total Joint Replacement Products

In 1985 ISO started work on a group of standards for Partial and Total Hip Joint Prostheses and in 1987 it published ISO 7206-2, which gives the requirements for articulating surfaces. Of course, this standard included no requirements for ceramic surfaces, but these were introduced in the 1996 revision. The current surface finish requirement for ceramic femoral heads is 0.02mm, while that for metal heads is 0.05mm, in other words, two and a half times rougher than the ceramic equivalent. This surface finish requirement is one important reason why ceramics have such a low wear rate (see Table 7). In 1995 FDA published a guidance document for "Ceramic Ball HIP Systems" and this adds two further requirements to the list, namely ball head burst strength and ball head fatigue strength. In the early 1990s the Committee for European Standards (CEN) started work on standards for non-active surgical implants and published its standards for joints replacement implants including hips and knees in 1998. These standards call for compliance with the new ISO standards for simulator wear testing. During this period attempts were made to standardize hip joint tapers. One such attempt resulted in ASTM F1636 and a further attempt is currently in development in CEN (see Table 8).

Table 7:
Evolution of surface finish requirements for articulating surfaces and BIOLOX forte value

Roughness (Ra)	Units	ISO 7206-2	ISO 7206-2	CeramTec
		1987	1996	BIOLOX forte
Metal	µm	<0.05	<0.05	NA
Ceramic	µm	NA	<0.02	<0.02

Table 8:
Standards and requirements applicable to the use of ceramic orthopaedic implant devices

1987:	ISO 7206-2, Articulating surfaces made of metallic and plastic materials
1995:	FDA Guidance for ceramic ball HIP systems
1996:	ISO 7206-2, Articulating surfaces made of metallic, ceramic and plastic materials
1998:	EN 12010, Joint Replacement Implants
1998:	EN 12563, Hip Replacement Implants
1998:	EN 12564, Knee Replacement Implants
1995:	ASTM F1636 Standard Specification for Bores and Cones for Modular Femoral Heads
2002:	ISO 14242 (and 3), Wear of Hip (and Knee) Joints

Conclusion

The development of legal and voluntary requirements is an on-going process. CeramTec actively supports these developments and is working hard to produce products which exceed all applicable requirements. CeramTec is confident that such products will be accepted in all markets worldwide and will perform with the safety and reliability required by its customers.

7.3 Improvements in Processing and Manufacturing at CeramTec

G. Griesmayr, M. Dietrich, J. Kasprowitsch and H. Dobbs

As many of you already know, with effect from February 2003 CeramTec together with two of its customers has been successful in obtaining FDA approval for the supply of ceramic inserts to the USA. Such approvals were not easy to obtain. This paper discusses what CeramTec has done to achieve these objectives.

Quality Philosophy

Every European medical device manufacturer which intends to sell its products in both Europe and the USA must meet both ISO 9000 and FDA requirements. In most respects these requirements are substantially similar, but in some important respects the FDA goes further than ISO. CeramTec had chosen to apply FDA standards to the manufacture of all its products no matter in what part of the world they will eventually be sold. In addition to external requirements, CeramTec endeavours to apply and maintain the highest levels of manufacturing control, for reasons of product safety and to avoid possible product-related complications.

Design Control

Today when a customer wants a new product or a change to an existing one, CeramTec must follow its Design Control procedures, which specify the new product development process. First a Project Leader must be assigned, who is responsible for the creation of the Project Plan. Depending on the complexity of the project, the plan will include

1) objectives based on customer requirements,
2) the required resources and responsibilities,
3) the required drawings, samples and prototypes,
4) the required laboratory and possibly clinical testing and the associated acceptance criteria,
5) the assessment of risk and risk reduction activities, if needed,
6) the transfer of the development to production and finally
7) the creation of appropriate records in a Design History File (DHF).

Before the project can begin, the plan must be approved by the Design Review Team, which includes representatives from product development, production, quality and sales plus at least one independent member. Once the plan is approved the work can begin, but before the product can be released to production the work must be reviewed and approved by the same Design Review Team to ensure that the desired objectives have been met.

Design Transfer and the development of a DHF are two areas where FDA requirements exceed ISO 9000 requirements. With respect to Design Transfer, FDA requires that "Each manufacturer shall establish and maintain procedures to ensure that the device design is correctly translated into production specifications." With respect to the DHF, FDA requires that "Each manufacturer shall establish and maintain a DHF for each type of device. The DHF shall contain or reference the records necessary to demonstrate that the design was developed in accordance with the approved design plan...".

The compilation of a retrospective DHF has occasionally been complicated by the fact that the original records may have been lost and may not be easily retrieved or recreated. To avoid this problem CeramTec systematically records all information exchanges with its customers. Similarly, it systematically informs its customers of all drawing changes for the purpose of prior approval and it logs both events (the request and the approval) in a dedicated database.

The design process has become a two way process in which there is an exchange of information in both directions. Not only must CeramTec (in this case a component supplier) work more closely than ever before with its customers (the prosthesis manufacturers), but also its customers must work more closely with CeramTec. Only in this way can both parties achieve the desired transparency and the deliverables needed to meet FDA requirements.

Process Validation

In addition to the ISO 9000 requirements, FDA requires the following: "Where the results of a process cannot be fully verified by subsequent inspection and test, the process shall be validated with a high degree of assurance and approved according to established procedures." In its guidance document entitled "General Principles of Process Validation" FDA specifies how this can be achieved. Also it specifies that revalidation must occur whenever processes are changed or after a specified time period.

To meet these requirements CeramTec developed a Master Validation Plan. This plan lists all the processes and equipment which it uses or plans to use and assigns a risk value to each. In all there were more than 120 items on the list. These ranged from low risk processes such as a surface polishing process to high risk processes such as a computerised dimensional measurement process or as a final cleaning process. Next CeramTec developed a validation procedure, which specifies the validation process as shown in Figure 1.

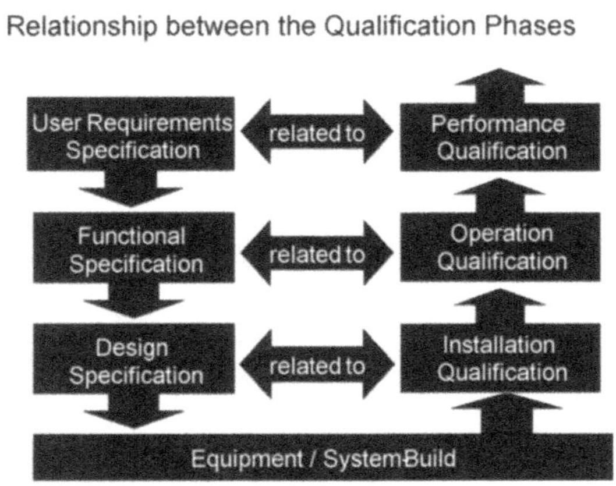

Figure 1:
Relationship between the qualification phases

Based on its risk assessment and following its validation procedure CeramTec has so far validated all high risk processes of which there were at least 60. This work has taken two years and has cost several million Euros. To complete the process and to validate all 120 processes will take another year.
CeramTec did this work because to do so was an external requirement, but the work has provided associated benefits for the company and its customers in the form of a significant improvement in product quality and process reliability. The following is an example of the benefits that can be obtained. When CeramTec attempted to validate its sintering ovens it found that it was not possible to achieve an improved temperature uniformity. To solve this problem CeramTec at first attempted to improve its existing ovens, but when this proved impossible, it purchased some new ones. Not only do the new ones maintain the required temperature with an accuracy of +/- 5 degrees, but also they are fully automated and provide further improvements in furnace control.

Software Validation

In addition to ISO 9000 requirements, FDA requires the validation of software as stated in the following: "When computers or automated data processing systems are used as part of production or the quality system, the manufacturer shall validate computer software for its intended use according to established protocol." In its guidance document entitled "General Principles of Software Validation" FDA specifies how this can be achieved. As a result of this requirement CeramTec is in the process of validating all its applicable software controlled equipment and business software. Take the example of its software controlled Laser Marking Equipment. Validation of this equipment required checking that the system limited user access to only specified users, that it accepted only data entries that were within specified ranges, that it correctly generated both the appropriate part number and the appropriate unique identification number, that it controlled the beam intensity so that the surface marking was visible, yet the surface impact did not exceed a specified amount and that it generated an adequate record of all parameters for every part all day long. This work was time-consuming, because all conceivable worst-case scenarios (data entries) had to be stress-tested (and there were hundreds of these), but the consequence of the work was the assurance that the system will perform reliably in all foreseeable circumstances.

Process Performance Qualification (PPQ)

A PPQ is the final part of the validation process. It is the part which is used to verify and document the ability of a process to consistently perform in accordance with established specifications and quality attributes. Specifically, with regard to the FDA-approved cup inserts, CeramTec had to verify that the final product, when processed and tested in accordance with CeramTec processes and procedures, conformed to the requirements and specifications of

CeramTec's customers. Before the PPQ could begin CeramTec had to successfully validated all the individual process steps, since a PPQ is in fact the final validation of the entire process chain. For CeramTec the process chain included all steps from raw material acceptance to final product release. FDA requires that this can be verified in three separate runs. This is what CeramTec did (see Figure 2).

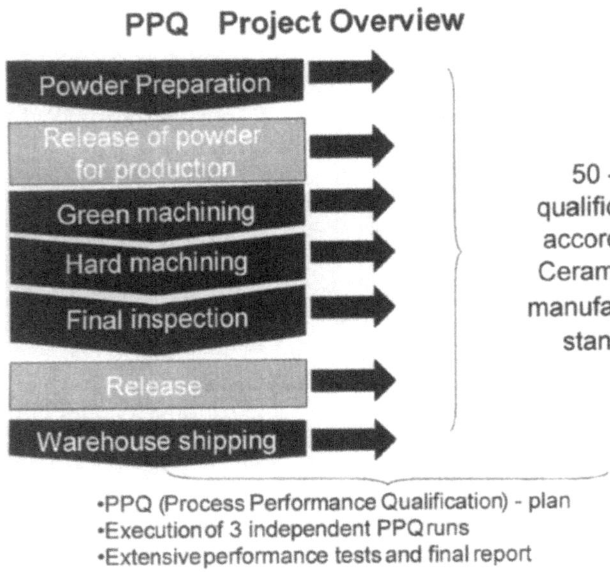

Figure 2:
PPQ Project Overview for ceramic insert

Improvements in Quality Assurance

Validation can also lead to quality assurance improvements. When CeramTec validated its Co-ordinate Measuring Machines (CMM) to measure the dimensions of its finished product, it conducted a process Failure Modes Effects Analysis (FMEA). It found that although the machines correctly identified parts which were out of tolerance, it was possible that the operator did not always correctly segregate these parts. Since no automated solution to this problem presented itself, CeramTec introduced the "four eyes principle", which requires that the segregation of parts is observed and checked by a second person, who must be trained and approved for this purpose. CeramTec now employs this principle for all critical manual processes which are performed by a single operator.

To ensure that the production process is properly controlled CeramTec introduced quality gates through which no product can pass unless it meets the required quality requirements (size, shape, strength, etc). In this way CeramTec can identify and quickly correct in-process quality problems and does not have to rely on final inspection, which would be less efficient and slower.

It is inevitable that from time to time there will be non-conformities or deviations of one kind or another. These may arise in-house, for example in production, or in the field, for example as a customer complaint. To manage such non-conformities, CeramTec has introduced a Corrective and Preventive Action (CAPA) system which records all such problems and with the help of a quality action team identifies appropriate solutions in a timely manner. Once these solutions have been identified and implemented, the system requires that their effectiveness is verified over a period of time. In this way, using its CAPA system, CeramTec is continuously working to improve quality.

An example of the functioning of the CAPA system is the following: before CeramTec installed its above-mentioned CMM machines it built a temperature and humidity controlled room, but once the machines were installed and validated it turned out that from time to time the required temperature and humidity limits were exceeded. Each time this happened the associated alarm went off and each time the alarm went off a process deviation report was raised and submitted to the quality department. Each report was analysed by the quality action team, whose job it was to determine the effect of the deviation on the product being measured, the cause of the problem and the most effective long term corrective action. The team determined that the existing air-conditioning and humidifying equipment was not powerful enough and that the best, quickest and cheapest solution was to install more powerful equipment. This was done at once and subsequently no further problems of this kind have occurred. Periodically the temperature and humidity readings are checked to verify the long-term effectiveness of the solution.

To ensure that all changes are correctly recorded and managed, CeramTec developed a change management system. This system includes all changes to quality documents, products and processes. Take the example of a change to a process step. First a change request has to be raised and submitted, then the change has to be evaluated by a project team, then tests have to be done to show the effect of the change on the process or the product. When this work is complete, the Change Committee reviews the work of the project team and if it is satisfactory then the customer has to be informed and in the case of critical changes the approval of the customer has to be obtained. Only when all these steps are complete can the change be implemented.

Conclusion

CT has made rapid progress in the development of systems to control design, development, production and quality assurance. It has successfully met external requirements which allow it to sell its products in the main markets world-wide. In the process it has benefited from associated quality and manufacturing improvements. However the process can never be allowed to stop, since in the future there will inevitably be new quality objectives. These could be new external requirements such as regulations or standards or new internally-driven needs such as scrap reduction or production process improvements. CeramTec is working to achieve these and other objectives in order to continue to supply its customers with the safest and most reliable products.

References

1. H-G Pfaff, GMP Compliant Quality Management Systems - A Contribution to Safety, in: Bioceramics in Joint Arthroplasty (eds JP Garino and G Willmann), pp Georg Thieme, Stuttgart, 2002.
2. FDA Quality System Regulation (21 CFR Part 820)
3. FDA Guidance Document on General Principles of Process Validation
4. FDA Guidance Document on General Principles of Software Validation

7.4 Review of Controlled Clinical Studies with Ceramic on Ceramic Total Hip Replacements in the United States of America

J. P. Garino

Introduction

Good quality clinical research in Orthopedic Surgery can be a difficult, expensive and lengthy process. Ideally, such clinical research should be randomized and prospective and should vary only one aspect in order to determine if the difference is responsible for better outcome verses more undesirable side effects (risk). This type of research is what was implemented with drugs due to the lack of science in the earlier part of the twentieth century. This initial lack of a demand for not only proof of efficacy for a new product, but there was often a lack of good safety testing which often meant that the product actually may have done some harm to its users. It was these safety issues that first lead to the development of the Food and Drug Administration (FDA) in the United States in 1930. Slowly and steadily over the course of that time frame, new acts and new parameters for the conduction of clinical research for pharmaceuticals came into being. The FDA was also given much power to enforce these new laws. Throughout this early time frame however, devices had been completely exempted from these laws and the FDA's scrutiny in terms of evaluating safety and efficacy.

Modern Device Evaluation Process in the USA

In 1976, the first device act was passed by Congress to bring devices under the offices of the FDA for efficacy and safety. All devices that have been manufactured and put into place prior to that time were exempted from this act. In addition, it allowed any future device that was proved to be substantially equivalent to a device already in use at the time before this act would not be evaluated at the most stringent standards that have been put forth by this new act. This new law came about due to problems and failures with primarily cardiac devices such as valves and pace makers. This act created a whole separate division of the FDA related to radiological treatments and devices. Under this new act, orthopaedic devices basically were put under either a Class 2 or Class 3 category. Class 2 devices were considered to be substantially equivalent to devices in current use and validation of the fact that the new device was "substantially equivalent" to an approved device is known as a 510K approval. From a manufacturer's standpoint to minimize the paperwork and expense of bringing a new product to market, obtaining the 510k approvals from the FDA in general was the way to go. In most cases, the manufacturer would slightly modify an existing implant or totally redesign an implant that in essence from a function and mechanical testing standpoint was "substantially equivalent" and therefore if it met the FDA criteria it could be brought to market without any clinical trials. Devices which may have a similar function to those already out on the market, but utilize a new material were often classified by the FDA as a Class 3 device, which means it was not substantially equivalent and therefore it needed to be restricted. A Class 3 assignment to a device meant that in order for this particular device to come to market it would have to undergo rigorous testing in a clinical setting to obtain clinical data regarding the safety and efficacy of the device and this is exactly what took place with the introduction of ceramic on ceramic hip replacement components in the United States [1].

Evaluation Of Ceramic-Ceramic THR (Fig. 1,2,3)

Although, ceramic on ceramic have been components in hip replacements and have been used for over 30 years in Europe[2], the same enthusiasm for this material did not reach the United States until the mid-1980s when the "Autofor" or Mittelmeier device finally received the appropriate approvals. The design of this device with its monoblock cementless screw in acetabular cup and cementless Femoral component without a biological coating lead to early failures due to loosening and the subsequent abandonment of the device[3]. In addition, it left some scars on the reputation of ceramic on ceramic total hip replacements, as in the eyes of many people evaluating this failure; failure was due to ceramic/ceramic articulation rather than the poor design of the components themselves. We know now that the ceramic/ceramic articulation of this device compared very well and that a hard on hard durable bearing was never going to be successful unless fixation of the components to the bone had first been established. However, the continued shortcomings of polyethylene lead to a continued interest in hard on hard bearings particularly for young patients[5]. The late 1980s – early 1990s demonstrated significant advances in obtaining improved and more durable fixations to bone with standard components particularly with cementless acetabular shells. The idea of now creating a ceramic liner for this metallic shell completely separated the fixation and bearing functions and optimized them. It is from this concept that the modern ceramic/ceramic devices evolved and began to take hold. Back in the United States, these ceramic/ceramic hip replacements, even though ceramic balls had now been in use and approved in the country for nearly eight years, the fact that the acetabular liner was also made of ceramic, represented a new material in a new role and the FDA gave it a Class 3 assignment. In order to get a ceramic/ceramic total hip replacement approved, a manufacturing company would have to go through an investigational device exemption (IDE) and perform extensive clinical studies using this device against a control. If the device through these trials proves to be both safe and effective for the purpose it was designed, then a pre-marketing application (PMA) could be submitted by the device company to the FDA for approval.

Although the ceramic/ceramic total hip replacement underwent all the mechanical testing required by devices that have been approved by the 510K route, that was the minimum criteria that the FDA would accept to even allow it to be classified as a Class 3 device. The new device had to at least meet those standards. Next in order to prove safety, the FDA required that clinical studies take place, so that unforeseen or unexpected problems with the device were identified in a small covert cohort of patients before the FDA would feel comfortable in releasing the device for general marketing. It is important to note that the FDA does have some input on the study designed and advises the company with regard to some of the aspects of their clinical to enhance the likelihood that the FDA will consider the data to be truly valid, but it makes no guarantees that following all aspects of the FDA's advice will automatically result in an approval. The IDE in many ways, it is very much like a drug study in so far as that all adverse events any untoward or unexpected complication or symptom needs to be reported regardless of whether or it is in anyway related to the device. This once again is the safety aspect of the trial and that more effective devices are not more valuable than less effective devices if they are not as safe. In general, the typical IDE study would require 300 or more patients at multiple centers and that those patients need to be followed for a minimum of two years before the FDA will consider a pre-marketing approval application. Informed consent is an extremely important aspect of the study. Investigations willing to participate in such a sponsored study must next obtain the approval from the hospital to conduct the research. This approval process is done through the Institutional Review Board (IRB). The mission of the IRB is to allow reasonable research to be conducted as long as there is no undue risk to the patient. The IRB is much more concerned with patient safety than study design although the latter is important. Finally, the IRB is responsible for the review of the informed consent to be sure that it contains all of the important information regarding the risk and benefit of being in the study and that the language is understandable (lay terminology). The consent must make clear that patients understand that they are participating in an experimental trial and that their cooperation is desired and that they are fully aware of any risks or benefits that may result from their participation in this trial. These complex research endeavors cost sponsoring companies several million dollars and represent a major investment in a new product, device or technology.

However, having a pre-marketing approval application accepted and successfully completing an IDE will allow for a manufacturer to now market this Class 3 device and all of this hard work and major investment then gives them edge over their competitors. Any other competitors wishing to produce a substantially equivalent device would need to go through the same IDE in order to market it to new patients in the United States. Although there are no rules regarding downclassification, in general, once four pre-marketing applications have been successfully granted then the device is considered for down classification to a Class 2. In many ways, this is similar to a patent expiring on a pharmaceutical, so that generic equivalents can be produced. Those generic equivalents produced by other companies, once the down classification occurs, would achieve approval by going through the 510K-approval process. That in general is how new devices get approved in the United States. It is a long, expensive and arduous process but it is a very effective way at optimizing the opportunity to provide effective devices that also are safe. For hip replacements, which have enjoyed tremendous durability and success with well over 80% lasting ten or more years, it becomes difficult to determine what devices are truly better than others unless randomized trials are performed and they are followed for significant periods of time. The IDE trials that have taken place for ceramic on ceramic devices will provide extensive information in the years to come as these extensively evaluated cohorts of patients are followed decades into the future, since most of the trials have been randomized against standard polyethylene. At least that comparison will be made in a very scientific matter. At the current time there are several IDE's that have completed enrollment with pre-marketing approval applications being submitted and others that are fulfilling their enrollment goals with pre-market approval applications to be filed in the near future.

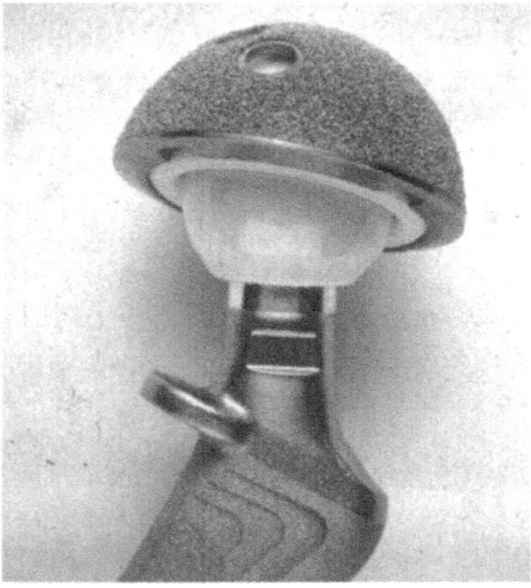

Figure 1:
Modern Ceramic-Ceramic THR: Courtesy of Wright Medical Technology

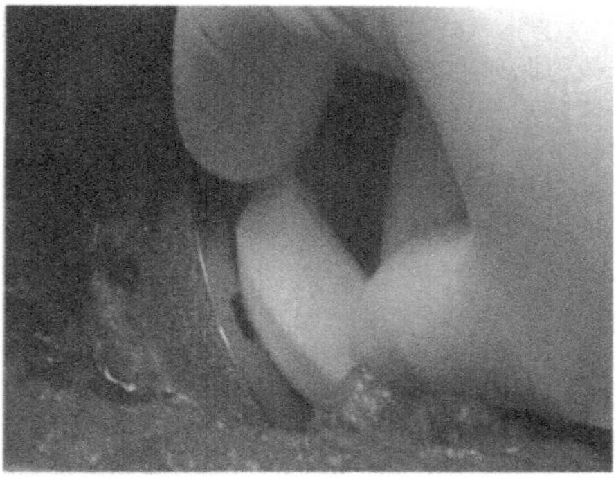

Figure 2:
Intraoperative view, Insertion of ceramic liner

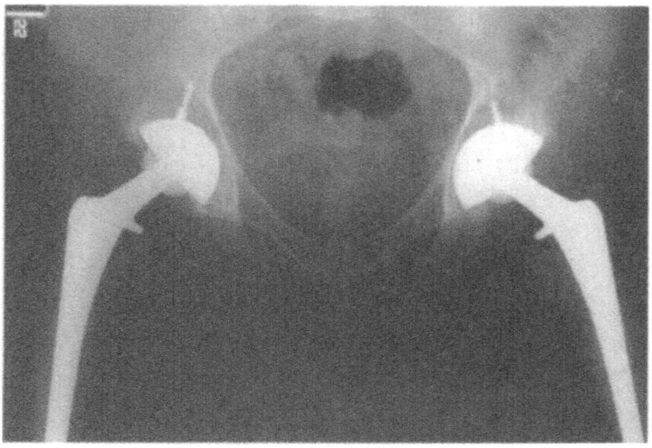

Figure 3:
Post-op view of patient with Bilateral Ceramic-Ceramic THR.

Brief Details On Ceramic Studies in Progress

The ceramic-ceramic study sponsored by Osteonics was the first to receive a clearance for their IDE and subsequently began enrollment in 1996. [5] That study was completed in early 1998 in terms of enrollment and those results are contained elsewhere in these proceedings. I brief, this study was a three armed IDE with two-thirds of the patients receiving a study ceramic insert and one-third of the patients receiving a standard polyethylene insert. Over 500 patients were enrolled. Following enrollment of this first cohort of patients and upon receiving a proper clearance from the FDA that this original cohort had no early and unexpected problems, the study was allowed to go forward in a non-randomized fashion (all patients receive the study device, a ceramic-ceramic total hip) by a mechanism known as continued access. Through this process, large numbers of patients could be enrolled, but they needed to be monitored to the fullest extent as any randomized patient in terms of scores, x-rays and adverse events. Wright Medical Technology was the next IDE to be approved. The enrollment for it's clinical cohort of over 300 patients plays between April of 1997 and August of 1998, and, like the previous study, after data from the original cohort was collected and there were no significant interoperative or immediate post-operative adverse events, the FDA approved that IDE to move forward with continued access. What is interesting and unique about the Wright Medical Technology (WMT) study, detailed data presented elsewhere in these proceedings, is that it was performed in a non-randomized fashion. The company took the position that it would utilize the ceramic liner in all patients and utilize any of its stems, while at the same time using historical controls. This was an easier trial to conduct from a logistical standpoint, because there was no randomization required, which is often a sticking point to enrolling patients who, at least in the case of ceramic on ceramic hip replacements were excited about the possibility of receiving the new technology, but were often disappointed if they were randomized to a polyethylene liner. This was a bit of a gamble on the part of WMT, because if the number of significant adverse events had been of substantial numbers and they were device related, such as dislocation, without a control arm one would never be able to determine for sure if that complication was a result of the ceramic/ceramic bearing or particular stem or surgeon for example. If that had been the case and the FDA had been alarmed by an excessive dislocation rate, once again for example, the FDA could have decided that the device was not safe enough for general use and the study would basically need to be started over again with controls. A very expensive and time costly situation. However, the device performed as expected and there were few device related complications and comparable to historical controls.

Encore Orthopaedics was the next IDE that came into being followed by Smith & Nephew. As of this moment, both have fulfilled their minimum number of patients in the original randomized cohort and have had continued access for a reasonable period of time. These sponsors are now gathering the two year data from the original cohort and will be submitting PMA's to the FDA probably within the next calendar year. Implex and BioMet are nearing the completion of their two-year time frame for data collection on the original cohort and may possibly submit PMA's by the end of the 2003 calendar year as well.

Since, the enrollment of the very first patient in the Osteonic IDE, nearly seven years have passed and the devices are not yet approved. Why is that? Back in the summer of 2000, the FDA's advisory board basically agreed that the ceramic/ceramic device data presented to them at that time should be eventually approved by the FDA. The subcommittee was impressed with the safety, efficacy and degree of follow up that had been obtained during that presentation. However, there was a problem with chipping due to the design of the ABG cup with its extended rim that allowed for slight initial mal-placement of the liner and subsequent chipping of the edges of the ceramic insert. This was improved by redesigning the cup, eliminating the elevated lip and putting a putting a metal jacket around the ceramic insert so that one would have a metal/metal taper locking the liner into the shell. These new shells have become an extention of the Osteonics IDE and no further chipping has been reported. In all of the other studies, containing several thousand patients, only 6 ceramic complications have been identified. Liners and ball heads have both been involved.

As things were moving toward an imminent approval, zirconia ceramic ball heads from a single, but popular manufacturer began to break at a high rate and a recall took place. This totally unexpected event sent a strong message to the FDA that ceramic devices must receive the most stringent evaluation possible. Prior to this recall, manufacturers that provided components to total hip replacement systems did not universally need to attain the same high level of good manufacturing practices that the FDA demanded of the American manufacturing companies that directly market their products to doctors, hospitals and patients. However since these ceramic components were now an integral part of the ceramic/ceramic system, the FDA modified its position to require even component providers to perform to the highest level of good manufacturing practice, which included, among other things, a quality improvement program and a complete and thorough documented validation of each and every step of its manufacturing process. To require this new standard of compliance of companies that have previously not needed to so, it would take a great deal of time and investment and the FDA would therefore approve no pre-marketing approval application until ceramic vendors had attained that high level of compliance that was now demanded. This new requirement therefore set back the ultimate approval and subsequent general marketing of ceramic/ceramic components in the United States probably many months. The FDA was in no need to quickly approve this new technology unless all the aspects of the approval process were thoroughly and totally in order. They had this luxury primarily due to the fact that safe and effective hip replacements were currently available.

The IDE's utilizing ceramic-ceramic hip replacements are doing well with only small numbers of complications and device failures. Whether they will truly prove to be vastly superior to standard THR technology remains to be seen, and will require the following of these original randomized cohorts well into the future.

Thus, the FDA is an organization dedicated to the safety and efficacy of many aspects of healthcare in the United States and specifically responsible for that of medical devices including orthopaedic implant. Although, it's high regulatory aspects can significantly slow the ability of new devices and technologies to come to the American marketplace. Unsafe and ineffective devices are unlikely to survive this rigorous process.

References

1. Garino, J.P: Medical device regulation by the FDA. Proceedings of the Second annual Symposia on the Wear Couple BIOLOX Forte, Stuttgart, Germany, February 1998

2. Boutin PM, Arthroplastic Total de hanche par prosthese en alumine fritte. Rev Chi Orthop 58:229-246

3. O'Leary JF, Mallory TH, Kraus TJ, et al: Mittelmeier ceramic total hip arthroplasty: A retrospective study. J Arthrop. 3:87-96, 1988.

4. Schmalzried TP, Jasty M, Harris WH: Periprosthetic bone loss in total hip arthroplasty: role of polyethylene wear debris and the concept of the effected joint space. JBJS 74A:849-863, 1992).

5. D'Antonio J. Capello W. Manley M. Bierbaum B. New experience with alumina-on-alumina ceramic bearings for total hip arthroplasty. [Clinical Trial. Journal Article. Multicenter Study. Randomized Controlled Trial] Journal of Arthroplasty. 17(4):390-7, 2002 Jun.

GPSR Compliance

The European Union's (EU) General Product Safety Regulation (GPSR) is a set of rules that requires consumer products to be safe and our obligations to ensure this.

If you have any concerns about our products, you can contact us on ProductSafety@springernature.com

In case Publisher is established outside the EU, the EU authorized representative is:

Springer Nature Customer Service Center GmbH
Europaplatz 3
69115 Heidelberg, Germany

Batch number: 10577876

Printed by Printforce, the Netherlands